T0259312

Cardiac Rhythm Disorders in Older Adults

Editors

MICHAEL W. RICH
WIN-KUANG SHEN

CLINICS IN GERIATRIC MEDICINE

www.geriatric.theclinics.com

November 2012 • Volume 28 • Number 4

ELSEVIER

1600 John F. Kennedy Blvd., Suite 1800. Philadelphia, Pennsylvania 19103-2899

http://www.theclinics.com

CLINICS IN GERIATRIC MEDICINE Volume 28, Number 4
November 2012 ISSN 0749-0690, ISBN-13: 978-1-4557-4934-8

Editor: Yonah Korngold

Clinics in Geriatric Medicine (ISSN 0749-0690) is published quarterly by Elsevier Inc., 360 Park Avenue South, New York, NY 10010-1710. Months of issue are February, May, August, and November. Business and Editorial Offices: 1600 John F. Kennedy Blvd., Suite 1800, Philadelphia, PA 191023-2899. Periodicals postage paid at New York, NY, and additional mailing offices. Subscription prices is $257.00 per year (US individuals), $448.00 per year (US institutions), $131.00 per year (US student/resident), $334.00 per year (Canadian individuals), $559.00 per year (Canadian institutions), $355.00 per year (foreign individuals) and $559.00 per year (foreign institutions). Foreign air speed delivery is included in all Clinics subscription prices. All prices are subject to change without notice. POSTMASTER: Send address changes to Clinics in Geriatric Medicine, Elsevier Health Sciences Division, Subscription Customer Service, 3251 Riverport Lane, Maryland Heights, MO 63043. Telephone: 1-800-654-2452 (U.S. and Canada); 314-447-8871 (outside U.S. and Canada). Fax: 314-447-8029. E-mail: journalscustomerservice-usa@elsevier.com (for print support) or journalsonlinesupport-usa@elsevier.com (for online support).

Reprints. For copies of 100 or more, of articles in this publication, please contact the Commercial Reprints Department, Elsevier Inc., 360 Park Avenue South, New York, New York 10010-1710. Tel.: (212) 633-3812; Fax: (212) 462-1935, email: reprints@elsevier.com.

Clinics in Geriatric Medicine is covered in MEDLINE/PubMed (Index Medicus), EMBASE/Excerpta Medica, Current Contents/Clinical Medicine (CC/CM), and the Cumulative Index to Nursing & Allied Health Literature.

Printed and bound by CPI Group (UK) Ltd, Croydon, CR0 4YY

Transferred to digital print 2012

Contributors

GUEST EDITORS

MICHAEL W. RICH, MD
Professor of Medicine, Cardiovascular Division, Washington University School of Medicine, St Louis, Missouri

WIN-KUANG SHEN, MD
Professor of Medicine, Mayo Clinic–Arizona, Scottsdale, Arizona

AUTHORS

WILBERT S. ARONOW, MD, FACC, FAHA
Professor of Medicine, Division of Cardiology, New York Medical College, Westchester Medical Center, Valhalla, New York

T. JARED BUNCH, MD
Intermountain Heart Rhythm Specialists and Cardiovascular Surgery, Intermountain Heart Institute; Department of Cardiology, Intermountain Medical Center, Murray, Utah

JANE CHEN, MD, FACC, FHRS
Associate Professor of Medicine, Cardiovascular Division, Washington University School of Medicine, St Louis, Missouri

GRANT V. CHOW, MD
Clinical Fellow (Cardiology), Division of Cardiology, Johns Hopkins Medical Institutions, Johns Hopkins University School of Medicine, Baltimore, Maryland

JOHN D. DAY, MD
Intermountain Heart Rhythm Specialists and Cardiovascular Surgery, Intermountain Heart Institute; Department of Cardiology, Intermountain Medical Center, Murray, Utah

JOHN R. DOTY, MD
Cardiovascular Surgery, Intermountain Heart Institute; Department of Cardiology, Intermountain Medical Center, Murray, Utah

ANDREW E. EPSTEIN, MD, FAHA, FACC, FHRS
Professor of Medicine, Electrophysiology Section, Division of Cardiovascular Medicine, Hospital of the University of Pennsylvania, Philadelphia, Pennsylvania

MARGARET C. FANG, MD, MPH
Associate Professor of Medicine, Division of Hospital Medicine, University of California, San Francisco, San Francisco, California

MICHAEL E. FIELD, MD
Assistant Professor of Medicine, Director of Cardiac Arrhythmia Service, University of Wisconsin, School of Medicine & Public Health, Madison, Wisconsin

JEROME L. FLEG, MD
Medical Officer, Division of Cardiovascular Sciences, National Heart, Lung, and Blood
Institute, Bethesda, Maryland

WILLIAM H. FRISHMAN, MD, MACP
Rosenthal Professor & Chair, Department of Medicine, Professor of Pharmacology,
New York Medical College, Director of Medicine and Acting Chief of Cardiology,
Westchester Medical Center, Valhalla, New York

NORA GOLDSCHLAGER, MD
Professor of Medicine, Cardiology Division, Department of Medicine, San Francisco
General Hospital; Department of Medicine, University of California, San Francisco,
California

BLAIR P. GRUBB, MD, FACC
Professor of Medicine and Pediatrics, College of Medicine and Life Sciences,
The University of Toledo, Toledo, Ohio

ARSHAD JAHANGIR, MD
Professor of Medicine, Center for Integrative Research on Cardiovascular Aging (CIRCA),
Aurora University of Wisconsin Medical Group, Aurora Health Care, Milwaukee,
Wisconsin

DAVID L. JOHNSON, MS, PAC
Intermountain Heart Rhythm Specialists and Cardiovascular Surgery, Intermountain Heart
Institute; Department of Cardiology, Intermountain Medical Center, Murray, Utah

BEVERLY KARABIN, RN, MSN, PhD
Associate Professor of Nursing, College of Nursing, The University of Toledo,
Toledo, Ohio

YUKI KOSHINO, MD, PhD
Research Associate, Division of Cardiovascular Diseases, Rochester, Minnesota

PREETHAM KUMAR, MD
Cardiology Fellow, Electrophysiology and Pacing Service, Division of Cardiovascular
Disease, Department of Medicine, Mayo Clinic, Jacksonville, Florida

FRED M. KUSUMOTO, MD
Associate Professor of Medicine, Mayo Clinic School of Medicine; Electrophysiology and
Pacing Service, Division of Cardiovascular Disease, Department of Medicine, Mayo
Clinic, Jacksonville, Florida

RACHEL LAMPERT, MD
Associate Professor of Medicine, Section of Cardiology, Department of Internal Medicine,
Yale University School of Medicine, New Haven, Connecticut

MIGUEL A. LEAL, MD
Assistant Professor of Medicine, University of Wisconsin, School of Medicine & Public
Health, Madison, Wisconsin

JONATHAN P. MAN, MD
Fellow, Cardiac Electrophysiology, Electrophysiology Section, Division of Cardiovascular
Medicine, Hospital of the University of Pennsylvania, Philadelphia, Pennsylvania

JOSEPH E. MARINE, MD
Associate Professor of Medicine, Division of Cardiology, Johns Hopkins Medical Institutions, Johns Hopkins University School of Medicine, Baltimore, Maryland

ROWLENS M. MELDUNI, MD, MPH
Assistant Professor of Medicine, Division of Cardiovascular Diseases, Mayo College of Medicine, Rochester, Minnesota

MAHEK MIRZA, MD
Center for Integrative Research on Cardiovascular Aging (CIRCA), Aurora University of Wisconsin Medical Group, Aurora Health Care, Milwaukee, Wisconsin

RICHARD L. PAGE, MD
George R. and Elaine Love Professor, Chair, Department of Medicine, University of Wisconsin, School of Medicine & Public Health, Madison, Wisconsin

GENE R. QUINN, MD, MS
Department of Medicine, University of California, San Francisco, San Francisco, California

WIN-KUANG SHEN, MD
Professor of Medicine, Mayo College of Medicine; Chair, Division of Cardiovascular Diseases, Mayo Clinic, Scottsdale, Arizona

ANTON STRUNETS, MD
Center for Integrative Research on Cardiovascular Aging (CIRCA), Aurora University of Wisconsin Medical Group, Aurora Health Care, Milwaukee, Wisconsin

Contents

> Normal aging is associated with a multitude of changes in the cardiovascular system, including decreased compliance of blood vessels, mild concentric left ventricular hypertrophy, an increased contribution of atrial contraction to left ventricular filling, and a higher incidence of many cardiac arrhythmias, both bradyarrhythmias and tachyarrhythmias. Conduction disorders also become more common with age, and may either be asymptomatic, or cause hemodynamic changes requiring treatment. The epidemiology of common arrhythmias and conduction disorders in the elderly is reviewed.

> Aging is associated with an increased prevalence of cardiac arrhythmias, which contribute to higher morbidity and mortality in the elderly. The frequency of cardiac arrhythmias, particularly atrial fibrillation and ventricular tachyarrhythmia, is projected to increase as the population ages, greatly impacting health care resource utilization. Several clinical factors associated with the risk of arrhythmias have been identified in the population, yet the molecular bases for the increased predisposition to arrhythmogenesis in the elderly are not fully understood. This review highlights the epidemiology of cardiac dysrhythmias, changes in cardiac structure and function associated with aging, and the basis for arrhythmogenesis in the elderly.

> Bradyarrhythmias and tachyarrhythmias are common in elderly patients as a result of aging and acquired cardiac disease. Antiarrhythmic drugs are effective in elderly patients for the management of supraventricular and ventricular arrhythmias; however, dosing of drugs must be performed with care because of age-related changes in drug pharmacokinetics, the presence of concomitant disease, and frequent drug-drug interactions. Despite the large number of antiarrhythmic drugs having different electrophysiologic actions, as described in this article, only the β-blockers have been shown to be effective in reducing mortality and to lack proarrhythmic actions.

> Atrial fibrillation (AF) is an increasingly prevalent disease in the elderly. Patients with AF are at increased risk of ischemic stroke, resulting in

significant morbidity and mortality. Warfarin is highly effective at reducing stroke risk, with a net clinical benefit favoring treatment in older individuals. The advent of newer oral anticoagulants provides promising alternatives to warfarin. Appropriate risk stratification for stroke should be performed for all patients with AF to guide antithrombotic therapy. For patients at lower stroke risk, bleeding risk stratification tools can also be used when the benefit of anticoagulant therapy is unclear.

Atrial fibrillation (AF) and atrial flutter (AFL) are common cardiac arrhythmias in older adults. Medical management focuses on rate and rhythm control of AF and AFL to promote symptomatic relief and avoid tachycardia-mediated cardiomyopathy. Pharmacologic treatment of AF and AFL is especially challenging in the elderly because of the presence of comorbidities that may affect drug kinetics, and polypharmacy, which may lead to drug interactions. The potential for complications from medications and procedures required to achieve and maintain sinus rhythm must be carefully balanced against the benefits of therapy. This article reviews medical management of AF and AFL specifically relating to rate and rhythm control. The controversy of rate versus rhythm control is also discussed.

As elderly patients present significant challenges for long-term pharmacologic management, nonpharmacologic treatment of atrial fibrillation (AF) will continue to be a vital option in improving the quality of life and function of these patients. This review discusses nonpharmacologic approaches for AF in the elderly. Observational studies of catheter ablation suggest similar long-term efficacy and safety rates in elderly and younger groups. Minimally invasive surgical approaches have distinct advantages in certain populations. Further research, adequately powered to assess age-related differences, is needed to confirm the findings of observational studies of elderly patients who have undergone nonpharmacologic approaches to rhythm control.

Ventricular arrhythmias constitute the main cause of sudden cardiac death. In the elderly, their presentation may be manifested by intermittent confusion or unexplained falls. In some cases, they may also be asymptomatic. The primary management goals are to identify and treat the underlying cause and prevent recurrence. With the exception of beta-blockers, none of the other antiarrhythmic drugs available reduce mortality associated with ventricular arrhythmias. In the elderly, these drugs are associated with a higher risk of adverse events. In this article, the authors review the data available regarding evaluation and management of ventricular arrhythmias in the elderly.

There are few randomized, well-controlled studies to guide decision making with respect to the treatment of ventricular arrhythmias in the elderly treated with either device implantation or catheter ablation. Although some data are conflicting, the elderly appear to have a greater degree of risk related to treatment compared with younger ones; however, this increased risk is in part a consequence of age itself and comorbid conditions. Conversely, in terms of benefit, although the data may again be mixed, there is ample information indicating that age should not contraindicate aggressive treatment when accepted indications for intervention exist.

This article provides an overview of quality of life (QOL) and end-of-life issues that pertain to older patients with implanted cardiac rhythm devices. Most patients with implantable cardioverter-defibrillators (ICDs) enjoy similar QOL to that of other patients with cardiac diseases, especially in the absence of ICD shocks. Conventional pacemakers, as well as devices incorporating cardiac resynchronization, can improve QOL in appropriately selected patients regardless of age. In patients approaching the end of life, all devices, but especially ICDs, can adversely impact QOL in patients and families. All patients should have the opportunity to discuss the option of device deactivation.

Over the next decade, there will be a dramatic increase in the number of elderly people in the United States and in most parts of the world. With this increase, there will be an accompanying increase in patients with sinus node dysfunction and atrioventricular block; therefore, it will be essential for health care personnel to have a basic knowledge of bradyarrhythmias and the considerations required for managing these rhythms in elderly patients. In particular, comprehensive assessment before decisions on medical and device-based management is critical and must take into account social issues and the presence of comorbid conditions.

Syncope is a common clinical problem accounting for 3% of all emergency room visits and 1% to 6% of all hospital admissions. Both a sign and a symptom, syncope can be caused by a wide variety of conditions. Syncope in the geriatric patient can be a particularly challenging problem because of the coexistence of multiple possible causative pathologic conditions in the same individual. This article reviews the causes, evaluation, and management of syncope in the elderly.

> Perioperative arrhythmias are a common complication of surgery, with incidence ranging from 4% to 20% for noncardiothoracic procedures, depending on the type of surgery performed. The immediate postoperative period is a dynamic time and is associated with many conditions conducive to the development of postoperative arrhythmias. The presence of postoperative atrial fibrillation is associated with increased morbidity, ICU stay, length of hospitalization, and hospital costs. The associated burdens are expected to rise in the future, given that the population undergoing cardiac surgery is getting older and sicker. Thousands of patients undergo major surgery each year and a major complication of these procedures is the occurrence of perioperative arrhythmia. It is imperative for clinicians to be up-to-date on current management of these arrhythmias.

CLINICS IN GERIATRIC MEDICINE

Preface

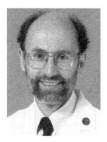 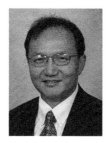

Michael W. Rich, MD   Win-Kuang Shen, MD
Guest Editors

The incidence and prevalence of heart rhythm disorders, including supraventricular and ventricular tachyarrhythmias, as well as bradyarrhythmias and conduction disorders, increase strikingly with age in both men and women. In this edition of the *Clinics in Geriatric Medicine*, the epidemiology, pathophysiology, diagnosis, and management of heart rhythm disorders commonly encountered in older adults are reviewed.

The first 2 articles provide essential background on the epidemiology and mechanisms of heart rhythm disorders in older adults. These are followed by an article devoted to the age-specific pharmacology of medications used in the treatment of common arrhythmias. Next are 3 articles that address various aspects of managing atrial fibrillation—arguably the quintessential heart rhythm disorder of aging—including stroke prevention, medical treatment, and device-based therapy. Similarly, 3 articles deal with ventricular arrhythmias in older patients, including medical management, device-based therapy, and quality-of-life and end-of-life issues in older adults with implanted cardiac devices. Bradyarrhythmias and conduction disorders are discussed in the next article, which is followed by an article on the evaluation and treatment of syncope. The monograph concludes with an article on the management of arrhythmias in the perioperative setting. All articles have been written by experts in the field and provide the most current information to guide clinical decision-making in older patients.

As editors of this volume, we are very pleased with how it has turned out, and we believe that you, the reader, will find it to be a useful addition to your library on the

Clin Geriatr Med 28 (2012) xiii–xiv
http://dx.doi.org/10.1016/j.cger.2012.09.001
0749-0690/12/$ – see front matter © 2012 Elsevier Inc. All rights reserved.

management of common conditions in our increasingly aging population. We would welcome any comments or suggestions you may have.

Sincerely,

Michael W. Rich, MD
Cardiovascular Division
Washington University School of Medicine
660 S. Euclid Avenue, Campus Box 8086
St Louis, MO 63110, USA

Win-Kuang Shen, MD
Mayo Clinic–Arizona
Scottsdale, AZ, USA

E-mail addresses:
mrich@wustl.edu (M.W. Rich)
wshen@mayo.edu (W.K. Shen)

Epidemiology of Arrhythmias and Conduction Disorders in Older Adults

Grant V. Chow, MD[a,1], Joseph E. Marine, MD[a,1],
Jerome L. Fleg, MD[b,*,1]

KEYWORDS

- Aging • Arrhythmia • Atrial fibrillation • Atrial flutter • Conduction disorders

KEY POINTS

- Changes in the cardiac conduction system include sinus node dysfunction, slowing of arterioventricular nodal conduction, left axis deviation, bundle branch blocks, and an increased prevalence of both supraventricular and ventricular premature beats and arrhythmias. Left bundle branch block, atrial fibrillation, and sustained ventricular tachycardia are particularly predictive of future adverse cardiac events, and frequently herald the presence of underlying cardiovascular disease.
- The prognostic significance of any given conduction abnormality or rhythm disturbance is dependent primarily on the presence and severity of any accompanying cardiac disease.
- Gaining an appreciation of the epidemiology of cardiac conduction disorders and arrhythmias in the elderly will assist the practitioner in differentiating electrocardiographic findings that represent normal aging from those suggesting a disease process requiring further evaluation.

EFFECTS OF AGING ON THE CONDUCTION SYSTEM, ASSOCIATED CONDUCTION DISORDERS, AND BRADYARRHYTHMIAS

Aging affects the cardiovascular system in multiple ways, including a decrease in compliance of blood vessels through arterial stiffening and thickening, mild left ventricular

Disclosures and financial support: The authors have no disclosures or financial conflicts of interest relevant to this manuscript to report. All authors contributed to the writing, editing, and content of this manuscript. The views expressed do not necessarily reflect those of the National Institutes of Health or the Department of Health and Human Services.

[a] Division of Cardiology, Johns Hopkins Medical Institutions, Johns Hopkins University School of Medicine, Carnegie 568, 600 N. Wolfe Street, Baltimore, MD 21287, USA; [b] Division of Cardiovascular Sciences, National Heart, Lung, and Blood Institute, Room 8150, 6701 Rockledge Drive, Bethesda, MD 20892, USA

[1] Author contributions: Grant Chow, MD, contributed in drafting and critical revision of the article. Joseph Marine, MD, and Jerome Fleg, MD, critically revised and approved the article for submission.

* Corresponding author.
E-mail address: flegj@nhlbi.nih.gov

thickening, and a shift in the balance of early versus late diastolic filling. Many of these changes result, in part, from cardiac cell enlargement with apoptosis of neighboring cells and subsequent fibrofatty infiltration of the myocardium.[1] The conduction system of the heart is also affected by the latter, producing changes that may result in conduction disorders or arrhythmia.

SINOATRIAL NODE

Aging is associated with increased fat and collagen deposition surrounding the sino-atrial (SA) node, which may result in delay of action potential propagation or even complete electrical separation of the node from surrounding tissue. During the course of normal aging, the number of pacemaker cells in the SA node declines significantly after age 60 years, with less than 10% of the cells seen in young adults remaining by age 75 years. Paradoxically, although older adults generally have fewer SA nodal pacemaker cells, they also have a lower prevalence of sinus bradycardia.[2] This counterintuitive observation is likely to the result of an offsetting age-related reduction in parasympathetic activity, which is also responsible for decreased heart rate variability and reduction in sinus arrhythmia.[3,4]

Although normal aging alone does not change the normal resting heart rate (HR) range of 60–80 beats per minute (bpm) in adults, it causes a predictable decrease in peak HR, with resultant decrease in maximal oxygen delivery during exercise. For each year following the onset of adulthood, the peak HR decreases at a rate of approximately 0.7 to 1.0 bpm per year. For routine stress testing, maximum age-predicted heart rate (MPHR) is commonly estimated as 220–age (years).[5] However, several groups[6–8] have recently called into question the accuracy of this formula, as its initial publication seems to have been based on a linear best fit to a series of observational data in 1971.[6] Several revised formulae for calculating MPHR are now available although none has yet been promoted in a widely recognized practice guideline.

Sinus Node Dysfunction

The umbrella terms sinus node dysfunction (SND) and sick sinus syndrome may be used in reference to any condition in which the atrial rate is inappropriate for physiologic requirements.[9] These include: (1) symptomatic sinus bradycardia, sinus pauses, or arrest; (2) chronotropic incompetence, and (3) alternating periods of atrial tachyarrhythmias and bradyarrhythmias (tachy-brady syndrome). Although the overall prevalence of SND in the elderly is unknown,[10] it is estimated that 70% to 80% of all pacemakers implanted for the indication of SND occur in patients more than 65 years of age.[11,12]

Sinus bradycardia

Sinus bradycardia is a common, usually normal and asymptomatic finding, defined by a sinus rate of less than 60 bpm. It should be recognized that this cutoff point is arbitrary. Although classified as an arrhythmia, it may be a normal variant in patients whose parasympathetic system is particularly dominant, such as competitive athletes. Although the prevalence of sinus bradycardia does not increase with age, symptomatic sinus bradycardia due to sick sinus syndrome occurs almost exclusively after the age of 65 years, at an estimated rate of 1 per 600 elderly cardiac patients.[9]

In the Baltimore Longitudinal Study of Aging (BLSA), 4.1% of 1172 healthy, nonendurance-trained, unmedicated participants aged 40 years or greater were found to have sinus bradycardia (defined as HR <50 bpm) on resting electrocardiography (ECG). Prevalence of unexplained sinus bradycardia was similar between men (3.9%) and women (4.5%), and was associated with an increased prevalence of conduction system abnormalities (43% vs 19%, $P<.05$), including first-degree atrioventricular (AV) block, left axis deviation, incomplete or complete right bundle branch block (RBBB); however, none experienced syncope, high-degree AV block, or symptomatic sinus node dysfunction.[13] There was no significant difference in major adverse cardiac events or deaths between groups during an average 5.4-year follow-up.

In 1987, Kannel and colleagues[14] reported results from the Framingham Heart Study, in which HR was determined from resting ECG examinations in a supine position. Of the 5070 individuals who entered the study without a history of cardiovascular disease, HR tended to increase with age in both men and women, with a linear increase in overall death rate observed with increasing baseline resting HR (**Table 1**). The prevalence of sinus bradycardia was low (<5%) for both men and women older than 65 years.

AV NODE AND THE HIS-PURKINJE SYSTEM

Aging results in varying degrees of calcification of the cardiac skeleton, particularly in the region including the central fibrous body and the left-sided valves (aortic and mitral valve rings). The AV node, AV bifurcation, as well as the proximal left and right bundle branches are located near the central fibrous body, and are thus vulnerable to slowed signal transmission with increasing age-related changes.

The PR interval undergoes a modest but significant prolongation with advancing age. In 46,129 study participants with very low probability of cardiovascular disease, an increase in mean PR interval occurred between the third and ninth decades of life, both in men (from 153 to 182 ms) and women (from 148 to 166 ms).[15] In the BLSA, a similar increase in PR interval prolongation was seen between the ages of 30 and 72 years, in both men (159–179 ms) and women (156–165 ms), due to prolongation of conduction proximal to the His bundle.[16] Although PR prolongation is often seen in normal aging, exaggeration of this phenomenon may clinically manifest as AV nodal block.

In contrast to the PR interval, QRS duration shows no significant age relationship, although the QRS axis does shift leftward with age. Mason and colleagues[15] reported a mean QRS axis shift from 56 to 8° between the third and ninth decades, with corresponding lower limits shifting from −3 to −60°. Thus, the prevalence of left axis deviation (defined as a QRS axis <−30°) increases to 20% by the tenth decade.[17] This age-associated leftward QRS axis shift may be due in part to increases in left ventricular wall thickness. Although some longitudinal studies have shown small increases in

Table 1				
Overall Framingham deaths by resting HR in the elderly, according to sex				
	Population At Risk (Person-Years)		**Age-Adjusted Annual Mortality Rate (per 1000)**	
Resting HR (bpm)	**Men**	**Women**	**Men**	**Women**
30–67	3660	3560	35	22
68–75	3646	6068	43	28
76–83	2172	4208	46	25
84–91	1572	3270	61	30
>91	1408	3264	64	35

A trend of increasing overall mortality was seen with stratification of the study population by resting HR. Higher HRs were associated with a higher age-adjusted annual mortality rate in both men and women. All trends were significant at P<.01.

Data from Kannel WB, Kannel C, Paffenbarger RS Jr, et al. Heart rate and cardiovascular mortality: The Framingham Study. Am Heart J 1987;113(6):1489–94.

cardiovascular mortality associated with this isolated ECG finding in the general population[18] or persons referred for exercise testing,[19] it remains unclear whether this increased risk extends to the elderly.

AV Nodal Block

First-degree AV block

First-degree AV block is defined as a PR interval of greater than 200 ms, representing a delay in AV conduction within the AV junction, usually within the AV node. The condition is usually asymptomatic and is associated with normal aging. The prevalence of first-degree AV block in healthy older men is approximately 3% to 4%, which is several-fold greater than in young men.[20] In 1986, the Manitoba study analyzed the resting ECGs of 3983 healthy airmen who were followed for 30 years, reporting percentage distribution of PR intervals according to age.[21] By the seventh decade, 20% of study participants had a PR interval of at least 200 ms but a PR interval of 220 ms or more was seen in only 4% of this group. No significant differences in cardiac morbidity or mortality were observed in these latter individuals compared with age-matched controls during 30 years of follow-up.[21]

Although previous cross-sectional and longitudinal studies have generally found no correlation between first-degree AV block and cardiac disease[22] or mortality,[21] a recent report using 20-year follow-up data from 7575 individuals in the Framingham Study (mean age 46 ± 15 years at baseline) demonstrated increased risks of atrial fibrillation, pacemaker implantation, and all-cause mortality associated with PR interval prolongation, even within the normal range.[23] In the Heart and Soul study representing 938 patients with known stable coronary disease and mean age 66 years, an association was found between first-degree AV block (defined as a PR interval ≥220 ms) and an increased risk of both heart failure hospitalization (odds ratio [OR] 2.33, 95% confidence interval [CI] 1.49–3.65; $P<.01$) and overall mortality (OR 1.58, 95% CI 1.13–2.20; $P<.01$) over a 5-year follow-up period.[24] Thus, the prognostic significance of first-degree AV block may differ, depending on whether cardiac disease is present.

Mobitz I second-degree AV block

Mobitz I second-degree AV block is characterized by a progressively lengthening PR interval until complete block occurs in the AV node, resulting in a nonconducted P wave. This conduction disorder is often asymptomatic and clinically silent.

Although no large population-based studies specifically report the prevalence of Mobitz I AV block, a study of 625 asymptomatic patients undergoing 24-hour ambulatory ECG monitoring showed transient Mobitz I block in 2.2% of individuals, occurring more frequently in those with a resting HR less than 60 bpm.[25] Of the 14 patients who experienced this conduction disorder, 64% were men, with a wide age distribution of 22 to 80 years (mean 42 ± 14 years). This wide age range likely encompasses both young individuals with AV block due to high vagal tone and older individuals with AV block due to AV nodal disease.

The natural history of Mobitz I block was examined in 147 patients from the Devon Heart Block and Bradycardia Survey found to have Mobitz I block on resting ECG. Professional athletes and patients with evidence of prior or coincidental Mobitz II or complete heart block, transient block following acute infarction, or drug-induced block were excluded.[26] Pacemakers were implanted in response to either significant symptoms associated with Mobitz I block (ie, presyncope, syncope, or confusion) or the subsequent development of higher degree block. After 1982, elderly patients were offered prophylactic pacemaker implantation if no contraindications existed. Of the 147 study patients, 90 (61%) received pacemakers. Patients aged 45 to 79 years who received a pacemaker enjoyed a significantly improved 5-year survival rate, whereas those more than 80 years of age showed a nonsignificant survival advantage over those who did not receive a pacemaker (**Table 2**).[26]

High-degree AV block

The term high-degree AV block (HAVB) encompasses both Mobitz II second-degree AV block and third-degree (or complete) AV block, both of which usually require a permanent pacemaker. HAVB may occur either as an isolated diagnosis in the elderly, often in the setting of hypertension and/or diabetes mellitus, accounting for approximately 40% of all implanted pacemakers in the United States,[27] or as a complication following acute myocardial infarction, cardiac surgery, endocarditis, or other cardiac injury.

The overall prevalence of HAVB in the general population is low. For the assessment of third-degree heart block, the Reykjavik Study prospectively evaluated 9139 men and 9773 women aged 33 to 79 years with baseline ECGs over a 24-year period.[28] Complete AV block was found in only 11 individuals (0.04%, mean age 55 years), and was transient in 7 (64%) of these 11 cases.

In the largest pacemaker and implantable cardioverter-defibrillator (ICD) survey ever performed, data on more than 80% of all devices implanted worldwide during 2009 were analyzed by Mond and colleagues.[29] Of the 61 countries participating in the survey, the United States implanted the most devices (n = 225,567), with Germany implanting the most devices per capita (927 devices per million population). In countries reporting the prevalence of pacemaker implantation for the indication of HAVB, results were highly variable between nations, from 15% (Greece) to 95% (Sudan) of all procedures performed. The mean age of patients receiving a pacemaker also varied significantly (men, mean 44 years [Qatar] to 78 years [Puerto Rico]; women, mean 47 years [Qatar] to 80 years [Italy]). Despite many differences in accessibility of health care and availability of pacemakers to the populations of the world, patients older than 60 years consistently comprised the largest group of pacemaker recipients, with the highest proportions in Uruguay (94%) and Italy (95%).

His-Purkinje Conduction Abnormalities

Right bundle branch block

Right bundle branch block increases in prevalence with age. In the Framingham Heart Study, the incidence of RBBB peaked in men in the seventh decade, whereas a continued increase occurred in women throughout the study period.[30] In total, 70 new cases of RBBB were detected during the 18-year follow-up period, representing 1.3% of the total study population. Although the initial appearance of RBBB was not associated with adverse clinical events, subsequent incidence of coronary artery disease was 2.5 times greater ($P<.001$) and congestive heart failure was almost 4 times greater ($P = .02$) in patients with RBBB compared with those without by the end of the study period.

In the BLSA, RBBB was observed in 39 of 1142 (3.4%) men on resting ECG, of whom 24 (2.1%) had no evidence of associated cardiac disease. Mean age on presentation with, or development of, RBBB was 64 ± 13.5 years. In both the BLSA and Framingham cohorts, the diagnosis of RBBB in persons without concurrent clinical heart disease was not associated with major adverse cardiac events.[31] In the Reykjavik Study, RBBB increased in prevalence from 0% in persons aged 30 to 39 years to 4.1% of men and 1.6% of women 75 to 79 years old. In men but not women, RBBB was associated with cardiomegaly, ischemic heart disease, and arrhythmias on resting ECG. However, neither total deaths nor cardiovascular deaths were associated with RBBB on multivariate analysis.[32]

Table 2
Survival of patients with Mobitz I second-degree heart block by age group, with and without a pacemaker

| Variable | Age Group (Years) | | | | | | | | | | All Patients | |
| | 20–44 | | 45–64 | | 65–79 | | 80+ | | | | | |
	Paced	Unpaced	Paced	Unpaced	Paced	Unpaced	Paced	Unpaced			Paced	Unpaced
Subjects (n)	5	10	18	7	52	18	15	22			90	57
Mean age (years)	34	32.6	57.1	58.1	72.9	72.2	85	85.9			69.6	68.8
5-year survival, % (SD)	100 (0)	100 (0)	94.4 (5.4)	57.1 (18.7)	76.6 (5.9)	50 (11.8)	45.9 (13)	33.4 (10.3)			76.3 (4.5)	53.5 (6.7)
P value	1		0.001[a]		0.003[a]		0.76[a]				0.0014[a]	

Patients between 45 and 79 years who received a pacemaker for the indications of symptomatic Mobitz I or subsequent high-degree AV block had a significant survival advantage over those who did not.

[a] Log rank test (age imbalances were sufficiently small to be negligible).

Data from Shaw DB, Gowers JI, Kekwick CA, et al. Is Mobitz type I atrioventricular block benign in adults? Heart 2004;90(2):169–74.

Left bundle branch block

In contrast to RBBB, left bundle branch block (LBBB) is more specific for the presence of cardiovascular disease (eg, antecedent hypertension, cardiac enlargement, cardiomyopathy, or coronary heart disease).[33,34] The prognosis of patients with LBBB, therefore, is closely tied to that of the underlying heart disease.

Both the incidence and prevalence of LBBB increase with age. In the Framingham Heart Study, 55 new cases (31 men, 24 women) of LBBB were detected during the 18-year follow-up period, representing 1.1% of the total study population.[33] Mean age at onset of LBBB was 62 years (range 36–78 years). Only 15 (27%) of the 55 new cases of LBBB were free from all previous cardiovascular abnormalities, although 5 (33%) of the 15 eventually developed coronary heart disease, a rate more than 3 times higher than control participants without LBBB.

The Irish Heart Foundation screened a large general population (n = 110,000) from 1968 to 1993 using a single resting ECG, revealing 112 individuals (0.1%) with LBBB and no prior history of hypertension or heart disease.[34] Follow-up of all cases and controls matched for age and sex was performed in 1993 via postal questionnaire, completed in 98% of cases and 97% of controls. Individuals with LBBB had a mean age of 51 ± 13 years and were predominantly male (73%). The prevalence of LBBB increased with age in both men and women (**Fig. 1**). Cardiovascular disease developed in more patients with LBBB than in controls (21% vs 11%; $P = .04$), although the incidence of cardiac death was not significantly increased. Two (1.9%) of the 112 individuals with new LBBB eventually required permanent pacemaker implantation.

TACHYARRHYTHMIAS

Tachyarrhythmias form a large heterogeneous group of disorders in older adults. The epidemiology of supraventricular and ventricular tachyarrhythmias in the elderly population is discussed in the following sections.

Supraventricular Tachyarrhythmias

Sinus tachycardia

Sinus tachycardia (ST) is common, may present without symptoms, and is usually a result of anxiety, fever, thyrotoxicosis, acute hypovolemia/anemia, or other acute

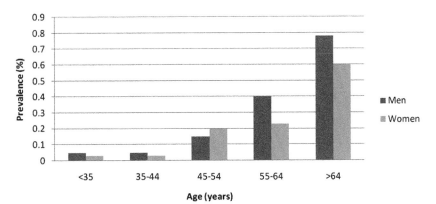

Fig. 1. Prevalence of LBBB in the Irish Heart Foundation study, according to age. The incidence and prevalence of LBBB increases with age, with highest levels seen in the elderly cohort. (*Data from* Fahy GJ, Pinski SL, Miller DP, et al. Natural history of isolated bundle branch block. Am J Cardiol 1996;77(14):1185–90.)

illness. Because sinus tachycardia generally results from increased sympathetic and/ or reduced parasympathetic tone, many texts classify this rhythm as a physiologic sign rather than a free-standing arrhythmia, just as fever is generally considered a symptom rather than a diagnosis. As such, its overall incidence and prevalence are difficult to ascertain, as there are a myriad of causes, and the condition is usually transient in nature.

Supraventricular premature beats

Supraventricular premature beats, including atrial premature beats (APB) and those of junctional origin, occur on resting ECG in 5% to 10% of all individuals older than 60 years and are commonly seen during ambulatory 24-hour monitoring. Among 1372 predominantly healthy individuals aged 65 years and older in the Cardiovascular Health Study (CHS), isolated APBs were seen in 97% in a 24-hour period.[35] In healthy BLSA volunteers older than 60 years, resting ECGs demonstrated APB in 6%, exercise stress testing provoked APB in 39%, and 24-hour ambulatory monitoring captured APB in 88%.[36] Even when frequent, supraventricular premature beats on ambulatory monitoring were not predictive of increased adverse cardiac outcomes over a 10-year mean follow-up period.[37]

Atrial fibrillation

Atrial fibrillation (AF) is the most prevalent clinically significant rhythm disorder in the elderly, affecting approximately 2.3 million Americans, comprising around 6% of those older than 65 years and 12% of individuals older than 85 years.[38] Furthermore, the prevalence of AF is projected to increase 2.5-fold over the next 50 years.[38] In 1995, Feinberg and colleagues[39] reported the combined age-specific prevalence of AF from 4 large studies: the Framingham,[40] Western Australia,[41] Rochester,[42] and CHS (**Fig. 2**).[43] The investigators found that the overall prevalence of AF was higher in men than in women for all age groups, but because there were almost twice the number of women than men older than 75 years in the general population, the absolute numbers of women and men with AF were similar. A recent meta-analysis[44] of 10 studies involving 1,031,351 participants found a markedly lower prevalence of AF in African Americans compared with whites (OR 0.51, 95% CI 0.44–0.59, P<.001) in both the general population and in those older than 60 years of age.

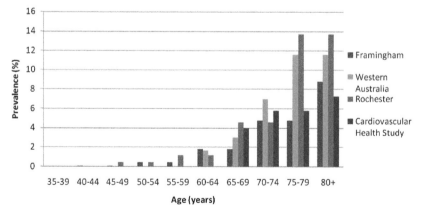

Fig. 2. Prevalence of AF in 4 population-based surveys. The incidence and prevalence of AF increase with age, with highest rates seen in the elderly. (*Data from* Feinberg WM, Blackshear JL, Laupacis A, et al. Prevalence, age distribution, and gender of patients with atrial fibrillation. Analysis and implications. Arch Intern Med 1995;155(3):469–73.)

Numerous factors likely contribute to the increase in AF prevalence with age, including an increased prevalence of comorbid conditions, such as hypertension, diabetes, thyrotoxicosis, and mitral valve disorders.[45] Increased left atrial size, which provides an anatomic substrate for wavelets of micro-reentry, is common among elderly individuals, and is an independent predictor of AF.[46] An age-related increase in left ventricular stiffness, with resulting diastolic dysfunction and increased left atrial pressure, may also serve as an important contributor.[47] AF may arise without obvious comorbidities (lone AF), accounting for 17% of men and 6% of women with this arrhythmia (mean ages 70.6 and 68.1 years, respectively) in the Framingham Study.[48] Lone AF was associated with a 4-fold higher rate of strokes but no increase in coronary events or heart failure over long-term follow-up. AF accompanying structural heart disease is associated with increased rates of heart failure, stroke, and cardiovascular death. AF accounts for nearly one-quarter of strokes occurring among octogenarians compared with only 1.5% in persons in their 50s.[49] AF is also a major predisposing factor to heart failure with preserved ejection fraction, the predominant form of heart failure in the elderly.[50]

Postoperative AF occurs in up to 40% of patients after cardiac surgery and is a major source of increased morbidity, hospital stay, and costs in these patients.[51] Advanced age is a potent risk factor for postoperative AF.[51,52]

Despite advances in blood pressure control and risk factor management over the past decade, the high incidence of AF in older adults continues unabated. Recent research indicates that approximately 10% of patients greater than 65 years of age who have a pacemaker or ICD had subclinical and previously undetected AF, discovered when their devices were routinely interrogated 3 months after implantation.[53]

Atrial flutter

Atrial flutter (AFL) is a relatively uncommon arrhythmia in adults, caused by a macro-reentrant loop in either the right or left atrium. In a recent population study of more than 54,000 individuals, the 4-year incidence of AFL was 0.14%, AF was 0.73%, and a combination of AFL and AF was 0.19%. The mean age of the AFL and AF cohorts were 70 and 72 years, respectively (P = NS).[54] Although many predisposing factors are shared between AFL and AF (with many patients affected by both arrhythmias), patients with AFL without concurrent AF were more likely to have had a history of obstructive lung disease (25% vs 12%, P = .006) and heart failure (28% vs 17%, P = .05), whereas hypertension was more common (63% vs 47%, P = .01) in the cohort with AF without concurrent AFL.[54]

Paroxysmal supraventricular tachycardia

Supraventricular tachycardia (SVT) is a general term encompassing the diagnoses of atrial tachycardia (AT), atrioventricular nodal reentrant tachycardia (AVNRT), and atrioventricular reciprocating tachycardia (AVRT). Short largely asymptomatic bursts of SVT have been observed in up to 50% of the normal elderly population in prior studies using 24-hour monitoring,[35,36] with increasing incidence associated with advanced age. Prevalence of clinically evident paroxysmal SVT also increases with age, occurring in an estimated 6.16 cases per 1000 population in patients more than 65 years of age.[55] In the BLSA, short bursts of paroxysmal SVT detected during exercise testing also became more prevalent with age, but did not presage increased risk of subsequent coronary events in clinically healthy older adults.[56] The prevalence of exercise-associated PSVT episodes steadily increased in men, but reached a plateau after the age of 60 years in women (**Fig. 3**).

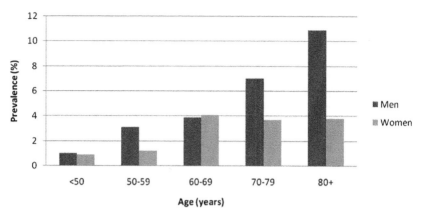

Fig. 3. Prevalence of exercise-associated PSVT in the BLSA, stratified by age group. The prevalence of PSVT increased steadily in men, whereas a plateau was seen in women after the age of 60 years. (*Data from* Maurer MS, Shefrin EA, Fleg JL. Prevalence and prognostic significance of exercise-induced supraventricular tachycardia in apparently healthy volunteers. Am J Cardiol 1995;75(12):788–92.)

Ventricular Tachyarrhythmias

Ventricular premature beats and nonsustained ventricular tachycardia

Ventricular premature beats (VPB) increase in prevalence with advancing age in both unselected patient populations and those clinically free of heart disease. An evaluation of approximately 2500 ECGs from elderly hospitalized patients revealed VPB in 8%,[57] whereas resting ECGs in apparently healthy BLSA volunteers with a normal ST-segment response to treadmill exercise showed isolated VPB in 8.6% of men more than 60 years of age, compared with only 0.5% in those aged 20 to 40 years.[58] There was no correlation of VPB prevalence with age in women.

Ambulatory 24-hour ECG recordings in multiple studies have shown a significantly higher prevalence of VPB, ranging from 69% to 96%, in the asymptomatic elderly compared with younger age groups.[35,36,59,60] In the CHS, VPB were found in 82% of 1372 elderly individuals, including 3-beat to 5-beat runs of nonsustained ventricular tachycardia (VT).[35] VPB was seen in 96% of individuals older than 80 years without clinical heart disease (n = 50).[59] In 98 asymptomatic BLSA participants older than 60 years, 35% had multiform VPB, 11% had VPB couplets, and 4% had brief bursts of nonsustained VT.[36] After a mean 10-year follow-up period, 14 (14.3%) of the 98 participants developed coronary events, with a virtually identical prevalence and complexity of VPB in those with and without events.[37] Thus, despite the presence of an increased prevalence and complexity of VPB in asymptomatic elderly, their prognostic significance seems minimal in the absence of clinical heart disease.

Exercise stress testing is also associated with a marked increase in the prevalence and complexity of VPB occurrence with age. In a comparison of apparently healthy BLSA volunteers between the third and ninth decade, isolated VPB during or after maximal treadmill stress testing increased in prevalence from 11% to 57% from the third to the ninth decade.[58] Asymptomatic exercise-associated runs of nonsustained VT (all ≤6 beats) were seen in 4% of BLSA volunteers aged 65 years or older, a rate 25-fold higher than that of younger persons.[61] Over a 2-year mean follow-up period, no study participant with nonsustained VT during exercise developed angina, myocardial infarction, syncope, or sudden death. In this same BLSA population, frequent or repetitive VPB during or after exercise testing was seen predominantly in older individuals, but was similarly unassociated with cardiovascular prognosis over a mean 5.6 years of follow-up.[62] However, in a younger French cohort of 6101 men (aged 48 ± 2 years) initially free of clinical cardiovascular disease, those who had frequent VPB during exercise had a 2.5-fold increased risk of cardiovascular death over 23 years of follow-up, independent of standard coronary risk factors.[63]

Although the occasional VPB on resting ECG or during exercise stress testing does not portend a poorer prognosis in apparently healthy individuals, in older patients with coronary disease, the presence of complex VPB is an adverse prognostic indicator. In 467 patients aged 62 to 102 years in a long-term care facility, complex VPB occurred in 21%.[64] In those without a history of coronary disease, the future coronary event rate (4%) was similar to that of the general nursing facility population, whereas in those with coronary disease and complex VPB, the future event rate was more than 11-fold higher (46%). Thus, it is important to ascertain the presence or absence of cardiovascular comorbidities in older persons with VPB.

Sustained ventricular tachycardia and sudden arrhythmic death

Sustained VT is a potentially life-threatening arrhythmia that occurs in 2 major forms: monomorphic (usually macro-reentrant and scar-related) and polymorphic (usually ischemia-related). Sudden arrhythmic death refers to hemodynamically unstable VT or ventricular fibrillation (VF), and accounts for most episodes of sudden cardiac death (SCD), a diagnosis that includes hemodynamically unstable VT, VF, asystole, and non-arrhythmic cardiac causes. SCD is responsible for an estimated 184,000 to 462,000 American deaths yearly, and is a major cause of mortality in the elderly.[65]

The Framingham Heart Study compared the incidence of SCD in women and men across all age groups (n = 5209), aged 30 to 62 years at study entry.[66] More than half of the study population were women (n = 2873, 55%), with a peak incidence of SCD which lagged that of men by more than 10 years. Congestive heart failure increased the risk of SCD by 5-fold in women and 16-fold in men. The incidence of SCD progressively increased with age, especially after age 74 years, reflecting the high prevalence of structural heart disease in the elderly (**Fig. 4**).

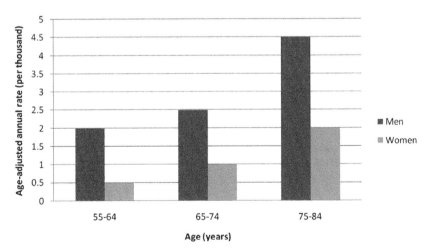

Fig. 4. Incidence of sudden death in the Framingham Study, grouped by age and sex. Incidence of sudden death increased progressively with increasing age, affecting men more frequently than women in each age group. (*Data from* Kannel WB, Wilson PW, D'Agostino RB, et al. Sudden coronary death in women. Am Heart J 1998;136(2):205–12.)

SUMMARY

Aging is associated with a myriad of changes in the cardiac conduction system, some of which manifest in association with cardiovascular disease, and others develop as part of normal aging. These changes include sinus node dysfunction, slowing of AV nodal conduction, left axis deviation, bundle branch blocks, and an increased prevalence of both supraventricular and ventricular premature beats and arrhythmias. LBBB, AF, and sustained VT are particularly predictive of future adverse cardiac events, and frequently herald the presence of underlying cardiovascular disease. The prognostic significance of any given conduction abnormality or rhythm disturbance is dependent primarily on the presence and severity of any accompanying cardiac disease. Gaining an appreciation of the epidemiology of cardiac conduction disorders and arrhythmias in the elderly will assist the practitioner in differentiating ECG findings that represent normal aging from those suggesting a disease process requiring further evaluation.

REFERENCES

1. Anversa P, Palackal T, Sonnenblick EH, et al. Myocyte cell loss and myocyte cellular hyperplasia in the hypertrophied aging rat heart. Circ Res 1990;67(4): 871–85.
2. Hiss RG, Lamb LE. Electrocardiographic findings in 122,043 individuals. Circulation 1962;25:947–61.
3. Schwartz J, Gibb WJ, Tran T. Aging effects on heart rate variation. J Gerontol 1991;46(3):M99–106.
4. Byrne EA, Fleg JL, Vaitkevicius PV, et al. Role of aerobic capacity and body mass index in the age-associated decline in heart rate variability. J Appl Physiol 1996; 81(2):743–50.
5. Shub C. Stable angina pectoris: 2. Cardiac evaluation and diagnostic testing. Mayo Clin Proc 1990;65(2):243–55.
6. Robergs RA, Landwehr R. The surprising history of the 'HRmax=220-age' equation. J Exerc Physiol Online 2002;5(2):1–10.
7. Tanaka H, Monahan KD, Seals DR. Age-predicted maximal heart rate revisited. J Am Coll Cardiol 2001;37(1):153–6.
8. Nes BM, Janszky I, Wisloff U, et al. Age-predicted maximal heart rate in healthy subjects: the HUNT fitness study. Scand J Med Sci Sports 2012. [Epub ahead of print].
9. Adan V, Owen LA. Diagnosis and treatment of sick sinus syndrome. Am Fam Physician 2003;67:1725–32.
10. Faddis MN, Rich MW. Pacing interventions for falls and syncope in the elderly. Clin Geriatr Med 2002;18(2):279–94.
11. Lamas GA, Prosser AP, Edery TP, et al. Age and sex bias in pacemaker selection. Circulation 1992;86(Suppl I):1–449.
12. Gregoratos G. Permanent pacemakers in older persons. J Am Geriatr Soc 1999; 47(9):1125–35.
13. Tresch DD, Fleg JL. Unexplained sinus bradycardia: clinical significance and long-term prognosis in apparently healthy persons older than 40 years. Am J Cardiol 1986;58(10):1009–13.
14. Kannel WB, Kannel C, Paffenbarger RS Jr, et al. Heart rate and cardiovascular mortality: the Framingham Study. Am Heart J 1987;113(6):1489–94.
15. Mason JW, Ramseth DJ, Chanter DO, et al. Electrocardiographic reference ranges derived from 79,743 ambulatory subjects. J Electrocardiol 2007;40(3):228–34.

16. Fleg JL, Das DN, Wright J, et al. Age-associated changes in the components of atrioventricular conduction in apparently healthy volunteers. J Gerontol 1990; 45(3):M95–100.

17. Golden GS, Golden LH. The "nona" electrocardiogram: findings in 100 patients of the 90 age group. J Am Geriatr Soc 1974;22(7):329–31.

18. Sox HC Jr, Garber AM, Littenberg B. The resting electrocardiogram as a screening test. A clinical analysis. Ann Intern Med 1989;111:489–502.

19. Gorodeski EZ, Ishwaran H, Blackstone EH, et al. Quantitative electrocardiographic measures and long-term mortality in exercise test patients with clinically normal electrocardiograms. Am Heart J 2009;158:61–70.e1.

20. Simonson E. The effect of age on the electrocardiogram. Am J Cardiol 1972;29(1): 64–73.

21. Mymin D, Mathewson FA, Tate RB, et al. The natural history of primary first-degree atrioventricular heart block. N Engl J Med 1986;315(19):1183–7.

22. Rodstein M, Brown M, Wolloch L. First-degree atrioventricular heart block in the aged. Geriatrics 1968;23(10):159–65.

23. Cheng S, Keyes MJ, Larson MG, et al. Long-term outcomes in individuals with prolonged PR interval or first-degree atrioventricular block. JAMA 2009;301(24): 2571–7.

24. Crisel RK, Farzaneh-Far R, Na B, et al. First-degree atrioventricular block is associated with heart failure and death in persons with stable coronary artery disease: data from the Heart and Soul Study. Eur Heart J 2011;32(15):1875–80.

25. DePaula RS, Antelmi I, Vincenzi MA, et al. Cardiac arrhythmias and atrioventricular block in a cohort of asymptomatic individuals without heart disease. Cardiology 2007;108(2):111–6.

26. Shaw DB, Gowers JI, Kekwick CA, et al. Is Mobitz type I atrioventricular block benign in adults? Heart 2004;90(2):169–74.

27. Parsonnet V, Bernstein AD, Galasso D. Cardiac pacing practices in the United States in 1985. Am J Cardiol 1988;62(1):71–7.

28. Kojic EM, Hardarson T, Sigfusson N, et al. The prevalence and prognosis of third-degree atrioventricular conduction block: the Reykjavik study. J Intern Med 1999; 246(1):81–6.

29. Mond HG, Proclemer A. The 11th world survey of cardiac pacing and implantable cardioverter-defibrillators: calendar year 2009 – a World Society of Arrhythmia's project. Pacing Clin Electrophysiol 2011;34(8):1013–27.

30. Schneider JF, Thomas HE, Kreger BE, et al. Newly acquired right bundle-branch block: the Framingham Study. Ann Intern Med 1980;92(1):37–44.

31. Fleg JL, Das DN, Lakatta EG. Right bundle branch block: long-term prognosis in apparently healthy men. J Am Coll Cardiol 1983;1(3):887–92.

32. Thrainsdottir IS, Hardarson T, Thorgeirsson G, et al. The epidemiology of right bundle branch block and its association with cardiovascular morbidity–The Reykjavik Study. Eur Heart J 1993;14:1590–6.

33. Schneider JF, Thomas HE Jr, Kreger BE, et al. Newly acquired left bundle-branch block: the Framingham study. Ann Intern Med 1979;90(3):303–10.

34. Fahy GJ, Pinski SL, Miller DP, et al. Natural history of isolated bundle branch block. Am J Cardiol 1996;77(14):1185–90.

35. Manolio TA, Furberg CD, Rautaharju PM, et al. Cardiac arrhythmias on 24-hour ambulatory electrocardiography in older women and men: the Cardiovascular Health Study. J Am Coll Cardiol 1994;23(4):916–25.

36. Fleg JL, Kennedy HL. Cardiac arrhythmias in a healthy elderly population: detection by 24-hour ambulatory electrocardiography. Chest 1982;81(3):302–7.

37. Fleg JL, Kennedy HL. Long-term prognostic significance of ambulatory electro-cardiographic findings in apparently healthy subjects 60 years of age. Am J Cardiol 1992;70(7):748–51.
38. Lakshminarayan K, Solid CA, Collins AJ, et al. Atrial fibrillation and stroke in the general Medicare population. A 10-year perspective (1992 to 2002). Stroke 2006; 37:1969–74.
39. Feinberg WM, Blackshear JL, Laupacis A, et al. Prevalence, age distribution, and gender of patients with atrial fibrillation. Analysis and implications. Arch Intern Med 1995;155(3):469–73.
40. Wolf PA, Benjamin EJ, Belanger AJ, et al. Secular trends in the prevalence of atrial fibrillation: the Framingham Study. Am Heart J 1996;131(4):790–5.
41. Lake RR, Cullen KJ, deKlerk NH, et al. Atrial fibrillation in an elderly population. Aust N Z J Med 1989;19(4):321–6.
42. Phillips SJ, Whisnant J, O'Fallon WM, et al. Prevalence of cardiovascular disease and diabetes in residents of Rochester, Minnesota. Mayo Clin Proc 1990;65(3): 344–59.
43. Furberg CD, Psaty BM, Manolio TA, et al. Prevalence of atrial fibrillation in elderly subjects: the Cardiovascular Health Study. Am J Cardiol 1994;74(3):238–41.
44. Hernandez MB, Asher CR, Hernandez AV, et al. African American race and prevalence of atrial fibrillation: a meta-analysis. Cardiol Res Pract 2012;2012:275624.
45. Schnabel RB. Can we predict the occurrence of atrial fibrillation? Clin Cardiol 2012;35(Suppl 1):5–9.
46. Psaty BM, Manolio TA, Kuller LH, et al. Incidence of and risk factors for atrial fibrillation in older adults. Circulation 1997;96:2455–61.
47. Tsang TS, Gersh BJ, Appleton CP, et al. Left ventricular diastolic dysfunction as a predictor of the first diagnosed nonvalvular atrial fibrillation in 840 elderly men and women. J Am Coll Cardiol 2002;40(9):1636–44.
48. Brand FN, Abbott RD, Kannel WB, et al. Characteristics and prognosis of lone atrial fibrillation 30-Year follow-up in the Framingham Study. JAMA 1985; 254(24):3449–53.
49. Wolf PA, Abbott RD, Kannel WB. Atrial fibrillation as an independent risk factor for stroke: the Framingham Study. Stroke 1991;22(8):983–8.
50. Kitzman DW, Gardin JM, Gottdiener JS, et al. Importance of heart failure with preserved systolic function in patients ≥65 years of age. Am J Cardiol 2001; 87:413–9.
51. Mathew JP, Fontes ML, Tudor JC, et al. A muklticenter risk index for atrial fibrillation after cardiac surgery. JAMA 2004;291:1720–9.
52. Amar D, Zhang H, Leung DH, et al. Older age is the strongest predictor of post-operative atrial fibrillation. Anesthesiology 2002;96(2):352–6.
53. Healey JS, Connolly SJ, Gold MR, et al. Subclinical atrial fibrillation and the risk of stroke. N Engl J Med 2012;366(2):120–9.
54. Mareedu RK, Abdalrahman IB, Dharmashankar KC, et al. Atrial flutter versus atrial fibrillation in a general population: differences in comorbidities associated with their respective onset. Clin Med Res 2010;8(1):1–6.
55. Orejarena LA, Vidaillet H Jr, DeStefano F, et al. Paroxysmal supraventricular tachycardia in the general population. J Am Coll Cardiol 1998;31(1):150–7.
56. Maurer MS, Shefrin EA, Fleg JL. Prevalence and prognostic significance of exercise-induced supraventricular tachycardia in apparently healthy volunteers. Am J Cardiol 1995;75(12):788–92.
57. Fisch C. Electrocardiogram in the aged. An independent marker of heart disease? Am J Med 1981;70(1):4–6.

58. Fleg JL. Epidemiology of ventricular arrhythmias in the elderly. In: Paciaroni E, editor. Proceedings of the 13th National Congress of Cardiology (Aging and Cardiac Arrhythmias) I.N.R.C.A. Ancona (Italy): Instituto a Carattere Scientifico; 1991. p. 26–30.

59. Kantelip JP, Sage E, Duchene-Marullaz P. Findings on ambulatory electrocardiologic monitoring in subjects older than 80 years. Am J Cardiol 1986;57(6): 398–401.

60. Camm AJ, Evans KE, Ward DE, et al. The rhythm of the heart in active elderly subjects. Am Heart J 1981;99(5):598–603.

61. Fleg JL, Lakatta EG. Prevalence and prognosis of exercise-induced nonsustained ventricular tachycardia in apparently healthy volunteers. Am J Cardiol 1984;54(7):762–4.

62. Busby MJ, Shefrin E, Fleg JL. Prevalence and long-term prognostic significance of exercise-induced frequent or repetitive ventricular ectopic beats in apparently healthy volunteers. J Am Coll Cardiol 1989;14:1659–65.

63. Jouven X, Zureik M, Desnos M, et al. Long-term outcome in asymptomatic men with exercise-induced premature ventricular depolarizations. N Engl J Med 2000;343(12):826–33.

64. Aronow WS, Epstein S, Koenigsberg M, et al. Usefulness of echocardiographic abnormal left ventricular ejection fraction, paroxysmal ventricular tachycardia, and complex ventricular arrhythmias in predicting new coronary events in patients over 62 years of age. Am J Cardiol 1988;61(15):1349–51.

65. Goldberger J, Cain M, Hohnloser S, et al. American Heart Association/American College of Cardiology Foundation/Heart Rhythm Society scientific statement on noninvasive risk stratification techniques for identifying patients at risk for sudden cardiac death: a scientific statement from the American Heart Association Council on Clinical Cardiology Committee on Electrocardiography and Arrhythmias and Council on Epidemiology and Prevention. Circulation 2008;118(14): 1497–518.

66. Kannel WB, Wilson PW, D'Agostino RB, et al. Sudden coronary death in women. Am Heart J 1998;136(2):205–12.

Mechanisms of Arrhythmias and Conduction Disorders in Older Adults

Mahek Mirza, MD[a], Anton Strunets, MD[a], Win-Kuang Shen, MD[b], Arshad Jahangir, MD[a],*

KEYWORDS

- Aging • Arrhythmias • Mechanisms • Elderly • Atrial fibrillation
- Ventricular fibrillation • Sudden cardiac death

KEY POINTS

- Aging is associated with an increased prevalence of cardiac arrhythmias, which contribute to higher morbidity and mortality in the elderly. The frequency of cardiac arrhythmias, particularly atrial fibrillation and ventricular tachyarrhythmia, is projected to increase as the population ages, greatly affecting health care resource utilization.
- Several clinical factors associated with the risk of arrhythmias have been identified in the population, yet the molecular bases for the increased predisposition to arrhythmogenesis in the elderly are not fully understood. Therefore, only limited therapeutic strategies directed at pathophysiologic processes that enhance cardiac vulnerability to arrhythmias are available.
- This is further compounded by the paucity of outcome studies providing evidence on which optimal management guidelines can be formulated for the very elderly.

INTRODUCTION

Aging is associated with an increased prevalence of cardiac arrhythmias, which contribute to higher morbidity and mortality in the elderly.[1–4] With the aging of the population, the frequency of cardiac arrhythmias, particularly atrial fibrillation (AF) and ventricular tachyarrhythmia, is projected to increase and thereby greatly affect health care resource utilization.[4–7] Several clinical factors associated with the risk of

Disclosures: None.

Funding sources: Drs Jahangir and Mirza's research effort was in part supported by National Heart, Lung, and Blood Institute grants R01 HL101240-03 and R01 HL089542-04.

[a] Center for Integrative Research on Cardiovascular Aging (CIRCA), Aurora University of Wisconsin Medical Group, Aurora Health Care, 3033 South 27th Street, Milwaukee, WI 53215, USA; [b] Division of Cardiovascular Diseases, Mayo Clinic, 13400 E. Shea Boulevard, Scottsdale, AZ 85259, USA

* Corresponding author.

E-mail address: arshad.jahangir@aurora.org

Clin Geriatr Med 28 (2012) 555–573

http://dx.doi.org/10.1016/j.cger.2012.08.005

arrhythmias have been identified in the population,[8,9] yet the molecular bases for the increased predisposition to arrhythmogenesis in the elderly are not fully understood. Therefore, only limited therapeutic strategies directed at pathophysiologic processes that enhance cardiac vulnerability to arrhythmias are available. This is further compounded by the paucity of outcome studies[10,11] that provide evidence on which optimal management guidelines can be formulated for the very elderly.[2,10,12–14] In this review, the authors highlight the epidemiology of cardiac dysrhythmias, changes in cardiac structure and function associated with aging, and the basis for arrhythmogenesis in the elderly, the understanding of which is critical to formulate preventive strategies.

EPIDEMIOLOGY

The incidence of cardiac dysrhythmias, both bradyarrhythmias and tachyarrhythmias, increases with advancing age.[12,15,16] The median age of pacemaker recipients for bradyarrhythmias in the United States is 75 years with more than 80% of pacemakers implanted in those 65 years or older.[16] The major indication for pacemaker implantation in the elderly is to relieve symptoms caused by bradycardia and/or chronotropic incompetency from sinus node dysfunction or His-Purkinje disease as a result of aging-related degenerative changes in the atrial pacemaker complex and conduction system that usually manifest in the seventh or eighth decade of life.[16–19]

Among tachyarrhythmias, AF is the most common arrhythmia encountered in clinical practice, with a 100-fold higher prevalence in octogenarians (8%–10%) compared to those younger than 55 years (<0.1%; **Fig. 1**).[2,12,20–22] With a 1-in-4 lifetime risk of development,[23] AF contributes to increased morbidity in the elderly, not only by adversely affecting quality of life but also by deterioration in myocardial function, which increases susceptibility to heart failure, stroke, hospitalization, and mortality.

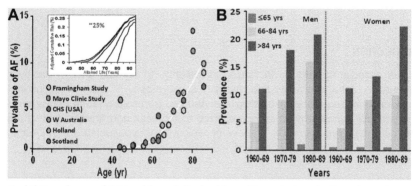

Fig. 1. (*A*) Prevalence of AF in older adults doubles with each decade. Prevalence increases 80- to 100-fold in the very elderly (0.1% at 40 years to ~8%–10% in ≥80 years). *Inset:* Cumulative lifetime risk for the development of AF (~25%) in the adult population. (*B*) Secular trends in prevalence of AF in Olmsted County, MN: 1960–1989. (*Data from* Feinberg WM, Blackshear JL, Laupacis A, et al. Prevalence, age distribution, and gender of patients with atrial fibrillation analysis and implications. Arch Int Med 1995;155: 469–73; Lloyd-Jones DM, Wang TJ, Leip EP, et al. Lifetime risk for development of atrial fibrillation: the Framingham Heart Study. Circulation 2004;110:1042–6; and Tsang TS, Petty GW, Barnes ME, et al. The prevalence of atrial fibrillation in incident stroke cases and matched population controls in Rochester, Minnesota: changes over three decades. J Am Coll Cardiol 2003;42:93–100.)

AF carries an annual health care cost exceeding $15 billion.[5,8,9,20,23–27] The median age of patients with AF is around 75 years, with 84% of the patients older than 65. With the rapid increase in the number of elderly[7] and concomitant cardiovascular comorbidities,[24,28] a 6-fold increase in the prevalence of AF (to 15.9 million) is projected,[20] highlighting the magnitude of the epidemic of AF and its far-reaching implications for the health and economics of the country.[20,24,29]

Aging is also associated with a progressive increase in the incidence of ventricular dysrhythmias, both benign and malignant, with or without structural heart disease. Unexpected death from cardiovascular causes occurs in 250,000 to 300,000 individuals annually with up to 75% to 80% resulting from ventricular fibrillation or tachycardia, more so in elderly patients with coronary artery disease, and may be the presenting event in 50% of patients.[2,3,30,31] In 15% to 20% of victims of sudden cardiac death (SCD), advanced atrioventricular (AV) block or asystole is documented.[32,33] However, an increase in pulseless electrical activity with a proportionate decrease in ventricular fibrillation as the presenting arrhythmia has been reported in more recent studies.[34,35] The true incidence of bradyarrhythmias causing sudden death in the elderly is not known because by the time the first rhythm is recorded, an arrhythmia beginning as ventricular tachyarrhythmia may degenerate into or appear as asystole. SCD accounts for 13% of all natural deaths and 50% of all deaths from cardiovascular causes.[15,36] Despite advancement in the management of cardiovascular disease, the incidence of SCD in the general population (0.1%–0.2% per year) has decreased only marginally and is expected to grow with the aging of the population.[11,15,30,31,34] The persistent dismal survival rate of 4% to 5% after an out-of-hospital cardiac arrest[37] calls for improvement in risk stratification and means to prevent SCD[15] by better defining mechanisms underlying aging-associated increase in the susceptibility to arrhythmogenesis and gathering evidence from clinical trials to develop cost-effective strategies to reduce the burden of arrhythmias in the elderly.[13]

STRUCTURAL AND FUNCTIONAL CHANGES IN THE AGING HEART

Structural and functional alterations in the mechanical and electrical cardiac system, as well as energetics and metabolism associated with the aging process, increase predisposition to cardiac arrhythmias.[1,38–40] Bradyarrhythmias, caused by reduced normal automaticity and delayed conduction, are common in the very elderly, even in the absence of apparent heart disease, and are further exacerbated by comorbidities or use of medications resulting in symptoms that require pacemaker implantation.[16,17,19,41,42] The intrinsic heart rate and heart rate reserve, as determined following cardiac parasympathetic and sympathetic blockade, decrease with aging.[43] This results from aging-associated replacement of pacemaker cells within the sinoatrial node and AV conduction fibers with an extracellular matrix composed of collagen and elastin fibers[44] and impairment of receptor and postreceptor signaling via β-adrenergic receptors contributing to the diminished heart rate response and heart rate variability, with resultant reduction in aerobic work capacity in the elderly.[16,44–46] In addition, amyloid, lipid, and lipofuscin deposition within the myocardium, particularly around the atrial pacemaker tissue, further contributes to bradyarrhythmias in the aging heart.[1,12,47,48] By age 75, the number of functional pacemaker cells decreases to less than 10% of those in young adults, which, along with the reduction in the expression of ion channels, promotes reduced automaticity.[49] Senescence-induced degenerative changes in the cardiac skeleton, particularly in areas close to the AV node, His-Purkinje tissue, and bundle branches, delay conduction and predispose elderly patients to dysrhythmias.[47,50] Electrical and structural remodeling with action potential duration prolongation and connexin remodeling increases the refractoriness of cardiac tissue and slows conduction.[51–53] These changes, along with a blunted response to neurohumoral activation, promote age-related increase in the propensity for chronotropic and dromotropic impairment and for the development of bradyarrhythmias and tachyarrhythmias.[1]

Susceptibility to both supraventricular and ventricular arrhythmogenesis is enhanced in the senescent heart even in the absence of apparent structural abnormalities and is further exaggerated with comorbidities accompanying the aging process.[12,15] This results from both structural and functional alterations – including cell loss, myocyte hypertrophy, and interstitial fibrosis – resulting in altered cellular coupling and exaggerated directional differences in conduction (anisotropy), increasing heterogeneity in impulse propagation properties and refractoriness of the myocardium. This creates zones of functional slowing or conduction block that stabilize reentry, enhancing susceptibility to arrhythmogenesis.[46,54–56] Changes in expression, distribution, and regulation of ion channels alter action potential waveforms and propagation, further enhancing vulnerability to dysrhythmias.[49,57] In the senescent heart, the action potential duration and repolarization are prolonged,[58–60] in part because of downregulation of K^+ currents, including the Ca^{2+}-activated K^+, transient outward (I_{to}), and adenosine triphosphate (ATP)-sensitive K^+ channels and partly because of delay in the inactivation of the Ca^{2+} current (I_{CaL}).[58,61,62] Along with an increase in sodium-Ca^{2+} exchanger, this delay increases predilection to Ca^{2+}-overload–mediated triggered activity and reentrant arrhythmias.[59,62–67] A reduction in the expression of the sarcoplasmic reticulum Ca^{2+}-ATPase[68,69] and post-translational modifications in the function of sarcoplasmic reticulum Ca^{2+}-ATPase, phospholamban, and the sarcoplasmic reticulum Ca^{2+}-release channel (ryanodine receptor 2) further alter Ca^{2+} homeostasis and susceptibility of the aging heart toward arrhythmogenesis.[60,70–74]

The heart, an aerobic organ with high energy demand, is dependent on adequate energy supply from mitochondrial oxidative phosphorylation, which provides more than 70% of ATP.[75] A decline in mitochondrial function including oxidative phosphorylation,[37,76–79] with reduction in the activity of respiratory chain components, adenine nucleotide translocase activity, and changes in mitochondrial matrix and membrane lipid pattern, occurs with the aging process and contributes to an enhanced susceptibility to myocardial dysfunction under conditions of increased energy demand, such as during tachyarrhythmias.[39,59,72,76,80–89] The contributions of age-related changes in cardiac microstructure, including sarcolemma, cytoskeleton, intercellular gap junctions, cellular geometry, and interstitium, as well as mitochondria[7,90] and other intracellular organelles, on the regulation of cardiac excitability or arrhythmogenesis are not well defined and warrant further studies.

ELECTROPHYSIOLOGIC SUBSTRATES FOR AF IN THE ELDERLY

AF is a heterogeneous disorder with variable causes, clinical profile, and natural history.[77] In most elderly patients, AF occurs in the setting of structural heart disease, with only a small percentage exhibiting AF as a primarily electrical disorder.[14,91–95] Aging is associated with changes in expression, distribution and/or function of ion channels that alter action potential waveforms, propagation, and Ca^{2+} handling, increasing vulnerability to AF.[46,78,79,96,97] In addition, aging-associated loss of atrial cardiomyocytes and increased interstitial fibrosis occurs even in the absence of structural heart disease and promotes the substrate for arrhythmogenesis. In humans, this can be demonstrated as fractionated electrocardiograms and low-voltage zones that increase with advancing age (**Fig. 2**).[38] Changes in hemodynamic, mechanical, neuro-humoral, metabolic, and inflammatory factors that accompany aging or aging-associated diseases, such as heart failure, valvular heart disease, hypertension, myocardial infarction and diabetes, contribute to the development of AF, yet the common mechanistic link between these factors and the development of the substrate for AF or its progression in the elderly is not fully understood.

The electrophysiologic basis for the initiation and/or maintenance of AF varies depending on the patient's age, underlying heart disease, or other electrophysiologic modulating factors.[8,9,98] Both enhanced impulse generation as a result of increased automaticity or triggered activity within the atria or pulmonary veins and conduction slowing are responsible for the initiation and maintenance of AF in the elderly. A range of adaptive and maladaptive processes in response to day-to-day stressors, such as volume or pressure overload, stretch, ischemia or rapid rates, contribute to triggers that further alter cellular excitability, cell-to-cell coupling, and anisotropy. This results in directional slowing of impulse propagation[54] and a source-sink mismatch,[53] creating a milieu that increases predisposition to AF in the senescent atria.[38,52–55,63,73,74,78,99–101]

AF may exist in paroxysmal (spontaneously terminates within 7 days), persistent (requires intervention for termination), or permanent forms, with one-fourth of patients with paroxysmal AF progressing to the permanent form,[9,14] which becomes resistant to pharmacologic and nonpharmacologic therapies.[102] Extended follow-up of a unique population of young patients (mean age 44 ± 11 years) with lone AF (in the absence

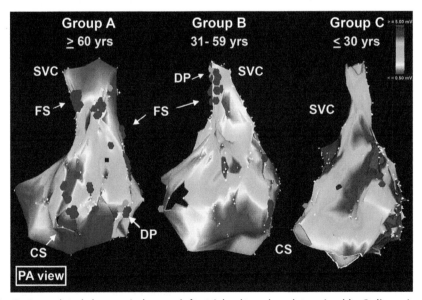

Fig. 2. Age-related changes in human left atrial voltage loss determined by 3-dimensional electroanatomic bipolar voltage mapping. Group A includes those ≥60 years of age; group B, 31–59 years; and group C, ≤30 years. Color annotation: bipolar voltages from 0.5 mV (*red*) to voltages 5 mV (*purple*). CS, coronary sinus; DP, double potentials; FS, fractionated signals; PA, posteroanterior; SVC, superior vena cava. (*Reproduced from* Kistler PM, Sanders P, Fynn SP, et al. Electrophysiologic and electroanatomic changes in the human atrium associated with age. J Am Coll Cardiol 2004;44:109–16; with permission from Elsevier.)

of structural heart disease or hypertension)[103] from Olmsted County, Minnesota, allowed assessment of the natural history of AF and determination of the effect of aging and aging-associated comorbidities on the progression of AF and subsequent risk of stroke, heart failure, and mortality.[14] The 30-year cumulative probability of development of permanent AF was 29% (95% confidence interval 16%–42%), with minimum risk of heart failure, stroke, or mortality. Older age at diagnosis or presence of QRS abnormalities on electrocardiography was a predictor of progression to permanent AF, whereas the presence of premature supraventricular complexes/tachycardia was protective and associated with decreased risk of permanent AF. These findings suggest that young patients with premature complexes and supraventricular arrhythmias in the absence of structural heart disease had a different electrophysiologic substrate, with a primary electrical disorder, compared to older patients or those with electrocardiographic or overt structural abnormalities[104] or with the development of hypertension, heart failure, diastolic dysfunction, or ischemic heart disease with advancing age,[9,14,105] resulting in different progression rates to permanent AF.[12,14]

Aging and its associated comorbidities have been known to increase the risk of progression of AF and its complications; however, the common link connecting these risk factors to the development or progression of AF is not fully understood. Myocardial fibrosis is a common factor associated with aging and comorbidities such as heart failure, ischemic or valvular heart disease, or other forms of cardiomyopathy and could contribute to aging-associated progression of AF. Further research in defining the role of myocardial cell loss and replacement fibrosis is warranted. In animal models, the facilitative role of rapid atrial rate in the initiation and maintenance of sustained AF has been demonstrated.[78,79,106] A progressive decrease in atrial refractoriness, increased heterogeneity and loss of the normal rate-dependent adaptation of refractoriness occurs in this animal model.[78] Slowing of the conduction velocity occurs within the atrium, although late. These changes in electrophysiologic properties of the atrium, termed "electrical remodeling," likely result from reduction in the L-type Ca^{2+} current and transient outward K^+ current, a progressive late reduction in the density of voltage-gated Na^+ channels, and gap junction redistribution that contributes to the slowing of conduction, thus increasing vulnerability of the atria to reentry and creating a condition in which AF perpetuates AF.[79,102,106,107] These electrophysiologic changes are different from structural changes that are observed in patients with heart failure or in the senescent atria with gradual loss of myofibrils, myocyte hypertrophy, fragmentation of sarcoplasmic reticulum, and fibrosis with changes in the structure and shape of mitochondria.[1,46,62,108–117] Changes in protein expression, similar to a de-differentiation process toward a partially fetal phenotype or that seen in hibernating myocardium, also take place with chronic AF.[108,110] The structural substrate with interstitial fibrosis and atrial enlargement seems to be more important in the pathogenesis of AF and its progression in humans than the electrical remodeling, as suggested by animal models in which AF was induced by heart failure or mitral regurgitation[78,111–113] and by its high prevalence in the elderly.[9,114] This is further supported by observations that despite reversibility of atrial refractoriness with restoration of sinus rhythm, AF inducibility or recurrences continued to be high,[115,116] indicating that strategy of prompt termination of AF to avoid adverse electrical remodeling is of little clinical benefit in the elderly.

The precise mechanisms underlying atrial structural remodeling in humans are not fully understood, but impaired intracellular Ca^{2+} handling, oxidative stress, and altered energetics seem to play an important role,[107] and mechanisms coupling Ca^{2+} loading to structural remodeling need to be further defined. Additional unknown factors are operative[102,112,117,118] and need to be elucidated for better understanding of the pathogenesis of AF in the elderly so effective strategies can be instituted for primary and secondary prevention of AF and thereby limit its burden on health care resources.

ELECTROPHYSIOLOGIC SUBSTRATES FOR VENTRICULAR ARRHYTHMIAS/SCD IN THE ELDERLY

The substrate for ventricular arrhythmias in the elderly varies depending on the presence of structural heart disease. The effect of aging on cardiac hemodynamics, structure, and function is complex and challenging to study in humans because of difficulty in isolating the effect of aging from diseases associated with the aging process. Ventricular dysfunction and fibrosis after myocardial infarction or with nonischemic cardiomyopathy predispose to ventricular arrhythmogenesis, which contributes to most cases of SCD in the elderly.[119–123] The risk factors for arrhythmias leading to SCD have been well described; however, precise mechanisms underlying the initiation and maintenance or prediction of timing for the development of dysrhythmias causing SCD in the elderly are not completely understood. This is because of the interactions between dynamic transient factors (ischemia, hypoxia, catecholamines, pH and electrolyte changes, stretch, or inflammation) on the underlying myocardial substrate that precipitate arrhythmias.[8,78,100] Ventricular tachyarrhythmias may be initiated by one mechanism, perpetuated by another, and then degenerate into a different mechanism. This is mainly because of the complex interactions between myocardial cellular and extracellular substrates and triggers that define the overall risk of arrhythmia susceptibility.[78,99–101]

Acute ischemia triggering lethal ventricular tachyarrhythmias contributes to most cases of SCD in the elderly.[124] In 50% of patients with coronary artery disease, sudden death is the initial manifestation.[37,125–127] Acute changes in coronary plaque morphology such as disruption or thrombus were found in more than 50% of the victims of sudden death.[128–130] Cardiac events caused by inherited arrhythmia syndromes, such as congenital long QT syndrome, short QT syndrome, Brugada syndrome or catecholaminergic polymorphic ventricular tachycardia, account for only a small percentage of sudden deaths in the elderly.[131,132] Familial clustering of cardiac events, however, does suggest a role of genetic factors in predisposition to sudden death,[133–135] which, in the elderly, seems to be caused by influences that increase the risk of a coronary event.[37,125,136–138] Patients with long QT syndrome maintain a high risk for life-threatening cardiac events even in later years, although the risk of aborted cardiac arrest or death conferred by long QT syndrome is attenuated, most likely because of the higher prevalence of comorbidities associated with senescence.[139–143]

Ventricular arrhythmias are common in the elderly, affecting more than 70% of individuals aged 60 years and older. With advancing age and presence of structural heart disease, not only do the prevalence and complexity of ventricular arrhythmias worsen but so does their prognostic significance.[15,144–147] Even in asymptomatic elderly, the prevalence of ventricular arrhythmias on ambulatory monitoring is as high as 60% to 90%. Complex premature beats, such as pairs and triplets, occur in up to 10% of such individuals and may be present in up to 60% of the older elderly during exercise. In the absence of heart disease, asymptomatic premature ventricular complexes presenting at rest are benign but, when elicited during exercise[148] or postexercise recovery period,[149] carry adverse prognosis and increased risk of cardiovascular death. In patients with reduced ventricular function, frequent premature ventricular complexes have poor prognostic significance.[147,150–156] The mechanisms underlying ventricular arrhythmogenesis are variable and depend on the underlying myocardial substrate. During ischemia or the acute phase of myocardial infarction, functional reentry can precipitate ventricular fibrillation, whereas reentry circuits around the scar tissue late after acute myocardial infarction result in ventricular tachycardia that degenerates into fibrillation. The vulnerability of the aging heart to arrhythmogenesis is increased during the peri-infarct period, with a higher likelihood of in-hospital cardiac arrest in those 75 years and older compared with younger patients.[157] Ventricular tachyarrhythmias occurring within 48 hours of an acute ischemic event are associated with an increase in hospital death; however, long-term mortality is not affected unless significant ventricular dysfunction persists.[158] The incidence of scar-related reentrant ventricular arrhythmias increases exponentially, with reduction in left ventricular ejection fraction to less than 30%.[125,159]

EVALUATION AND MANAGEMENT OF ELDERLY PATIENTS WITH CARDIAC ARRHYTHMIAS

Several noninvasive and invasive risk stratification protocols have been developed for patients at risk for cardiac arrhythmias who may benefit from interventions to reduce complications and risk of life-threatening events.[15,16,77] A simple 12-lead electrocardiogram allows identification of the underlying structural or functional substrate, such as conduction system abnormalities, prior infarction, ventricular hypertrophy, arrhythmogenic right ventricular cardiomyopathy, or primary electrical disorders like long or short QT syndrome and Brugada syndrome. A prolonged QTc interval in the elderly and a QRS duration longer than 150 ms in patients with severely depressed ventricular function predicts a higher risk of SCD.[3,16,160] A prolonged PR interval or delayed conduction in the atria increases the risk of AF.[77] On signal-averaged electrocardiogram, the absence of late potentials has a high negative predictive value in excluding wide complex tachycardia as a cause of unexplained syncope in the elderly patient with coronary artery disease.[161,162] Appearance of exercise-induced complex ventricular ectopy or ventricular tachycardia in the elderly during exercise testing may predict an increased risk of mortality compared with patients with simple ectopy observed at rest only.[148,149,163] Microvolt fluctuation in the amplitude or morphology of T waves during rest,[164] exercise testing, or atrial pacing may identify high-risk postinfarction or cardiomyopathy patients.[165,166] Assessments of atrial and ventricular dimensions and contractile function with imaging techniques such as echocardiogram are an essential part of cardiac evaluation of patients at risk for arrhythmias.[16,77,167] In patients suspected of ventricular arrhythmias triggered by ischemia,[168] exercise or pharmacologic testing to detect ischemia can be performed with imaging using echocardiography, magnetic resonance imaging, or nuclear perfusion scanning.[169,170] In patients with ventricular arrhythmias or aborted sudden death, coronary angiography is useful to assess for coronary artery disease. Invasive electrophysiology testing is useful for risk stratification for SCD in elderly patients with ischemic heart disease and moderate left ventricular dysfunction or syncope but is of limited utility for patients with dilated cardiomyopathy or inherited arrhythmia syndromes.[171–179] Use of multiple risk markers in combination may better predict arrhythmogenic events than a single parameter given the complexity and variability of the underlying substrates predisposing to arrhythmogenesis and SCD.[31]

Discussion of the management of cardiac dysrhythmias is beyond the scope of this article but can be obtained from recent guidelines.[15,16,31,77,180–186] However, little information is available from clinical trials focusing on the efficacy of various therapeutic modalities in the older-elderly such as antiarrhythmic agents, ablation procedures for atrial and ventricular tachyarrhythmias, or implantable cardioverter-defibrillators.[13,98] Information about the efficacy of therapies for cardiac arrhythmias in the very elderly with limited life expectancy is difficult to assess, especially because only a select few individuals older than 80 years were included in randomized clinical trials and nonrandomized data suffer from selection bias.[129] A diminished benefit of therapies such as implantable cardioverter-defibrillators has been demonstrated with pooled analysis of SCD prevention trials because of an increased number of nonarrhythmic cardiac and noncardiac deaths in the very elderly with multiple comorbidities.[130]

SUMMARY

Cardiac dysrhythmias are common in the elderly, and their overall prevalence and impact on health care costs are expected to increase with the changing population demographics. Despite an increase in the number of elderly persons with atrial and ventricular arrhythmias, only limited insight into mechanisms underlying aging-associated increase in the susceptibility of the heart to arrhythmogenesis is available. In addition, evidence from well-designed clinical trials in the very elderly supporting safer and effective management decisions is lacking, which limits specific practice guidelines. Ongoing research to fulfill this unmet need may provide novel insights into the pathogenesis of cardiac arrhythmias and improvement in preventive and therapeutic strategies.[13]

ACKNOWLEDGMENTS

The authors gratefully acknowledge Joe Grundle and Katie Klein for editorial preparation of the article.

REFERENCES

1. Strait JB, Lakatta EG. Aging-associated cardiovascular changes and their relationship to heart failure. Heart Fail Clin 2012;8:143–64.
2. Roger VL, Go AS, Lloyd-Jones DM, et al. Heart disease and stroke statistics-2012 update: a report from the American Heart Association. Circulation 2012;125:e2–220.
3. Chugh SS, Jui J, Gunson K, et al. Current burden of sudden cardiac death: multiple source surveillance versus retrospective death certificate-based review in a large U.S. community. J Am Coll Cardiol 2004;44:1268–75.
4. Piccini JP, Hammill BG, Sinner MF, et al. Incidence and prevalence of atrial fibrillation and associated mortality among medicare beneficiaries, 1993-2007. Circ Cardiovasc Qual Outcomes 2012;5:85–93.
5. Go AS, Hylek EM, Phillips KA, et al. Prevalence of diagnosed atrial fibrillation in adults: national implications for rhythm management and stroke prevention: the Anticoagulation and Risk Factors in Atrial Fibrillation (ATRIA) Study. JAMA 2001; 285:2370–5.
6. Jahangir A, Shen WK. Pacing in elderly patients. Am Heart J 2003;146:750–3.
7. Jahangir A, Sagar S, Terzic A. Aging and cardioprotection. J Appl Physiol 2007; 103:2120–8.
8. Jahangir A, Munger T, Packer D, et al. Atrial fibrillation. In: Potrid PJ, Kowey PR, editors. Cardiac arrhythmia: mechanisms, diagnosis, and management. 2nd edition. Philadelphia: Lippincott Williams & Wilkins; 2001. p. 457–99.
9. Fuster V, Ryden LE, Cannom DS, et al. ACC/AHA/ESC 2006 guidelines for the management of patients with atrial fibrillation: a report of the American College

of Cardiology/American Heart Association Task Force on Practice Guidelines and the European Society of Cardiology Committee for Practice Guidelines (Writing Committee to Revise the 2001 Guidelines for the Management of Patients With Atrial Fibrillation): developed in collaboration with the European Heart Rhythm Association and the Heart Rhythm Society. Circulation 2006; 114:e257–354.

10. Aronow WS. Heart disease and aging. Med Clin North Am 2006;90:849–62.

11. Adabag AS, Luepker RV, Roger VL, et al. Sudden cardiac death: epidemiology and risk factors. Nat Rev Cardiol 2010;7:216–25.

12. Fuster V, Ryden LE, Cannom DS, et al. 2011 ACCF/AHA/HRS focused updates incorporated into the ACC/AHA/ESC 2006 guidelines for the management of patients with atrial fibrillation: a report of the American College of Cardiology Foundation/American Heart Association Task Force on Practice Guidelines. Circulation 2011;123:e269–367.

13. Liu XK, Jahangir A, Shen WK. Cardiac arrhythmias. In: Halter JB, Ouslander JG, Tinetti ME, et al, editors. Hazzard's geriatric medicine and gerontology. 6th edition. New York: McGraw-Hill; 2009. p. 951–65.

14. Jahangir A, Lee V, Friedman PA, et al. Long-term progression and outcomes with aging in patients with lone atrial fibrillation: a 30-year follow-up study. Circulation 2007;115:3050–6.

15. Zipes DP, Camm AJ, Borggrefe M, et al. ACC/AHA/ESC 2006 guidelines for management of patients with ventricular arrhythmias and the prevention of sudden cardiac death: a report of the American College of Cardiology/American Heart Association Task Force and the European Society of Cardiology Committee for Practice Guidelines (Writing Committee to Develop Guidelines for Management of Patients With Ventricular Arrhythmias and the Prevention of Sudden Cardiac Death). J Am Coll Cardiol 2006;48:e247–346.

16. Epstein AE, DiMarco JP, Ellenbogen KA, et al. ACC/AHA/HRS 2008 guidelines for device-based therapy of cardiac rhythm abnormalities: a report of the American College of Cardiology/American Heart Association Task Force on Practice Guidelines (Writing Committee to Revise the ACC/AHA/NASPE 2002 Guideline Update for Implantation of Cardiac Pacemakers and Antiarrhythmia Devices) developed in collaboration with the American Association for Thoracic Surgery and Society of Thoracic Surgeons. J Am Coll Cardiol 2008;51:e1–62.

17. Rosenqvist M, Obel IW. Atrial pacing and the risk for AV block: is there a time for change in attitude? Pacing Clin Electrophysiol 1989;12(1 Pt 1):97–101.

18. Lamas GA, Lee KL, Sweeney MO, et al. Ventricular pacing or dual-chamber pacing for sinus-node dysfunction. N Engl J Med 2002;346:1854–62.

19. Vlietstra RE, Jahangir A, Shen WK. Choice of pacemakers in patients aged 75 years and older: ventricular pacing mode vs. dual-chamber pacing mode. Am J Geriatr Cardiol 2005;14:35–8.

20. Miyasaka Y, Barnes ME, Gersh BJ, et al. Secular trends in incidence of atrial fibrillation in Olmsted County, Minnesota, 1980 to 2000, and implications on the projections for future prevalence. Circulation 2006;114:119–25.

21. Mozaffarian D, Furberg CD, Psaty BM, et al. Physical activity and incidence of atrial fibrillation in older adults: the Cardiovascular Health Study. Circulation 2008;118:800–7.

22. Kim MH, Johnston SS, Chu BC, et al. Estimation of total incremental health care costs in patients with atrial fibrillation in the United States. Circ Cardiovasc Qual Outcomes 2011;4:313–20.

23. Lloyd-Jones DM, Wang TJ, Leip EP, et al. Lifetime risk for development of atrial fibrillation: the Framingham Heart Study. Circulation 2004;110:1042–6.
24. Lloyd-Jones D, Adams R, Carnethon M, et al. Heart disease and stroke statistics–2009 update: a report from the American Heart Association Statistics Committee and Stroke Statistics Subcommittee. Circulation 2009;119:480–6.
25. Wattigney WA, Mensah GA, Croft JB. Increased atrial fibrillation mortality: United States, 1980-1998. Am J Epidemiol 2002;155:819–26.
26. Wattigney WA, Mensah GA, Croft JB. Increasing trends in hospitalization for atrial fibrillation in the United States, 1985 through 1999: implications for primary prevention. Circulation 2003;108:711–6.
27. Ozcan C, Jahangir A, Friedman PA, et al. Long-term survival after ablation of the atrioventricular node and implantation of a permanent pacemaker in patients with atrial fibrillation. N Engl J Med 2001;344:1043–51.
28. Tsang TS, Petty GW, Barnes ME, et al. The prevalence of atrial fibrillation in incident stroke cases and matched population controls in Rochester, Minnesota: changes over three decades. J Am Coll Cardiol 2003;42:93–100.
29. Wu EQ, Birnbaum HG, Mareva M, et al. Economic burden and co-morbidities of atrial fibrillation in a privately insured population. Curr Med Res Opin 2005;21: 1693–9.
30. Myerburg RJ, Hendel RC. Expanding risk-profiling strategies for prediction and prevention of sudden cardiac death. J Am Coll Cardiol 2010;56:215–7.
31. Fishman GI, Chugh SS, Dimarco JP, et al. Sudden cardiac death prediction and prevention: report from a National Heart, Lung, and Blood Institute and Heart Rhythm Society Workshop. Circulation 2010;122:2335–48.
32. Luu M, Stevenson WG, Stevenson LW, et al. Diverse mechanisms of unexpected cardiac arrest in advanced heart failure. Circulation 1989;80:1675–80.
33. Bayés de Luna A, Coumel P, Leclercq JF. Ambulatory sudden cardiac death: mechanisms of production of fatal arrhythmia on the basis of data from 157 cases. Am Heart J 1989;117:151–9.
34. Cobb LA, Fahrenbruch CE, Olsufka M, et al. Changing incidence of out-of-hospital ventricular fibrillation, 1980-2000. JAMA 2002;288:3008–13.
35. Herlitz J, Andersson E, Bang A, et al. Experiences from treatment of out-of-hospital cardiac arrest during 17 years in Göteborg. Eur Heart J 2000;21:1251–8.
36. Gillum RF. Geographic variation in sudden coronary death. Am Heart J 1990; 119:380–9.
37. Nichol G, Thomas E, Callaway CW, et al. Regional variation in out-of-hospital cardiac arrest incidence and outcome. JAMA 2008;300:1423–31.
38. Kistler PM, Sanders P, Fynn SP, et al. Electrophysiologic and electroanatomic changes in the human atrium associated with age. J Am Coll Cardiol 2004;44: 109–16.
39. Preston CC, Oberlin AS, Holmuhamedov EL, et al. Aging-induced alterations in gene transcripts and functional activity of mitochondrial oxidative phosphorylation complexes in the heart. Mech Ageing Dev 2008;129:304–12.
40. Roberts-Thomson KC, Kistler PM, Sanders P, et al. Fractionated atrial electrograms during sinus rhythm: relationship to age, voltage, and conduction velocity. Heart Rhythm 2009;6:587–91.
41. Rodriguez RD, Schocken DD. Update on sick sinus syndrome, a cardiac disorder of aging. Geriatrics 1990;45:26–30, 33–6.
42. Dobrzynski H, Boyett MR, Anderson RH. New insights into pacemaker activity: promoting understanding of sick sinus syndrome. Circulation 2007;115: 1921–32.

43. Jose AD. Effect of combined sympathetic and parasympathetic blockade on heart rate and cardiac function in man. Am J Cardiol 1966;18:476–8.
44. Lakatta EG. Cardiovascular regulatory mechanisms in advanced age. Physiol Rev 1993;73:413–67.
45. Fleg JL, O'Connor F, Gerstenblith G, et al. Impact of age on the cardiovascular response to dynamic upright exercise in healthy men and women. J Appl Physiol 1995;78:890–900.
46. Dun W, Boyden PA. Aged atria: electrical remodeling conducive to atrial fibrillation. J Interv Card Electrophysiol 2009;25:9–18.
47. Lie JT, Hammond PI. Pathology of the senescent heart: anatomic observations on 237 autopsy studies of patients 90 to 105 years old. Mayo Clin Proc 1988;63:552–64.
48. Olivetti G, Melissari M, Capasso JM, et al. Cardiomyopathy of the aging human heart. Myocyte loss and reactive cellular hypertrophy. Circulation Res 1991;68:1560–8.
49. Tellez JO, McZewski M, Yanni J, et al. Ageing-dependent remodelling of ion channel and Ca2+ clock genes underlying sino-atrial node pacemaking. Exp Physiol 2011;96:1163–78.
50. Cheitlin MD. Cardiovascular physiology-changes with aging. Am J Geriatr Cardiol 2003;12:9–13.
51. Huang C, Ding W, Li L, et al. Differences in the aging-associated trends of the monophasic action potential duration and effective refractory period of the right and left atria of the rat. Circ J 2006;70:352–7.
52. Liu XK, Jahangir A, Terzic A, et al. Age- and sex-related atrial electrophysiologic and structural changes. Am J Cardiol 2004;94:373–5.
53. Spach MS, Heidlage JF, Dolber PC, et al. Mechanism of origin of conduction disturbances in aging human atrial bundles: experimental and model study. Heart Rhythm 2007;4:175–85.
54. Koura T, Hara M, Takeuchi S, et al. Anisotropic conduction properties in canine atria analyzed by high-resolution optical mapping: preferential direction of conduction block changes from longitudinal to transverse with increasing age. Circulation 2002;105:2092–8.
55. de Bakker JM, van Rijen HM. Continuous and discontinuous propagation in heart muscle. J Cardiovasc Electrophysiol 2006;17:567–73.
56. Hao X, Zhang Y, Zhang X, et al. TGF-beta1-mediated fibrosis and ion channel remodeling are key mechanisms in producing the sinus node dysfunction associated with SCN5A deficiency and aging. Circ Arrhythm Electrophysiol 2011;4:397–406.
57. Nerbonne JM, Kass RS. Physiology and molecular biology of ion channels contributing to ventricular repolarization. In: Gussak I, Antzelevitch C, editors. Contemporary cardiology: cardiac repolarization: bridging basic and clinical science. Totowa (NJ): Humana Press; 2003. p. 25–62.
58. Josephson IR, Guia A, Stern MD, et al. Alterations in properties of L-type Ca channels in aging rat heart. J Mol Cell Cardiol 2002;34:297–308.
59. Jahangir A, Holmuhamedov EL, Cabrera Aguilera CC, et al. Molecular basis for the increased vulnerability of the aging heart to injury (abstract). Eur Heart J 2006;27(Suppl 1):5101.
60. Lakatta EG, Maltsev VA, Vinogradova TM. A coupled system of intracellular Ca2+ clocks and surface membrane voltage clocks controls the time-keeping mechanism of the heart's pacemaker. Circulation Res 2010;106:659–73.

61. Janczewski AM, Spurgeon HA, Lakatta EG. Action potential prolongation in cardiac myocytes of old rats is an adaptation to sustain youthful intracellular Ca2+ regulation. J Mol Cell Cardiol 2002;34:641–8.

62. Walker KE, Lakatta EG, Houser SR. Age associated changes in membrane currents in rat ventricular myocytes. Cardiovasc Res 1993;27:1968–77.

63. Jahangir A, Terzic A. KATP channel therapeutics at the bedside. J Mol Cell Cardiol 2005;39:99–112.

64. Toro L, Marijic J, Nishimaru K, et al. Aging, ion channel expression, and vascular function. Vascul Pharmacol 2002;38:73–80.

65. Zhou YY, Lakatta EG, Xiao RP. Age-associated alterations in calcium current and its modulation in cardiac myocytes. Drugs Aging 1998;13:159–71.

66. Xiao RP, Zhu W, Zheng M, et al. Subtype-specific [alpha]1- and [beta]-adrenoceptor signaling in the heart. Trends Pharmacol Sci 2006;27:330–7.

67. Morita N, Lee JH, Bapat A, et al. Glycolytic inhibition causes spontaneous ventricular fibrillation in aged hearts. Am J Physiol Heart Circ Physiol 2011; 301:H180–91.

68. Lompré AM, Lambert F, Lakatta EG, et al. Expression of sarcoplasmic reticulum Ca2+-ATPase and calsequestrin genes in rat heart during ontogenic development and aging. Circ Res 1991;69:1380–8.

69. Taffet GE, Tate CA. CaATPase content is lower in cardiac sarcoplasmic reticulum isolated from old rats. Am J Physiol 1993;264:H1609–14.

70. Koban MU, Moorman AF, Holtz J, et al. Expressional analysis of the cardiac Na-Ca exchanger in rat development and senescence. Cardiovasc Res 1998;37:405–23.

71. Xu A, Narayanan N. Effects of aging on sarcoplasmic reticulum Ca2+-cycling proteins and their phosphorylation in rat myocardium. Am J Physiol 1998;275:H2087–94.

72. Finkel T, Holbrook NJ. Oxidants, oxidative stress and the biology of ageing. Nature 2000;408:239–47.

73. Anyukhovsky EP, Sosunov EA, Chandra P, et al. Age-associated changes in electrophysiologic remodeling: a potential contributor to initiation of atrial fibrillation. Cardiovasc Res 2005;66:353–63.

74. Kawamura S, Takahashi M, Ishihara T, et al. Incidence and distribution of isolated atrial amyloid: histologic and immunohistochemical studies of 100 aging hearts. Pathol Int 1995;45:335–42.

75. Saraste M. Oxidative phosphorylation at the fin de siecle. Science 1999;283:1488–93.

76. Loeb LA, Wallace DC, Martin GM. The mitochondrial theory of aging and its relationship to reactive oxygen species damage and somatic mtDNA mutations. Proc Natl Acad Sci U S A 2005;102:18769–70.

77. Fuster V, Ryden LE, Cannom DS, et al. 2011 ACCF/AHA/HRS focused updates incorporated into the ACC/AHA/ESC 2006 guidelines for the management of patients with atrial fibrillation: a report of the American College of Cardiology Foundation/American Heart Association Task Force on Practice Guidelines developed in partnership with the European Society of Cardiology and in collaboration with the European Heart Rhythm Association and the Heart Rhythm Society. J Am Coll Cardiol 2011;57:e101–98.

78. Nattel S, Shiroshita-Takeshita A, Brundel BJ, et al. Mechanisms of atrial fibrillation: lessons from animal models. Prog Cardiovasc Dis 2005;48:9–28.

79. Finet JE, Rosenbaum DS, Donahue JK. Information learned from animal models of atrial fibrillation. Cardiol Clin 2009;27:45–54, viii.

80. Di Lisa F, Bernardi P. A CaPful of mechanisms regulating the mitochondrial permeability transition. J Mol Cell Cardiol 2009;46:775–80.
81. Murphy MP. How mitochondria produce reactive oxygen species. Biochem J 2009;417:1–13.
82. Seppet E, Eimre M, Peet N, et al. Compartmentation of energy metabolism in atrial myocardium of patients undergoing cardiac surgery. Mol Cell Biochem 2005;270:49–61.
83. Navarro A, Boveris A. The mitochondrial energy transduction system and the aging process. Am J Physiol Cell Physiol 2007;292:C670–86.
84. Hagen TM. Oxidative stress, redox imbalance, and the aging process. Antioxid Redox Signal 2003;5:503–6.
85. Bak MI, Wei JY, Ingwall JS. Interaction of hypoxia and aging in the heart: analysis of high energy phosphate content. J Mol Cell Cardiol 1998;30:661–72.
86. Chicco AJ, Sparagna GC. Role of cardiolipin alterations in mitochondrial dysfunction and disease. Am J Physiol Cell Physiol 2007;292:C33–44.
87. Lesnefsky EJ, Gudz TI, Migita CT, et al. Ischemic injury to mitochondrial electron transport in the aging heart: damage to the iron-sulfur protein subunit of electron transport complex III. Arch Biochem Biophys 2001;385:117–28.
88. Pepe S. Effect of dietary polyunsaturated fatty acids on age-related changes in cardiac mitochondrial membranes. Exp Gerontol 2005;40:751–8.
89. Lesnefsky EJ, Minkler P, Hoppel CL. Enhanced modification of cardiolipin during ischemia in the aged heart. J Mol Cell Cardiol 2009;46:1008–15.
90. Jahangir A, Ozcan C, Holmuhamedov EL, et al. Increased calcium vulnerability of senescent cardiac mitochondria: protective role for a mitochondrial potassium channel opener. Mech Ageing Dev 2001;122:1073–86.
91. Darbar D, Herron KJ, Ballew JD, et al. Familial atrial fibrillation is a genetically heterogeneous disorder. J Am Coll Cardiol 2003;41:2185–92.
92. Olson TM, Alekseev AE, Liu XK, et al. Kv1.5 channelopathy due to KCNA5 loss-of-function mutation causes human atrial fibrillation. Hum Mol Genet 2006;15:2185–91.
93. Olson TM, Alekseev AE, Moreau C, et al. KATP channel mutation confers risk for vein of Marshall adrenergic atrial fibrillation. Nat Clin Pract Cardiovasc Med 2007;4:110–6.
94. Ellinor PT, Yoerger DM, Ruskin JN, et al. Familial aggregation in lone atrial fibrillation. Hum Genet 2005;118:179–84.
95. Andalib A, Brugada R, Nattel S. Atrial fibrillation: evidence for genetically determined disease. Curr Opin Cardiol 2008;23:176–83.
96. Jahangir A, Sattiaraju S, Shen WK. Senescence and arrhythmogenesis. In: Gussak I, Antzelevitch C, editors. Electrical disease of the heart: genetics, mechanisms, treatment, and prevention. London: Springer; 2008. p. 247–60.
97. Kléber AG, Rudy Y. Basic mechanisms of cardiac impulse propagation and associated arrhythmias. Physiol Rev 2004;84:431–88.
98. Mirza M, Shen WK, Jahangir A. Senescence and arrhythmogenesis. In: Gussak I, Antzelevitch C, editors. Electrical disease of the heart: genetics, mechanisms, treatment, and prevention. 2nd edition. London: Springer, in press.
99. Bonnema DD, Webb CS, Pennington WR, et al. Effects of age on plasma matrix metalloproteinases (MMPs) and tissue inhibitor of metalloproteinases (TIMPs). J Card Fail 2007;13:530–40.
100. Adamson PB, Barr RC, Callans DJ, et al. The perplexing complexity of cardiac arrhythmias: beyond electrical remodeling. Heart Rhythm 2005;2:650–9.
101. Polyakova V, Miyagawa S, Szalay Z, et al. Atrial extracellular matrix remodelling in patients with atrial fibrillation. J Cell Mol Med 2008;12:189–208.

102. Allessie M. The "second factor": a first step toward diagnosing the substrate of atrial fibrillation? J Am Coll Cardiol 2009;53:1192–3.
103. Kopecky SL, Gersh BJ, McGoon MD, et al. The natural history of lone atrial fibrillation. A population-based study over three decades. N Engl J Med 1987;317: 669–74.
104. Osranek M, Bursi F, Bailey KR, et al. Left atrial volume predicts cardiovascular events in patients originally diagnosed with lone atrial fibrillation: three-decade follow-up. Eur Heart J 2005;26:2556–61.
105. Nieuwlaat R, Eurlings LW, Cleland JG, et al. Atrial fibrillation and heart failure in cardiology practice: reciprocal impact and combined management from the perspective of atrial fibrillation: results of the Euro Heart Survey on Atrial Fibrillation. J Am Coll Cardiol 2009;53:1690–8.
106. Wijffels MC, Kirchhof CJ, Dorland R, et al. Atrial fibrillation begets atrial fibrillation. A study in awake chronically instrumented goats. Circulation 1995;92: 1954–68.
107. Nattel S, Maguy A, Le Bouter S, et al. Arrhythmogenic ion-channel remodeling in the heart: heart failure, myocardial infarction, and atrial fibrillation. Physiol Rev 2007;87:425–56.
108. Ausma J, Coumans WA, Duimel H, et al. Atrial high energy phosphate content and mitochondrial enzyme activity during chronic atrial fibrillation. Cardiovasc Res 2000;47:788–96.
109. Ausma J, Dispersyn GD, Duimel H, et al. Changes in ultrastructural calcium distribution in goat atria during atrial fibrillation. J Mol Cell Cardiol 2000;32: 355–64.
110. Dispersyn GD, Ausma J, Thone F, et al. Cardiomyocyte remodelling during myocardial hibernation and atrial fibrillation: prelude to apoptosis. Cardiovasc Res 1999;43:947–57.
111. Knackstedt C, Gramley F, Schimpf T, et al. Association of echocardiographic atrial size and atrial fibrosis in a sequential model of congestive heart failure and atrial fibrillation. Cardiovasc Pathol 2008;17:318–24.
112. Corradi D, Callegari S, Maestri R, et al. Structural remodeling in atrial fibrillation. Nat Clin Pract Cardiovasc Med 2008;5:782–96.
113. Burstein B, Nattel S. Atrial fibrosis: mechanisms and clinical relevance in atrial fibrillation. J Am Coll Cardiol 2008;51:802–9.
114. Xu J, Cui G, Esmailian F, et al. Atrial extracellular matrix remodeling and the maintenance of atrial fibrillation. Circulation 2004;109:363–8.
115. Fynn SP, Garratt CJ. The effectiveness of serial cardioversion therapy for recurrence of atrial fibrillation. Eur Heart J 2002;23:1487–9.
116. Everett TH 4th, Li H, Mangrum JM, et al. Electrical, morphological, and ultrastructural remodeling and reverse remodeling in a canine model of chronic atrial fibrillation. Circulation 2000;102:1454–60.
117. Lin CS, Pan CH. Regulatory mechanisms of atrial fibrotic remodeling in atrial fibrillation. Cell Mol Life Sci 2008;65:1489–508.
118. Lin PH, Lee SH, Su CP, et al. Oxidative damage to mitochondrial DNA in atrial muscle of patients with atrial fibrillation. Free Radic Biol Med 2003;35:1310–8.
119. Myerburg RJ. Sudden cardiac death: exploring the limits of our knowledge. J Cardiovasc Electrophysiol 2001;12:369–81.
120. Geelen P, Lorga Filho A, Primo J, et al. Experience with implantable cardioverter defibrillator therapy in elderly patients. Eur Heart J 1997;18:1339–42.
121. Panotopoulos M, Panagiotis T, Axtell K, et al. Efficacy of the implantable cardioverter-defibrillator in the elderly. J Am Coll Cardiol 1997;29:556–60.

122. Saksena S, Mathew P, Giorgberidze I, et al. Implantable defibrillator therapy for the elderly. Am J Geriatr Cardiol 1998;7:11–3.
123. Wilkoff BL, Cook JR, Epstein AE, et al. Dual-chamber pacing-or ventricular backup pacing in patients with an implantable defibrillator: the Dual Chamber and VVI Implantable Defibrillator (DAVID) Trial. JAMA 2002;288:3115–23.
124. Penn J, Goldenberg I, Moss AJ, et al. Improved outcome with preventive cardiac resynchronization therapy in the elderly: a MADIT-CRT substudy. J Cardiovasc Electrophysiol 2011;22:892–7.
125. Myerburg RJ, Castellanos A. Emerging paradigms of the epidemiology and demographics of sudden cardiac arrest. Heart Rhythm 2006;3:235–9.
126. Bardy GH, Lee KL, Mark DB, et al. Amiodarone or an implantable cardioverter-defibrillator for congestive heart failure. N Engl J Med 2005;352:225–37.
127. Cleland JG, Daubert JC, Erdmann E, et al. The effect of cardiac resynchroniza-tion on morbidity and mortality in heart failure. N Engl J Med 2005;352:1539–49.
128. van Rees JB, Borleffs CJ, Thijssen J, et al. Prophylactic implantable cardioverter-defibrillator treatment in the elderly: therapy, adverse events, and survival gain. Europace 2012;14:66–73.
129. Jahangir A, Shen WK, Neubauer SA, et al. Relation between mode of pacing and long-term survival in the very elderly. J Am Coll Cardiol 1999;33:1208–16.
130. Krahn AD, Connolly SJ, Roberts RS, et al. Diminishing proportional risk of sudden death with advancing age: implications for prevention of sudden death. Am Heart J 2004;147:837–40.
131. Grimm W. Outcomes of elderly heart failure recipients of ICD and CRT. Int J Cardiol 2008;125:154–60.
132. Kocovic DZ. Cardiac resynchronization therapy and other new approaches for the treatment of heart failure in the elderly. Am J Geriatr Cardiol 2006;15:108–13.
133. Foley PW, Chalil S, Khadjooi K, et al. Long-term effects of cardiac resynchroni-zation therapy in octogenarians: a comparative study with a younger population. Europace 2008;10:1302–7.
134. Silva RM, Mont L, Nava S, et al. Radiofrequency catheter ablation for arrhythmic storm in patients with an implantable cardioverter defibrillator. Pacing Clin Elec-trophysiol 2004;27:971–5.
135. Scheinman MM. NASPE survey on catheter ablation. Pacing Clin Electrophysiol 1995;18:1474–8.
136. Tchou P, Jazayeri M, Denker S, et al. Transcatheter electrical ablation of right bundle branch. A method of treating macroreentrant ventricular tachycardia attributed to bundle branch reentry. Circulation 1988;78:246–57.
137. Stevenson WG, Khan H, Sager P, et al. Identification of reentry circuit sites during catheter mapping and radiofrequency ablation of ventricular tachycardia late after myocardial infarction. Circulation 1993;88:1647–70.
138. Gurevitz OT, Glikson M, Asirvatham S, et al. Use of advanced mapping systems to guide ablation in complex cases: experience with noncontact mapping and electroanatomic mapping systems. Pacing Clin Electrophysiol 2005;28:316–23.
139. Joshi S, Wilber DJ. Ablation of idiopathic right ventricular outflow tract tachy-cardia: current perspectives. J Cardiovasc Electrophysiol 2005;16:S52–8.
140. Pedrinazzi C, Durin O, Agricola P, et al. Efficacy and safety of radiofrequency catheter ablation in the elderly. J Interv Card Electrophysiol 2007;19:179–85.
141. Inada K, Roberts-Thomson KC, Seiler J, et al. Mortality and safety of catheter ablation for antiarrhythmic drug-refractory ventricular tachycardia in elderly patients with coronary artery disease. Heart Rhythm 2010;7:740–4.

142. Kelly P, Ruskin JN, Vlahakes GJ, et al. Surgical coronary revascularization in survivors of prehospital cardiac arrest: its effect on inducible ventricular arrhythmias and long-term survival. J Am Coll Cardiol 1990;15:267–73.

143. Brugada J, Aguinaga L, Mont L, et al. Coronary artery revascularization in patients with sustained ventricular arrhythmias in the chronic phase of a myocardial infarction: effects on the electrophysiologic substrate and outcome. J Am Coll Cardiol 2001;37:529–33.

144. Fleg JL, Kennedy HL. Cardiac arrhythmias in a healthy elderly population: detection by 24-hour ambulatory electrocardiography. Chest 1982;81:302–7.

145. Kennedy HL, Whitlock JA, Sprague MK, et al. Long-term follow-up of asymptomatic healthy subjects with frequent and complex ventricular ectopy. N Engl J Med 1985;312:193–7.

146. Hinkle LE Jr, Carver ST, Stevens M. The frequency of asymptomatic disturbances of cardiac rhythm and conduction in middle-aged men. Am J Cardiol 1969;24:629–50.

147. Kannel WB, Cupples LA, D'Agostino RB. Sudden death risk in overt coronary heart disease: the Framingham Study. Am Heart J 1987;113:799–804.

148. Jouven X, Zureik M, Desnos M, et al. Long-term outcome in asymptomatic men with exercise-induced premature ventricular depolarizations. N Engl J Med 2000;343:826–33.

149. Frolkis JP, Pothier CE, Blackstone EH, et al. Frequent ventricular ectopy after exercise as a predictor of death. N Engl J Med 2003;348:781–90.

150. Messerli FH, Ventura HO, Elizardi DJ, et al. Hypertension and sudden death: increased ventricular ectopic activity in left ventricular hypertrophy. Am J Med 1984;77:18–22.

151. Bigger JT Jr, Fleiss JL, Kleiger R, et al. The relationships among ventricular arrhythmias, left ventricular dysfunction, and mortality in the 2 years after myocardial infarction. Circulation 1984;69:250–8.

152. Huikuri HV, Mäkikallio TH, Raatikainen MJ, et al. Prediction of sudden cardiac death: appraisal of the studies and methods assessing the risk of sudden arrhythmic death. Circulation 2003;108:110–5.

153. Stevenson WG, Stevenson LW, Middlekauff HR, et al. Sudden death prevention in patients with advanced ventricular dysfunction. Circulation 1993;88:2953–61.

154. Aronow WS, Ahn C, Mercando AD, et al. Prevalence and association of ventricular tachycardia and complex ventricular arrhythmias with new coronary events in older men and women with and without cardiovascular disease. J Gerontol A Biol Sci Med Sci 2002;57:M178–80.

155. Volpi A, Cavalli A, Turato R, et al. Incidence and short-term prognosis of late sustained ventricular tachycardia after myocardial infarction: results of the Gruppo Italiano per lo Studio della Sopravvivenza nell'Infarto Miocardico (GISSI-3) Data Base. Am Heart J 2001;142:87–92.

156. Trusty JM, Beinborn DS, Jahangir A. Dysrhythmias and the athlete. AACN Clin Issues 2004;15:432–48.

157. Ornato JP, Peberdy MA, Tadler SC, et al. Factors associated with the occurrence of cardiac arrest during hospitalization for acute myocardial infarction in the second national registry of myocardial infarction in the US. Resuscitation 2001;48:117–23.

158. Behar S, Goldbourt U, Reicher-Reiss H, et al. Prognosis of acute myocardial infarction complicated by primary ventricular fibrillation. Am J Cardiol 1990;66:1208–11.

159. Huikuri HV, Castellanos A, Myerburg RJ. Medical progress: sudden death due to cardiac arrhythmias. N Engl J Med 2001;345:1473–82.

160. Schouten EG, Dekker JM, Meppelink P, et al. QT interval prolongation predicts cardiovascular mortality in an apparently healthy population. Circulation 1991; 84:1516–23.

161. Steinberg JS, Berbari EJ. The signal-averaged electrocardiogram: update on clinical applications. J Cardiovasc Electrophysiol 1996;7:972–88.

162. Cook JR, Flack JE, Gregory CA, et al. Influence of the preoperative signal-averaged electrocardiogram on left ventricular function after coronary artery bypass graft surgery in patients with left ventricular dysfunction. The CABG Patch Trial. Am J Cardiol 1998;82:285–9.

163. Podrid PJ, Graboys TB. Exercise stress testing in the management of cardiac rhythm disorders. Med Clin North Am 1984;68:1139–52.

164. Couderc JP, Zareba W, McNitt S, et al. Repolarization variability in the risk stratification of MADIT II patients. Europace 2007;9:717–23.

165. Bloomfield DM, Bigger JT, Steinman RC, et al. Microvolt T-wave alternans and the risk of death or sustained ventricular arrhythmias in patients with left ventricular dysfunction. J Am Coll Cardiol 2006;47:456–63.

166. Chow T, Kereiakes DJ, Bartone C, et al. Prognostic utility of microvolt T-wave alternans in risk stratification of patients with ischemic cardiomyopathy. J Am Coll Cardiol 2006;47:1820–7.

167. Cheitlin MD, Armstrong WF, Aurigemma GP, et al. ACC/AHA/ASE 2003 guideline update for the clinical application of echocardiography: summary article: a report of the American College of Cardiology/American Heart Association Task Force on Practice Guidelines (ACC/AHA/ASE Committee to Update the 1997 Guidelines for the Clinical Application of Echocardiography). J Am Coll Cardiol 2003;42:954–70.

168. Klocke FJ, Baird MG, Lorell BH, et al. ACC/AHA/ASNC guidelines for the clinical use of cardiac radionuclide imaging–executive summary: a report of the American College of Cardiology/American Heart Association Task Force on Practice Guidelines (ACC/AHA/ASNC Committee to Revise the 1995 Guidelines for the Clinical Use of Cardiac Radionuclide Imaging). J Am Coll Cardiol 2003;42:1318–33.

169. Azaouagh A, Churzidse S, Konorza T, et al. Arrhythmogenic right ventricular cardiomyopathy/dysplasia: a review and update. Clin Res Cardiol 2011;100:383–94.

170. Marcus FI, McKenna WJ, Sherrill D, et al. Diagnosis of arrhythmogenic right ventricular cardiomyopathy/dysplasia: proposed modification of the task force criteria. Circulation 2010;121:1533–41.

171. Wilber DJ, Garan H, Finkelstein D, et al. Out-of-hospital cardiac arrest. Use of electrophysiologic testing in the prediction of long-term outcome. N Engl J Med 1988;318:19–24.

172. Chen LY, Jahangir A, Decker WW, et al. Score indices for predicting electrophysiologic outcomes in patients with unexplained syncope. J Interv Card Electrophysiol 2005;14:99–105.

173. Bachinsky WB, Linzer M, Weld L, et al. Usefulness of clinical characteristics in predicting the outcome of electrophysiologic studies in unexplained syncope. Am J Cardiol 1992;69:1044–9.

174. Priori SG, Schwartz PJ, Napolitano C, et al. Risk stratification in the long-QT syndrome. N Engl J Med 2003;348:1866–74.

175. Moya A, Sutton R, Ammirati F, et al. Guidelines for the diagnosis and management of syncope (version 2009). Eur Heart J 2009;30:2631–71.

176. Priori SG, Napolitano C, Gasparini M, et al. Natural history of Brugada syndrome: insights for risk stratification and management. Circulation 2002;105:1342–7.

177. Brugada J, Brugada R, Brugada P. Determinants of sudden cardiac death in individuals with the electrocardiographic pattern of Brugada syndrome and no previous cardiac arrest. Circulation 2003;108:3092–6.
178. Nienaber CA, Hiller S, Spielmann RP, et al. Syncope in hypertrophic cardiomyopathy: multivariate analysis of prognostic determinants. J Am Coll Cardiol 1990;15:948–55.
179. Buxton AE, Lee KL, Hafley GE, et al. Relation of ejection fraction and inducible ventricular tachycardia to mode of death in patients with coronary artery disease: an analysis of patients enrolled in the multicenter unsustained tachycardia trial. Circulation 2002;106:2466–72.
180. Calkins H, Kuck KH, Cappato R, et al. 2012 HRS/EHRA/ECAS expert consensus statement on catheter and surgical ablation of atrial fibrillation: recommendations for patient selection, procedural techniques, patient management and follow-up, definitions, endpoints, and research trial design. J Interv Card Electrophysiol 2012;33:171–257.
181. Patel MR, Bailey SR, Bonow RO, et al. ACCF/SCAI/AATS/AHA/ASE/ASNC/HFSA/HRS/SCCM/SCCT/SCMR/STS 2012 appropriate use criteria for diagnostic catheterization: a report of the American College of Cardiology Foundation Appropriate Use Criteria Task Force, Society for Cardiovascular Angiography and Interventions, American Association for Thoracic Surgery, American Heart Association, American Society of Echocardiography, American Society of Nuclear Cardiology, Heart Failure Society of America, Heart Rhythm Society, Society of Critical Care Medicine, Society of Cardiovascular Computed Tomography, Society for Cardiovascular Magnetic Resonance, and Society of Thoracic Surgeons. J Am Coll Cardiol 2012;59:1995–2027.
182. Skanes AC, Healey JS, Cairns JA, et al. Focused 2012 update of the Canadian Cardiovascular Society atrial fibrillation guidelines: recommendations for stroke prevention and rate/rhythm control. Can J Cardiol 2012;28:125–36.
183. Camm AJ, Kirchhof P, Lip GY, et al. Guidelines for the management of atrial fibrillation: the task force for the management of atrial fibrillation of the European Society of Cardiology (ESC). Europace 2010;12:1360–420.
184. Dubner S, Auricchio A, Steinberg JS, et al. ISHNE/EHRA expert consensus on remote monitoring of cardiovascular implantable electronic devices (CIEDs). Europace 2012;14:278–93.
185. Curtis AB. Update on the clinical management of atrial fibrillation: guidelines and beyond. Postgrad Med 2011;123:7–20.
186. Savelieva I, Kakouros N, Kourliouros A, et al. Upstream therapies for management of atrial fibrillation: review of clinical evidence and implications for European Society of Cardiology guidelines. Part I: primary prevention. Europace 2011;13:308–28.

Pharmacology of Antiarrhythmic Drugs in Elderly Patients

William H. Frishman, MD[a],*, Wilbert S. Aronow, MD[b]

KEYWORDS

- Antiarrhythmic drugs • Arrhythmias • Tachyarrhythmias • Bradyarrhythmias
- Pharmacokinetics • Pharmacotherapy • Elderly

KEY POINTS

- Bradyarrhythmias and tachyarrhythmias are common in elderly patients as a result of aging and acquired cardiac disease.
- Antiarrhythmic drugs are effective in elderly patients for the management of supraventricular and ventricular arrhythmias; however, dosing of drugs must be performed with care because of age-related changes in drug pharmacokinetics, the presence of concomitant disease, and frequent drug-drug interactions.
- Despite the large number of antiarrhythmic drugs having different electrophysiologic actions, as described in this article, only the β-blockers have been shown to be effective in reducing mortality and to lack proarrhythmic actions.

Cardiac arrhythmias are common in elderly patients and are often a cause of serious morbidity and mortality.[1] This article reviews the pathophysiology of arrhythmias in elderly patients and the antiarrhythmic pharmacologic modalities used in treatment.

PATHOPHYSIOLOGY OF ARRHYTHMIAS
Bradyarrhythmias

The cardiac conduction system undergoes multiple changes with age that can affect its electrical properties, and when exaggerated, can cause clinical diseases such as sick sinus syndromes, atrioventricular (AV) conduction abnormalities, bundle branch block, and complete heart block.[2] These cardiac irregularities are usually associated with fatigue and lightheadedness.[2] Often, these rhythm abnormalities are brought out by drugs used to treat other arrhythmias. Diseases of cardiac conduction are usually

---

Nothing to disclose.
[a] Department of Medicine, New York Medical College, Westchester Medical Center, Munger 263, Valhalla, NY 10595, USA; [b] Division of Cardiology, New York Medical College, Westchester Medical Center, Macy Pavilion 138, Valhalla, NY 10595, USA
* Corresponding author.
E-mail address: William_Frishman@nymc.edu

Clin Geriatr Med 28 (2012) 575–615
http://dx.doi.org/10.1016/j.cger.2012.07.001   **geriatric.theclinics.com**

treated with pacemakers. Atropine can be used for the treatment of transient bradyarrhythmias.

Tachyarrhythmias

An increase in the prevalence and incidence of supraventricular and ventricular arrhythmias is a characteristic of human aging.[2] The resting heart rate is usually not affected by aging.[1] However, isolated atrial ectopic beats are commonly found in older patients during rest and exercise. These increased beats are not often associated with underlying cardiac disease and usually do not require treatment.

Atrial fibrillation is found in approximately 10% of patients older than 80 years, and is associated with an increased risk of embolic stroke.[3] The arrhythmia is often seen in patients with increased left atrial size, often caused by left ventricular (LV) diastolic dysfunction, which can impair atrial emptying. Apathetic hyperthyroidism may also cause atrial fibrillation in elderly patients. Chronic atrial fibrillation is usually treated with drugs to reduce rapid ventricular rates and with anticoagulation.[3]

Short bursts of supraventricular tachycardia are often seen in many elderly patients.[3] Unless associated with symptoms, these transient arrhythmias are not treated. A β-blocker is the usual treatment of choice when therapy is needed.[4]

The finding of premature ventricular beats increases in frequency with advancing age, both at rest and with exercise, and the need to treat them remains controversial.[1] Sustained ventricular arrhythmias need to be treated with drugs or devices.[5]

Other more commonly found cardiac abnormalities that may increase the frequency of arrhythmias in elderly patients are problems associated with myocardial stiffening and ventricular filling (diastolic dysfunction), problems with myocardial contraction (systolic dysfunction), alular heart disease, hypertensive heart disease, and coronary artery disease.

PHARMACOKINETIC CONSIDERATIONS WITH ANTIARRHYTHMIC DRUG USE IN ELDERLY PATIENTS

Age-related physiologic changes may affect the absorption, bioavailability, drug distribution, metabolism, and drug excretion of antiarrhythmic drugs (**Table 1**).[6] Despite these physiologic changes, the oral absorption of cardiovascular drugs is not significantly affected by aging.[6] However, the bioavailability of certain antiarrhythmic drugs depends on the extent of drug absorption on first-pass metabolism by the liver or the wall of the gastrointestinal (GI) tract. In elderly patients, the absolute bioavailability of drugs such as propranolol and verapamil is increased because of reduced first-pass hepatic metabolism.[6]

With aging, there is a reduction in lean body mass[7] and in total body water,[8] causing a decrease in volume of distribution (V_d) of hydrophilic drugs. This decrease leads to higher plasma concentrations of hydrophilic drugs such as digoxin and angiotensin-converting enzyme (ACE) inhibitors with the first dose in elderly patients.[9] The increased proportion of body fat that occurs with aging also causes an increased V_d for lipophilic drugs. This increase leads to lower initial plasma concentrations for lipophilic drugs such as most β-blockers, antihypertensive drugs, and central α agonists.

The level of α_1-acid glycoprotein increases in elderly patients.[10] Weak bases, such as disopyramide, lidocaine, and propranolol, bind to α_1-acid glycoprotein. This situation may cause a reduction in the free fraction of these drugs in the circulation, a decreased V_d, and a higher initial plasma concentration.[11] In elderly patients, there is also a tendency for plasma albumin concentration to be reduced.[12] Weak acids,

Table 1
Physiologic changes with aging potentially affecting antiarrhythmic drug kinetics

Process	Physiologic Change	Result	Drugs Affected
Absorption	Reduced gastric acid production	Reduced tablet dissolution and decreased solubility of basic drugs	
	Reduced gastric emptying rate	Decreased absorption for acidic drugs	
	Reduced GI mobility, GI blood flow, absorptive surface	Less opportunity for drug absorption	
Distribution	Decreased total body mass. Increased proportion of body fat	Increased V_d of highly lipid-soluble drugs	↓ β-blockers
	Decreased proportion of body water	Decreased V_d of hydrophilic drugs	↑ digoxin
	Decreased plasma albumin, disease-related increased $α_1$-acid glycoprotein, altered relative tissue perfusion	Changed % of free drug, V_d, and measured levels of bound drugs	↑ disopyramide, lidocaine, propranolol
Metabolism	Reduced liver mass, liver blood flow, and hepatic metabolic capacity	Accumulation of metabolized drugs	↑ propranolol, lidocaine, diltiazem, labetalol, verapamil, mexiletine
Excretion	Reduced glomerular filtration, renal tubular function, and renal blood flow	Accumulation of renally cleared drugs	Digoxin, antiarrhythmic, drugs, atenolol, sotalol, nadolol

Abbreviations: GI, gastrointestinal; V_d, volume of distribution.
  Data from Hui KK. Gerontologic considerations in cardiovascular pharmacology and therapeutics. In: Singh BN, Dzau VJ, Vanhoutte PM, et al, editors. Cardiovascular pharmacology and therapeutics. New York: Churchill-Livingstone; 1994.

such as salicylates and warfarin, bind extensively to albumin. Decreased binding of drugs such as warfarin to plasma albumin may result in increased free-drug concentrations, resulting in more intense drug effects.[13]

The half-life of a drug (or of its major metabolite) is the length of time in hours that it takes for the serum concentration of that drug to decrease to half of its peak level. This definition can be described by the kinetic equation: $t½ = 0.693 × V_d/Cl$, where $t½$ is directly related to drug distribution and inversely to clearance (Cl). Therefore, changes in V_d or Cl because of aging, as previously mentioned, can affect the half-life of a drug. In elderly patients, an increased half-life of a drug means a longer time until steady-state conditions are achieved. With a prolonged half-life of a drug, there may be an initial delay in maximum effects of the drug and prolonged adverse effects. **Table 2** lists the pharmacokinetic changes, routes of elimination, and dosage adjustment for selected antiarrhythmic drugs that can be used in elderly patients.[14]

Decreased hepatic blood flow, liver mass, liver volume, and hepatic metabolic capacity occur in elderly patients.[15] There is a reduction in the rate of many drug oxidation reactions (phase 1) and little change in drug conjugation reactions (phase 2). These changes in elderly patients may result in higher serum concentrations of

Table 2
Pharmacokinetic changes, route of elimination, and dosage adjustment of selected antiarrhythmic drugs in elderly patients

Drug	T½	V_d	Cl	Primary Route(s) of Elimination	Dosage Adjustment
Class I					
Disopyramide	↑	—	↓	Renal	Initiate at lowest dose; titrate to response
Flecainide	↑	↑	↓	Hepatic/renal	Initiate at lowest dose; titrate to response
Lidocaine	↑	↑	NS	Hepatic	Initiate at lowest dose; titrate to response
Mexilitine	—	—	—	Hepatic	No adjustment needed
Moricizine	—	—	—	Hepatic	No adjustment needed
Procainamide	—	—	↓	Renal	Initiate at lowest dose; titrate to response
Propafenone	—	—	—	Hepatic	No adjustment needed
Quinidine	↑	NS	↓	Hepatic	Initiate at lowest dose; titrate to response
Tocainide	↑	—	↓	Hepatic/renal	No adjustment needed
Class II (β-Adrenergic Blockers)					
Nonselective without ISA					
Nadolol	NS	—	—	Renal	Initiate at lowest dose; titrate to response
Propranolol	↑	NS	↓	Hepatic	Initiate at lowest dose; titrate to response
Timolol	—	—	—	Hepatic	Initiate at lowest dose; titrate to response
β₁ Selective Without ISA					
Atenolol	↑	NS	↓	Renal	Initiate at lowest dose; titrate to response
Bisoprolol	—	—	—	Hepatic/renal	Initiate at lowest dose; titrate to response
Esmolol	—	—	—	Erythrocytes	Use usual dose with caution
Metoprolol	NS	NS	NS	Hepatic	Initiate at lowest dose; titrate to response
β1 Selective with ISA					
Acebutolol	↑	↓	—	Hepatic/biliary	Initiate at lowest dose; titrate to response
Nonselective with ISA					
Pindolol	—	—	—	Hepatic/renal	Initiate at lowest dose; titrate to response
Dual-Acting					
Carvedilol	—	—	—	Hepatic/biliary	Initiate at lowest dose; titrate to response
Labetalol	—	—	NS	Hepatic	Initiate at lowest dose; titrate to response
Class III					
Amiodarone	—	—	—	Hepatic/biliary	No adjustment needed
Bretylium	—	—	—	Renal	Initiate at lowest dose; titrate to response
Dofetilide	—	—	—	Renal	Adjust dose based on renal function
Ibutilide	—	—	—	Hepatic	No adjustment needed
Sotalol	—	—	—	Renal	Adjust dose based on renal function
Class IV (Calcium Channel Blockers)					
Diltiazem	↑	NS	↓	Hepatic	Initiate at lowest dose; titrate to response
Verapamil	↑	NS	↓	Hepatic	Initiate at lowest dose; titrate to response
Other Antiarrhythmics					
Adenosine	—	—	—	Erythrocytes/vascular endothelial cells	No adjustment needed
Atropine	—	—	—	Hepatic/renal	Use usual dose with caution
Digoxin	↑	↓	↓	Renal	Initiate at lowest dose; titrate to response

Abbreviations: Cl, clearance; ISA, intrinsic sympathomimetic activity; NS, no significant change; T½, half-life; V_d, volume of distribution; ↑, increase; ↓, decrease; —, no information or not relevant.
  Increase in Cl is small compared with increase in V_d.
  Data from Cheng-Lai A, Frishman WH. Appendices. In: Frishman WH, Sica DA, editors. Cardiovascular pharmacotherapeutics. 3rd edition. Minneapolis (MN): Cardiotext; 2011. p. 746–7.

cardiovascular drugs that are metabolized in the liver, including propranolol, lidocaine, labetalol, verapamil, diltiazem, nitrates, warfarin, and mexiletine.

With aging, there is a reduction in the total number of functioning nephrons and thereby a parallel decline in both glomerular filtration rate and renal plasma flow.[16,17] The age-related decline in renal function is likely the single most important physiologic change causing pharmacokinetic alterations in elderly patients.[6] The change in renal function with aging is insidious and poorly characterized by serum creatinine determinations, although serum creatinine measurements remain one of the most widely used tests for gauging renal function. Estimating renal function from a serum creatinine value requires its being indexed for muscle mass, which is difficult in even the most skilled hands. Creatinine is a by-product of creatine metabolism in muscle and its daily production correlates closely with muscle mass. Thus, the greater the muscle mass, the higher the normal serum creatinine level. For example, in a heavily muscled man, a serum creatinine value of 1.4 mg/dL might be considered normal, although such a value may be considered grossly abnormal in an individual with less muscle, such as an aged individual. A safer way to estimate renal function in elderly patients is by use of a urine-free formula, such as the Cockcroft-Gault formula[18]:

$$\text{Creatinine clearance (mL/min)} = (140 - \text{age}) \times \text{body weight (kg)}/72 \times \text{Screat (mg/dL)}$$

For women, the results of this equation can be multiplied by 0.85 to account for the small muscle mass in most women. Creatinine clearance is reciprocally related to serum creatinine concentrations, such that a doubling of serum creatinine represents an approximate halving of renal function. The axiom that glomerular filtration rate is reciprocally related to serum creatinine is most important with the first doubling of serum creatinine. For example, a serum creatinine value of 0.6 mg/dL in an elderly patient doubles to 1.2 mg/dL, and with this doubling creatinine clearance decreases from 80 mL/min to about 40 mL/min.

The National Kidney Foundation guidelines use the Modification of Diet in Renal Disease (MDRD) equation to estimate the glomerular filtration rate.[19] The MDRD equation is

$$\text{Glomerular filtration rate (mL/min/1:73 m}^2) = 186 \times \text{Screat}^{-1.154} \times \text{age}^{-0.203} \times 0.742$$
$$\text{if female, } \times 1.210 \text{ if Black}^{19}$$

The reduced clearance of many drugs primarily excreted by the kidneys causes their half-life to be increased in elderly patients. Cardiovascular drugs known to be excreted by the kidney, via various degrees of filtration and tubular secretion, include digoxin, diuretics, ACE inhibitors, antiarrhythmic medications (bretylium, disopyramide, flecainide, procainamide, and tocainide), and the β-blockers (atenolol, bisoprolol, carteolol, nadolol, and sotalol). Typically, a renally cleared compound begins to accumulate when creatinine clearance values decrease less than 60 mL/min.

USE OF CARDIOVASCULAR DRUGS IN ELDERLY PATIENTS

Antiarrhythmic drugs described in this article are classified using the Vaughn Williams classification (see **Table 2**).

Class IA agents block the sodium channel and fast response, predominantly in atrial ventricular and Purkinje tissues. The maximum rate of phase 0 of the action potential is depressed, slowing conduction velocity.[20] The potency of sodium channel blockade is moderate, and repolarization (action potential) duration is prolonged. There is also some potassium channel blockade of the 1A drugs. Class IA antiarrhythmic drugs are effective for treating many atrial and ventricular tachyarrhythmias.

Teo and colleagues[21] analyzed 59 randomized controlled trials comprising 23,229 patients that investigated the use of class I antiarrhythmic drugs after acute myocardial infarction (MI). Patients receiving class I antiarrhythmic drugs had a significantly higher mortality than patients receiving no antiarrhythmic drugs. None of the 59 trials showed that a class I antiarrhythmic drug decreased mortality in postinfarction patients. Therefore, it is not recommended that class I antiarrhythmic drugs be used for the treatment of ventricular tachycardia or complex ventricular arrhythmias associated with heart disease. Class IA agents can prolong the QT interval versus IB and IC agents and can increase the risk of torsades de pointes.

Quinidine suppresses a wide variety of supraventricular and ventricular arrhythmias.[20] GI side effects are common, and the drug can decrease digoxin clearance, leading to digoxin toxicity. Quinidine may also interfere with the metabolism of encainide and propafenone.

Procainamide is a local anesthetic agent that can effectively suppress a wide variety of atrial, AV nodal and ventricular tachyarrhythmias.[20] It can cause a drug-induced lupus syndrome, with increased levels of lupus anticoagulants.

Disopyramide has electrophysiologic effects similar to quinidine and procainide.[20] Disopyramide significantly depresses myocardial contractility and must be used with caution in elderly patients with LV dysfunction.

Class IB agents also block sodium channels, but to a lesser degree than class IA drugs.[20] As a subclass, they are generally ineffective for the treatment of supraventricular arrhythmias and are only occasionally effective as a monotherapy for ventricular arrhythmias.

Lidocaine can be effective for the treatment of ventricular tachyarrhythmias, particularly in patients with myocardial ischemia.[5] Prophylactic use of lidocaine after MI has been abandoned as a clinical practice. Drugs that alter hepatic metabolism can influence the pharmacokinetics of lidocaine.

Intravenous lidocaine may be used to treat complex ventricular arrhythmias during acute MI.[22] Lidocaine toxicity is more common in elderly patients, and older patients should be monitored for dose-related confusion, tinnitus, paresthesias, slurred speech, tremors, seizures, delirium, respiratory depression, and hypotension. Older patients with congestive heart failure (CHF) or impaired liver function are also at an increased risk for developing adverse effects from lidocaine.[23] In these patients, the loading dose should be decreased by 25% to 50%, and any maintenance infusion should be initiated at a rate of 0.5 to 2.5 mg/min, with the patient monitored closely for adverse effects. The dose of lidocaine should also be reduced if the patient is receiving β-blockers[24] or cimetidine, because these drugs reduce the metabolism of lidocaine.

In elderly patients, the adverse effects of lidocaine can be eliminated by reducing the lidocaine dose or by discontinuing the drug.

Mexilitine is closely related in structure to lidocaine.[20] The drug can be used to suppress frequent and high-grade ventricular arrhythmias. Adverse effects are common and include those related to the GI tract and central nervous system (CNS).

Class IC antiarrhythmic drugs are potent sodium-channel–blocking agents.[20] They have little action on repolarization. They have rapid actions for both atrial and ventricular arrhythmias, especially ventricular ectopy. They are associated with a ventricular proarrhythmic effect, especially in patients with structural heart disease.[20]

Flecainide is a derivative of procainamide and is approved for the treatment of both ventricular and superventricular arrhythmias. It can cause depression of cardiac contractility and cardiac output. Other adverse reactions are blurred vision, headache, dizziness, paresthesias, and tremor.[20]

Propafenone is an antiarrhythmic agent that is structurally similar to β-blocking drugs. It is approved in the United States for treatment of both life-threatening ventricular and supraventricular arrhythmias in patients without structural heart disease. Similar to flexainide, the drug is potentially proarrhythmic and associated with GI and neurologic side effects. Similar to flecainide, it should be used with caution in patients with a history of recent MI.[19]

Class II agents are the β-adrenergic–blocking drugs. Their effects on arrhythmias have been well documented (**Box 1**) and they are the only antiarrhythmic drug class that is not proarrhythmic. β-Adrenergic blocking drugs have shown efficacy in reducing mortality and sudden death in survivors of MI and in patients with LV dysfunction.[25] β-Blockers are especially useful in the treatment of hypertension in older patients who have had a previous MI, angina pectoris, silent myocardial ischemia, complex ventricular arrhythmias, supraventricular tachyarrhythmias, or hypertrophic cardiomyopathy. β-Blockers decrease complex ventricular arrhythmias, including ventricular tachycardia.[26–29] β-Blockers also increase the ventricular fibrillation threshold in animal models and have been shown to reduce the incidence of ventricular fibrillation in patients with acute MI.[30] A randomized, double-blind, placebo-controlled study of propranolol in high-risk survivors of acute MI at 12 Norwegian hospitals reported that patients treated with propranolol for 1 year had a statistically significant 52% decrease in sudden cardiac death.[27] In addition, β-blockers

---

Box 1
Effects of β-blockers in various arrhythmias

Supraventricular

Sinus tachycardia: treat underlying disorder; excellent response to β-blocker if need to control rate (eg, ischemia, heart failure).

Atrial fibrillation: β-blockers reduce rate, rarely restore sinus rhythm, may be useful in combination with digoxin or verapamil and diltiazem. Atrial flutter: β-blockers reduce rate, sometimes restore sinus rhythm.

Atrial tachycardia: effective in slowing ventricular rate, may restore sinus rhythm; useful in prophylaxis.

Maintain patients in normal sinus rhythm after electrocardioversion of atrial and ventricular arrhythmias.

Ventricular

Premature ventricular contractions: good response to β-blockers, especially digitalis-induced, exercise (ischemia-induced, mitral valve prolapse, or hypertrophic cardiomyopathy).

Ventricular tachycardia: effective as quinidine, most effective in digitalis toxicity or exercise (ischemia)-induced.

Ventricular fibrillation: electrical defibrillation is treatment of choice. β-Blockers can be used to prevent recurrence in cases of excess digitalis or sympathomimetic amines; seem to be effective in reducing the incidence of ventricular fibrillation and sudden death after MI.

Reprinted from Frishman WH. Clinical pharmacology of the β-adrenoceptor blocking drugs. 2nd edition. Norwalk (CT): Appleton-Century-Crofts; 1984; with permission.

decrease myocardial ischemia,[28,29,31] which may reduce the likelihood of ventricular fibrillation.

Studies have shown that β-blockers reduce mortality in older and younger patients with complex ventricular arrhythmias and heart disease.[28,29,32–35] In the β-Blocker Heart Attack Trial (BHAT) of 3290 patients comparing propranolol with placebo, propranolol reduced sudden cardiac death by 28% in patients with complex ventricular arrhythmias and by 16% in patients without ventricular arrhythmias.[25,32]

Hallstrom and colleagues[33] performed a retrospective analysis of the effect of anti-arrhythmic drug use in 941 patients resuscitated from prehospital cardiac arrest caused by ventricular fibrillation between 1970 and 1985. β-Blockers were adminis-tered to 28% of the patients, and no antiarrhythmic drug to 39%. There was a reduced incidence of death or recurrent cardiac arrest in patients treated with β-blockers versus no antiarrhythmic drug (relative risk 0.47; adjusted relative risk 0.62).

In a retrospective analysis of data from the Cardiac Arrhythmia Suppression Trial (CAST), Kennedy and colleagues[35] found that 30% of patients with an LV ejection frac-tion less than 40% were receiving β-blockers. Forty percent of these 1735 patients were between 66 and 79 years old. Patients on β-blockers had a significant reduction in all-cause mortality of 43% within 30 days, 46% at 1 year, and 33% at 2 years. Patients receiving β-blockers also had a significant decrease in arrhythmic death or cardiac arrest of 66% at 30 days, 53% at 1 year, and 36% at 2 years. Multivariate anal-ysis showed that β-blockers were an independent factor for reducing arrhythmic death or cardiac arrest by 40%, for decreasing all-cause mortality by 33%, and for reducing the occurrence of new or worsening CHF by 32%. From these data,[26,27,30–33] β-blockers can be used in the treatment of older and younger patients with ventricular tachycardia or complex ventricular arrhythmias associated with ischemic or nonische-mic heart disease, and with normal or abnormal LV ejection fraction, if there are no absolute contraindications to the drugs. β-blockers are also useful in the treatment of supraventricular tachyarrhythmias in older and younger patients.[22–36] If a rapid ventricular rate associated with atrial fibrillation persists at rest or during exercise despite digoxin therapy, then verapamil,[37] diltiazem,[38] or a β-blocker [39] should be added to the therapeutic regimen. These drugs act synergistically with digoxin to depress conduction through the AV junction. The initial oral dose of propranolol is 10 mg every 6 hours, which can be increased to a maximum of 80 mg every 6 hours if necessary.

Contraindications to β-blocker use include bradyarrhythmias or heart blocks, when an implantable pacemaker may be needed if β-blockers are to be continued.

Class III antiarrhythmic drugs prolong the duration of the action potential and increase refractoriness. This effect is mediated by blockade of potassium channels during phase 2 or 3 of the action potential.

Amiodarone is effective in suppressing ventricular tachycardia and complex ventricular arrhythmias. However, there are conflicting data about the effect of amiodarone on mortality.[40–47] The Veterans Administration Cooperative Study comparing amiodarone versus placebo in patients with heart failure with malignant ventricular arrhythmias recently showed that amiodarone was effective in decreasing ventricular tachycardia and complex ventricular arrhythmias, but it did not affect mortality.[46]

In the Sudden Cardiac Death in Heart Failure Trial, 2521 patients, mean age 60 years, with New York Heart Association class II or III heart failure, an LV ejection frac-tion of 35% or less and a mean QRS duration on the resting electrocardiogram (ECG) of 120 milliseconds, were randomized to placebo, amiodarone, or an implantable cardioverter-defibrillator (ICD).[47] At 46-month median follow-up, compared with placebo, amiodarone insignificantly increased mortality by 6% but ICD therapy significantly reduced all-cause mortality by 23%.[47]

The incidence of adverse effects from amiodarone has been reported to approach 90% after 5 years of treatment.[48] In the Cardiac Arrest in Seattle: Conventional versus Amiodarone Drug Evaluation study, the incidence of pulmonary toxicity was 10% at 2 years in patients receiving an amiodarone dose of 158 mg daily.[49] From these data, the use of amiodarone should be reserved for the treatment of life-threatening ventricular tachyarrhythmias or in patients who cannot tolerate or who do not respond to β-blocker therapy.

Amiodarone is also the most effective drug for treating refractory atrial fibrillation in terms of converting atrial fibrillation to sinus rhythm. However, because of the high incidence of adverse effects caused by amiodarone, it should be used in low doses in patients with atrial fibrillation when life-threatening atrial fibrillation is refractory to other therapy.[50]

Sotalol is a nonselective β-blocker with class III antiarrhythmic activity. It is effective for the treatment of supraventricular and ventricular arrhythmias. It should be used with caution with other drugs that prolong the QT interval. Dose adjustment may be required based on renal function.[51]

Ibutilide has a structure similar to sotalol, but has no β-adrenergic–blocking activity. It is indicated in intravenous form only for the acute treatment of recent-onset atrial flutter or atrial fibrillation. The drug can cause polymorphic ventricular tachycardia. No dose adjustment is required in elderly patients.

Dofetilide, an oral formulation, decreases the action potential in a predictable concentration-dependent manner. It is effective for treating atrial fibrillation or flutter. The dose needs to be regulated according to the creatinine clearance. The drug can also cause polymorphic ventricular tachycardia, especially in patients with chronic heart failure.[52] Dose adjustment may be required in elderly patients based on renal function.

The placebo-controlled Danish Investigations of Arrhythmia and Mortality on Dofetilide (DIAMOND) Study Group trial showed that dofetilide did not affect all-cause mortality, cardiac mortality, or total arrhythmic deaths, and showed effectiveness in treating atrial fibrillation and flutter in patients with recent MI and LV dysfunction.[53] In another placebo-controlled DIAMOND study, dofetilide was shown to be safe and effective in reducing the incidence of atrial fibrillation in patients with either heart failure or acute MI and LV dysfunction.[54] Dofetilide is one of the antiarrhythmic agents of choice in patients with LV dysfunction.[55]

Dronedarone has a structure similar to amiodarone, but may have fewer adverse effects. It is approved for the suppression of atrial flutter/fibrillation; however, it may increase mortality in patients with heart failure.[56–58] No dose adjustment is required in elderly patients.

Vernakalant is a new antiarrhythmic drug that targets atrial-specific channels: the Kv1.5 channel, which carries $I_{K(ur)}$, and the Kir3.1/3.4 channel, which carries $I_{K(Ach)}$. Vernakalant can also work to block I_{to}, late I_{na}, with minor blockade of I_{Kr} currents. Vernakalant is available in both intravenous and oral forms. In phase II and phase III trials, intravenous vernakalant was shown to be effective in terminating acute-onset atrial fibrillation with duration greater than 3 hours and less than 7 days (~50% efficiency vs 10% for placebo). It does not seem to be effective for atrial fibrillation with duration greater than 7 days, nor does it seem to be effective for atrial flutter. Studies with oral vernakalant have been designed to evaluate its efficacy and safety in the prevention of atrial fibrillation recurrence.[59] The drug is available in intravenous form in Europe for rapid conversion of atrial fibrillation to sinus rhythm in adult nonsurgical patients with atrial fibrillation of 7 days' duration or less.[60] However, the United States sponsor has discontinued development of the drug in both intravenous and oral formulations because of safety issues.

Class IV antiarrhythmic agents are the calcium channel blockers (**Box 2**).[61]

Verapamil is a synthetic papaverine and the first calcium channel–blocking drug to be used clinically.[20,61] It is used for the treatment and prevention of supraventricular arrhythmias and for the control of ventricular rate at rest and during exercise in patients with rapid atrial fibrillation and flutter. The drug works by slowing the slow inward calcium ion current. The drug is contraindicated for chronic use in patients with LV dysfunction, and in patients with sinus node or AV sinus dysfunction. The drug can cause sinus bradycardia and sinus and AV node blocks when used concomitantly with β-blockers. The drug also does not prolong life in survivors of MI with LV dysfunction.

In elderly patients, the oral formulation should be initiated at a lower dose. Intravenous injections should be given slowly over a longer period.[61]

Diltiazem is a benzothiazepine derivative that blocks the inward calcium ion current.[20,61] Similar to verapamil, it is indicated for the treatment of supraventricular tachycardias and for slowing down rapid ventricular rates in patients with atrial fibrillation or flutter. Similar to verapamil, it should not be used chronically in patients with sinus node or AV node dysfunction unless a pacemaker is in place. The drug should also not be used in patients with LV dysfunction or in survivors of an acute MI with LV dysfunction. Also similar to verapamil, the drug can cause serious sinus node and AV blocks when used concomitantly with β-blockers.

Box 2
Effects of diltiazem and verapamil in treatment of common arrhythmias

Effective

Sinus tachycardia

Supraventricular tachycardia

    AV nodal reentrant paroxysmal supraventricular tachycardia (PSVT)

    Accessory pathway reentrant

    PSVT sinoatrial-nodal reentrant PSVT

    Atrial reentrant PSVT

Atrial flutter (ventricular rate decreases but arrhythmia only occasionally converts)

Atrial fibrillation (ventricular rate decreases but arrhythmia only occasionally converts)

Ineffective

Nonparoxysmal automatic atrial tachycardia

Atrial fibrillation and flutter in Wolff-Parkinson-White syndrome (ventricular rate may not decrease)

Ventricular tachyarrhythmias[a]

[a] There is only limited experience in this area.

  Reproduced from Frishman WH, LeJemtel TH. Electropharmacology of the slow channel inhibitors in the management of cardiac arrhythmias: verapamil. Pace 1982;5:402; with permission.

Other Antiarrhythmic Drugs

Digoxin is used to slow the rapid ventricular rate in patients with supraventricular tachyarrhythmias such as atrial fibrillation, and treating patients with CHF in sinus rhythm associated with abnormal LV ejection fraction that does not respond to diuretics, ACE inhibitors, and β-blockers.[62] Digoxin should not be used to treat patients with CHF in sinus rhythm associated with normal LV ejection fraction.[63] By increasing contractility through increasing intracellular calcium ion concentration, digoxin may increase LV stiffness and increase LV filling pressures, adversely affecting LV diastolic dysfunction. Because almost half the elderly patients with CHF have normal LV ejection fractions,[64,65] the LV ejection fraction should be measured in all older patients with CHF so that appropriate therapy may be given.[66] Many older patients with compensated CHF who are in sinus rhythm and are on digoxin may have the drug withdrawn without decompensation in cardiac function.[67,68]

Therapeutic levels of digoxin do not reduce the frequency or duration of episodes of paroxysmal atrial fibrillation detected by 24-hour ambulatory ECGs.[69] In addition, therapeutic concentrations of digoxin do not prevent the occurrence of a rapid ventricular rate in patients with paroxysmal atrial fibrillation.[69,70] Many elderly patients are able to tolerate atrial fibrillation without the need for digoxin therapy because the ventricular rate is slow as a result of concomitant AV nodal disease.

Digoxin has a narrow toxic/therapeutic ratio, especially in elderly patients.[71] Decreased renal function and lean body mass may increase serum digoxin levels in this population. Serum creatinine levels may be normal in elderly persons despite a marked reduction in creatinine clearance, thereby decreasing digoxin clearance and increasing serum digoxin levels. Older persons are also more likely to take drugs that interact with digoxin (**Table 3**) by interfering with bioavailability or elimination. Quinidine, cyclosporin, itraconazole, calcium preparations, verapamil, amiodarone, diltiazem, triamterene, spironolactone, tetracycline, erythromycin, propafenone, and propantheline can increase serum digoxin levels. Hypokalemia, hypomagnesemia, hypercalcemia, hypoxia, acidosis, acute and chronic lung disease, hypothyroidism, and myocardial ischemia may also cause digitalis toxicity despite normal serum digoxin levels. Digoxin may also cause visual disturbances,[72] depression, and confusional states in older persons, even with therapeutic blood levels.

Adenosine is an endogenous compound, and as an intravenous drug it can exert a negative chronotropic effect on the sinus and AV nodes. It is used as a parenteral drug to treat supraventricular arrhythmias.[20] Dose adjustment is not required in elderly patients.

Atropine is the best known of the muscarinic receptor antagonists. With increasing doses, atropine causes a progressive vasolytic effect with an increase in heart rate, a decrease in the refractory period of the AV node, and increased AV conduction.[73] Atropine is indicated for use in severe symptomatic bradycardia, specifically in the context of acute MI. The drug can precipitate ventricular tachyarrhythmias and symptoms of systemic vagotonia (eg, drug mouth). Use the usual dose with caution in elderly patients.

DRUG-DRUG INTERACTIONS

Drug-drug interactions with antiarrhythmic agents are common in elderly patients and are listed in **Table 3**.[74]

Table 3
Selected drug-drug interactions with antiarrhythmic agents[a]

Interactions with Class I Antiarrhythmic Agents

Primary Drugs	Interacting Drugs	Proposed Mechanism of Interaction	Possible Effects	Clinical Management
Quinidine	Antiarrhythmics (procainamide, disopyramide)	Additive cardiac effects	Increased risk of cardiotoxicity (QT prolongation, torsades de pointes, cardiac arrest)	Monitor blood pressure and ECG; concurrent use of 2 or more class IA antiarrhythmic agents is generally not recommended
	Antiarrhythmics (amiodarone, dofetilide, dronedarone, ibutilide, sotalol)	Additive effects on QT prolongation	Increased risk of cardiotoxicity (QT prolongation, torsades de pointes, cardiac arrest)	If concurrent use of quinidine and a class III antiarrhythmic is necessary, monitor ECG carefully
	Amiodarone	Additive cardiac toxicity; additive effects on QT prolongation	May increase serum quinidine concentration Increased risk of cardiotoxicity (QT prolongation, torsades de pointes, cardiac arrest)	The concurrent use of a class Ia and a class III antiarrhythmic agent is generally not recommended; if concurrent use is deemed necessary, quinidine dose should be reduced by one-third, and the patient should be monitored for signs of arrhythmias
	Disopyramide	Additive cardiac effects	Slight increase in disopyramide concentrations	Monitor for disopyramide toxicity (dosage adjustment for both drugs may be needed)
	Flecainide, propafenone, methadone	Additive effects on QT prolongation	Increased risk of cardiotoxicity (QT prolongation, torsades de pointes, cardiac arrest)	Concurrent use of 2 or more drugs that prolong QT interval is generally not recommended
	Mexiletine	Inhibition of CYP2D6 hepatic enzymes by quinidine results in decreased metabolism of mexiletine	Increased serum mexiletine concentration	Monitor for mexiletine toxicity

Drug	Mechanism	Effect	Management
Procainamide	Additive cardiac effects; interference with renal procainamide clearance	Increased risk of cardiotoxicity (QT prolongation, torsades de pointes, cardiac arrest)	Monitor ECG and procainamide concentrations and adjust dosage as needed
Propafenone	Hepatic metabolism of propafenone may decrease	Increased plasma propafenone concentrations	Monitor for propafenone toxicity and adjust dosage of propafenone as needed
Antibacterials (ciprofloxacin, clarithromycin, cotrimoxazole, erythromycin, gatifloxacin, levofloxacin, moxifloxacin)	Additive effects on QT prolongation; clarithromycin and erythromycin may decrease metabolism of quinidine	Increased risk of cardiotoxicity (QT prolongation, torsades de pointes, cardiac arrest); increased quinidine plasma concentration by clarithromycin and erythromycin	Concurrent use of 2 or more drugs that prolong QT interval is generally not recommended; monitor for quinidine toxicity
Antifungals (fluconazole)	Additive effects on QT prolongation	Increased risk of cardiotoxicity (QT prolongation, torsades de pointes, cardiac arrest)	Concurrent use of 2 or more drugs that prolong QT interval is generally not recommended
Antifungals (itraconazole, ketoconazole)	Decreased quinidine metabolism	Increased plasma quinidine concentration	Monitor for quinidine toxicity; concurrent use of itraconazole and quinidine is contraindicated
Antifungals (posaconazole, voriconazole)	Inhibition of quinidine metabolism	Increase risk of QT prolongation and torsades de pointes; increased quinidine plasma concentration	Concurrent use of posaconazole or voriconazole and quinidine is contraindicated
Antipsychotics (thioridazine, ziprasidone)	Additive cardiac effects	Increased risk of cardiotoxicity (QT prolongation, torsades de pointes, cardiac arrest)	Concurrent use of quinidine and thioridazine or ziprasidone is contraindicated
Antiretrovirals (amprenavir, atazanavir, darunavir, fosamprenavir, lopinavir)	Inhibition of quinidine metabolism	Increased quinidine plasma concentration; increased risk of quinidine toxicity	Monitor for quinidine toxicity and adjust dosage of quinidine as needed

(continued on next page)

Table 3
(continued)

Primary Drugs	Interacting Drugs	Proposed Mechanism of Interaction	Possible Effects	Clinical Management
	Antiretrovirals (ritonavir, nelfinavir, saquinavir, tipranavir)	Inhibition of quinidine metabolism	Increased quinidine plasma concentration; increased risk of quinidine toxicity	Concurrent use of these antiretroviral agents and quinidine is contraindicated
	β-blockers (atenolol, metoprolol, propranolol, timolol)	Additive cardiovascular effects Possible decreased β-blocker metabolism and clearance	Augmentation of β-blocker effects (bradycardia, hypotension)	Monitor blood pressure, heart rate, and adjust dosages as needed
	Calcium antagonists (verapamil, diltiazem)	Inhibition of quinidine metabolism	Increased plasma quinidine concentrations	Monitor for quinidine toxicity
	Digoxin	Decreased renal and nonrenal clearance of digoxin	Increased plasma digoxin concentrations and increased risk of digoxin toxicity	Monitor for signs and symptoms of digoxin toxicity, check digoxin level, and decrease dose of digoxin as needed
	Enzyme inducers (carbamazepine, phenytoin, phenobarbital, rifampin)	Increase quinidine metabolism and elimination	Decreased plasma quinidine concentration; decreased quinidine effectiveness	Assess the therapeutic efficacy of quinidine and adjust dosage as needed
	Neuromuscular blockers (succinylcholine, atracurium, pancuronium, vecuronium)	Altered metabolism of succinylcholine by quinidine; additive effects of pancuronium or vecuronium with quinidine	Increased toxicity of interacting drugs (respiratory depression, apnea, prolonged neuromuscular blockade)	Monitor for respiratory depression and prolonged neuromuscular blockade; respiratory support should be provided as needed
	Tricyclic antidepressants (amitriptyline, desipramine, imipramine, nortriptyline)	Decreased antidepressant metabolism; additive cardiac effects	Increased adverse effects from antidepressants (dry mouth, urinary retention, sedation) and increased risk of cardiotoxicity (QT prolongation, torsades de pointes, cardiac arrest)	Monitor for increased antidepressant adverse effects and signs and symptoms of additive cardiac effects (changes in ECG); concurrent use of a class Ia antiarrhythmic and a tricyclic antidepressant is generally not recommended

	Interacting agent	Mechanism	Possible result	Management
	Urinary alkalinizers (acetazolamide, antacids)	Increase in urinary pH may result in a significant decrease in quinidine renal elimination	Possible increased serum quinidine concentrations and quinidine toxicity	Monitor for quinidine toxicity and adjust dosage of quinidine as needed
	Warfarin	Decreased clotting factor synthesis	Increased bleeding risk from warfarin	Monitor INR; adjust warfarin dose as needed
Procainamide	Antiarrhythmics (disopyramide, quinidine)	Additive cardiac effects; quinidine also decreases procainamide clearance via competition for renal tubular secretion	Increased risk of cardiotoxicity (QT prolongation, torsades de pointes, cardiac arrest)	Monitor blood pressure and ECG; concurrent use of 2 or more class IA antiarrhythmic agents is generally not recommended
	Antiarrhythmics (amiodarone, dofetilide, dronedarone, ibutilide, sotalol)	Additive effects on QT prolongation	Increased risk of cardiotoxicity (QT prolongation, torsades de pointes, cardiac arrest)	If concurrent use of procainamide and a class III antiarrhythmic is absolutely necessary, monitor ECG carefully
	Amiodarone	Decreased procainamide clearance	May increase serum procainamide concentration and lead to procainamide toxicity	Monitor for signs of procainamide toxicity (QT prolongation, torsades de pointes), assess procainamide levels, and reduce procainamide dose accordingly
	Flecainide, propafenone	Additive effects on QT prolongation	Increased risk of cardiotoxicity (QT prolongation, torsades de pointes, cardiac arrest)	Concurrent use of 2 or more drugs that prolong QT interval is generally not recommended
	Antibacterials (ciprofloxacin, clarithromycin, cotrimoxazole, erythromycin, gatifloxacin, levofloxacin, moxifloxacin, ofloxacin)	Additive effects on QT prolongation; Ofloxacin inhibits the active renal tubular secretion of procainamide	Increased risk of cardiotoxicity (QT prolongation, torsades de pointes, cardiac arrest) Increased procainamide plasma concentration by ofloxacin	Concurrent use of 2 or more drugs that prolong QT interval is generally not recommended; monitor ECG and procainamide serum concentration and adjust procainamide dose as needed

(continued on next page)

Table 3
(continued)

Primary Drugs	Interacting Drugs	Proposed Mechanism of Interaction	Possible Effects	Clinical Management
	Antifungals (fluconazole)	Additive effects on QT prolongation	Increased risk of cardiotoxicity (QT prolongation, torsades de pointes, cardiac arrest)	Concurrent use of 2 or more drugs that prolong QT interval is generally not recommended
	Antipsychotics (haloperidol, quetiapine, risperidone, thioridazine, ziprasidone)	Additive cardiac effects	Increased risk of cardiotoxicity (QT prolongation, torsades de pointes, cardiac arrest)	Concurrent use of a class IA antiarrhythmic and an antipsychotic is generally not recommended; concurrent use of procainamide and thioridazine or ziprasidone is contraindicated
	Histamine (H$_2$) antagonists (cimetidine, ranitidine)	Decreased procainamide renal clearance as a result of competition for active tubular secretion	Increase risk of procainamide toxicity (cardiac arrhythmias, hypotension, CNS depression)	Monitor for signs and symptoms of procainamide toxicity; monitor procainamide plasma concentration; decrease dose of procainamide as needed
	Neuromuscular blockers (succinylcholine, atracurium, pancuronium, vecuronium)	Reduction of acetylcholine release by procainamide	Excessive neuromuscular blockade	Monitor for prolonged neuromuscular blockade, adjust doses of neuromuscular blocker as needed
	Tricyclic antidepressants (amitriptyline, desipramine, imipramine, nortriptyline)	Additive cardiac effects	Increased risk of cardiotoxicity (QT prolongation, torsades de pointes, cardiac arrest)	Monitor for signs and symptoms of additive cardiac effects (changes in ECG); concurrent use of a class IA antiarrhythmic and a tricyclic antidepressant is generally not recommended

Disopyramide			
	Antiarrhythmics (procainamide, quinidine)	Additive cardiac effects	Increased risk of cardiotoxicity (QT prolongation, torsades de pointes, cardiac arrest)	Monitor blood pressure and ECG; concurrent use of 2 or more class Ia antiarrhythmic agents is generally not recommended
	Antiarrhythmics (amiodarone, dofetilide, dronedarone, ibutilide, sotalol)	Additive effects on QT prolongation	Increased risk of cardiotoxicity (QT prolongation, torsades de pointes, cardiac arrest)	If concurrent use of disopyramide and a class III antiarrhythmic is necessary, monitor ECG carefully
	Flecainide, propafenone	Additive effects on QT prolongation	Increased risk of cardiotoxicity (QT prolongation, torsades de pointes, cardiac arrest)	Concurrent use of 2 or more drugs that prolong QT interval is generally not recommended
	Antibacterials (azithromycin, ciprofloxacin, clarithromycin, cotrimoxazole, erythromycin, gatifloxacin, levofloxacin, moxifloxacin)	Additive effects on QT prolongation; azithromycin, clarithromycin, and erythromycin may decrease metabolism of disopyramide	Increased risk of cardiotoxicity (QT prolongation, torsades de pointes, cardiac arrest) Increased disopyramide plasma concentration by azithromycin, clarithromycin, and erythromycin	Concurrent use of 2 or more drugs that prolong QT interval is generally not recommended; monitor for signs and symptoms of disopyramide toxicity (anticholinergic effects, hypotension, heart failure, cardiac arrhythmias)
	Antifungals (fluconazole)	Additive effects on QT prolongation	Increased risk of cardiotoxicity (QT prolongation, torsades de pointes, cardiac arrest)	Concurrent use of 2 or more drugs that prolong QT interval is generally not recommended
	Antifungals (itraconazole)	Decreased disopyramide metabolism	Increased plasma disopyramide concentration and risk of disopyramide toxicity	Monitor for signs and symptoms of disopyramide toxicity; adjust dose of disopyramide as needed

(continued on next page)

Table 3
(continued)

Primary Drugs	Interacting Drugs	Proposed Mechanism of Interaction	Possible Effects	Clinical Management
	Antipsychotics (haloperidol, quetiapine, risperidone, thioridazine, ziprasidone)	Additive cardiac effects	Increased risk of cardiotoxicity (QT prolongation, torsades de pointes, cardiac arrest)	Concurrent use of a class IA antiarrhythmic and an antipsychotic is generally not recommended; concurrent use of disopyramide and thioridazine is contraindicated
	Antiretrovirals (atazanavir, ritonavir, saquinavir)	Inhibition of disopyramide metabolism	Increased disopyramide plasma concentration and increased risk of disopyramide toxicity	Monitor for signs and symptoms of disopyramide toxicity and adjust dose of disopyramide as needed
	β-blockers (atenolol, betaxolol, propranolol)	Additive cardiovascular effects	Bradycardia, hypotension, decreased cardiac output	Monitor blood pressure, heart rate, and cardiac function and adjust dosages as needed
	Digoxin	Unknown	Increased plasma digoxin concentrations and increased risk of digoxin toxicity	Monitor for signs and symptoms of digoxin toxicity, check digoxin level, and decrease dose of digoxin as needed
	Enzyme inducers (phenytoin, phenobarbital, rifampin)	Increase disopyramide metabolism and elimination	Decreased plasma disopyramide concentration; decreased disopyramide effectiveness	Assess the therapeutic efficacy of disopyramide and adjust dosage as needed
	Tricyclic antidepressants (amitriptyline, desipramine, imipramine, nortriptyline)	Additive cardiac effects	Increased risk of cardiotoxicity (QT prolongation, torsades de pointes, cardiac arrest)	Monitor for signs and symptoms of additive cardiac effects (changes in ECG); concurrent use of a class Ia antiarrhythmic and a tricyclic antidepressant is generally not recommended

Lidocaine	Amiodarone	Decreased lidocaine metabolism	Increased serum lidocaine concentration; increased lidocaine toxicity	Monitor for signs and symptoms of lidocaine toxicity (neurotoxicity, cardiac arrhythmias, hypotension, seizures) and reduce lidocaine dose as needed
	Antiretrovirals (amprenavir, atazanavir, darunavir, fosamprenavir, lopinavir, ritonavir)	Inhibition of lidocaine metabolism	Increased lidocaine plasma concentration; increased risk of lidocaine toxicity	Monitor for signs and symptoms of lidocaine toxicity and adjust dosage of lidocaine accordingly
	β-blockers (metoprolol, nadolol, propranolol)	Decreased lidocaine metabolism	Increased lidocaine plasma concentration; increased risk of lidocaine toxicity	Monitor for signs and symptoms of lidocaine toxicity and adjust dosage of lidocaine accordingly
	Cimetidine	Decreased lidocaine metabolism possibly caused by decreased hepatic blood flow	Increased lidocaine plasma concentration; increased risk of lidocaine toxicity	Monitor for signs and symptoms of lidocaine toxicity and adjust dosage of lidocaine accordingly
	Phenytoin	Increased lidocaine metabolism and elimination Phenytoin also has additive cardiac depressive effects with lidocaine	Decreased plasma lidocaine concentration and decreased lidocaine effectiveness	Assess the therapeutic efficacy of lidocaine and adjust dosage as needed
	Succinylcholine	Unknown	Increased toxicity of neuromuscular blockers (respiratory depression, apnea, prolonged neuromuscular blockade)	Monitor for respiratory depression and prolonged neuromuscular blockade; respiratory support should be provided as needed
Mexiletine	Antiarrhythmics (amiodarone, quinidine)	Decreased metabolism of mexiletine	Increased mexiletine plasma concentration; increased risk of mexiletine toxicity (nausea, dizziness, cardiac arrhythmias)	Monitor for signs and symptoms of mexiletine toxicity and adjust dosage of mexiletine accordingly

(continued on next page)

Table 3
(continued)

Primary Drugs	Interacting Drugs	Proposed Mechanism of Interaction	Possible Effects	Clinical Management
	Enzyme inducers (phenytoin, rifampin)	Increased mexiletine metabolism and elimination	Decreased plasma mexiletine concentration and decreased mexiletine effectiveness	Assess the therapeutic efficacy of mexiletine and adjust dosage as needed
	Ritonavir	Inhibition of mexiletine metabolism	Increased mexiletine plasma concentration; increased risk of mexiletine toxicity	Monitor for signs and symptoms of mexiletine toxicity and adjust dosage of mexiletine accordingly
	Theophylline	Mexiletine inhibits the CYP1A2 metabolism of theophylline	Increased theophylline plasma concentration; increased risk of theophylline toxicity (nausea, vomiting, palpitation, seizures)	Monitor for signs and symptoms of theophylline toxicity, check theophylline serum concentration, and adjust dose of theophylline as needed
Flecainide	Amiodarone	Amiodarone inhibits CYP2D6 and decreases metabolism of flecainide; additive effects on QT prolongation	Increased flecainide plasma concentration; increased risk of flecainide toxicity (cardiac arrhythmias, neurologic effects, exacerbation of heart failure)	Monitor ECG and monitor for signs and symptoms of flecainide toxicity and reduce dosage of flecainide accordingly
	Antibacterials (ciprofloxacin, clarithromycin, cotrimoxazole, erythromycin, gatifloxacin, levofloxacin, moxifloxacin)	Additive effects on QT prolongation	Increased risk of cardiotoxicity (QT prolongation, torsades de pointes, cardiac arrest)	Concurrent use of 2 or more drugs that prolong QT interval is generally not recommended
	Antifungals (fluconazole)	Additive effects on QT prolongation	Increased risk of cardiotoxicity (QT prolongation, torsades de pointes, cardiac arrest)	Concurrent use of 2 or more drugs that prolong QT interval is generally not recommended

Drug	Interacting drug	Mechanism	Effect	Recommendation
	Antipsychotics (thioridazine, ziprasidone)	Additive cardiac effects	Increased risk of cardiotoxicity (QT prolongation, torsades de pointes, cardiac arrest)	Concurrent use of flecainide and thioridazine or ziprasidone is contraindicated
	Antiretrovirals (darunavir, delavirdine ritonavir, saquinavir, tipranavir)	Inhibition of flecainide metabolism	Increased flecainide plasma concentration; increased risk of flecainide toxicity	Monitor for signs and symptoms of flecainide toxicity and reduce dosage of flecainide accordingly; concurrent use of flecainide and ritonavir or saquinavir or tipranavir is contraindicated
	Cimetidine	Decreased flecainide renal clearance	Increased flecainide plasma concentration; increased risk of flecainide toxicity	Monitor for signs and symptoms of flecainide toxicity and reduce dosage accordingly
	Selective serotonin inhibitors (fluoxetine, sertraline)	Decreased metabolism of flecainide	Increased flecainide plasma concentration; increased risk of flecainide toxicity	Monitor for signs and symptoms of flecainide toxicity and reduce dosage accordingly
Propafenone	Amiodarone	Decreased metabolism of propafenone; additive effects on QT prolongation	Increased propafenone plasma concentration; increased risk of propafenone toxicity (blurred vision, CNS depression, tachycardia)	Monitor ECG and monitor for signs and symptoms of propafenone toxicity and reduce dosage of propafenone accordingly
	Antibacterials (ciprofloxacin, clarithromycin, cotrimoxazole, erythromycin, gatifloxacin, levofloxacin, moxifloxacin)	Additive effects on QT prolongation	Increased risk of cardiotoxicity (QT prolongation, torsades de pointes, cardiac arrest)	Concurrent use of 2 or more drugs that prolong QT interval is generally not recommended
	Antifungals (fluconazole)	Additive effects on QT prolongation	Increased risk of cardiotoxicity (QT prolongation, torsades de pointes, cardiac arrest)	Concurrent use of 2 or more drugs that prolong QT interval is generally not recommended

(continued on next page)

Table 3
(continued)

Primary Drugs	Interacting Drugs	Proposed Mechanism of Interaction	Possible Effects	Clinical Management
	Antipsychotics (risperidone, thioridazine, ziprasidone)	Additive cardiac effects	Increased risk of cardiotoxicity (QT prolongation, torsades de pointes, cardiac arrest)	Concurrent use of propafenone and thioridazine or ziprasidone is contraindicated
	Antiretrovirals (darunavir, delavirdine ritonavir, saquinavir, tipranavir)	Inhibition of propafenone metabolism	Increased propafenone plasma concentration; increased risk of propafenone toxicity	Monitor for signs and symptoms of propafenone toxicity and reduce dosage of propafenone accordingly; concurrent use of propafenone and ritonavir or saquinavir or tipranavir is contraindicated
	β-blockers (metoprolol, propranolol)	Decreased β-blocker metabolism	Increased β-blocker adverse effects (fatigue, bradycardia, hypotension)	Monitor heart rate and blood pressure; decrease dose of β-blocker as needed
	Cyclosporine	Decreased metabolism or increased gastrointestinal absorption of cyclosporine	Increased risk of cyclosporine toxicity (renal dysfunction, cholestasis, paresthesias)	Monitor cyclosporine concentration and adjust dosage of cyclosporine as needed
	Cimetidine	Decreased propafenone metabolism	Increased propafenone plasma concentration; increased risk of propafenone toxicity	Monitor for signs and symptoms of propafenone toxicity and reduce dosage of propafenone accordingly
	Digoxin	Decreased digoxin volume of distribution and decreased nonrenal clearance of digoxin	Increased digoxin plasma concentration; increased risk of digoxin toxicity	Monitor for signs and symptoms of digoxin toxicity, check digoxin concentration, and reduce dosage of digoxin accordingly

Enzyme inducers (rifampin, phenobarbital)	Increased propafenone metabolism and elimination	Decreased plasma propafenone concentration and decreased propafenone effectiveness	Assess the therapeutic efficacy of propafenone and adjust dosage as needed
Quinidine	Decreased propafenone metabolism	Increased propafenone plasma concentration; increased risk of propafenone toxicity	Monitor for signs and symptoms of propafenone toxicity and reduce dosage of propafenone accordingly
Selective serotonin inhibitors (fluoxetine, sertraline)	Decreased metabolism of propafenone	Increased propafenone plasma concentration; increased risk of propafenone toxicity	Monitor for signs and symptoms of propafenone toxicity and reduce dosage of propafenone accordingly
Theophylline	Decreased theophylline metabolism	Increased theophylline plasma concentration; increased risk of theophylline toxicity (nausea, vomiting, palpitation, seizures)	Monitor for signs and symptoms of theophylline toxicity, check theophylline serum concentration, and adjust dose of theophylline as needed
Warfarin	Decreased warfarin clearance	Increased bleeding risk from warfarin	Monitor INR; adjust warfarin dose as needed
Interactions with Class III Antiarrhythmic Agents			
Amiodarone			
Antiretrovirals (amprenavir, atazanavir, darunavir, delavirdine, fosamprenavir, lopinavir, nelfinavir, ritonavir, saquinavir, tipranavir)	Inhibition of CYP3A4-mediated amiodarone metabolism by antiretrovirals	Increased amiodarone plasma concentration; increased risk of amiodarone toxicity (hypotension, bradycardia, sinus arrest)	Monitor for signs and symptoms of amiodarone toxicity, check amiodarone concentration, and reduce dosage of amiodarone accordingly; concurrent use of amiodarone and ritonavir or nelfinavir or tipranavir is contraindicated
β-blockers (metoprolol, propranolol)	Additive cardiac effects; possible inhibition of β-blocker metabolism by amiodarone	Hypotension, bradycardia, cardiac arrest	Monitor cardiac function (especially heart rate); adjust dosages of β-blockers accordingly

(continued on next page)

Table 3
(continued)

Primary Drugs	Interacting Drugs	Proposed Mechanism of Interaction	Possible Effects	Clinical Management
	Cholestyramine	Decreased bioavailability of amiodarone	Decreased plasma amiodarone concentration and decreased amiodarone effectiveness	Administer amiodarone 2 h before or 4 h after cholestyramine
	Calcium antagonists (diltiazem, verapamil)	Additive calcium channel blocker activity caused by inhibition of metabolism of either agent through CYP3A4	Additive reduction in heart rate and myocardial contractility	Monitor for bradycardia and signs and symptoms of reduced cardiac output
	Cyclosporine	Inhibition of CYP3A4-mediated cyclosporine metabolism	Increased cyclosporine plasma concentration; increased risk of cyclosporine toxicity (renal dysfunction, cholestasis, paresthesias)	Monitor for signs or symptoms of cyclosporine toxicity, check serum cyclosporine concentrations, and adjust cyclosporine dose as needed
	Digoxin	Inhibition of P-glycoprotein by amiodarone; reduced digoxin clearance	Increased digoxin plasma concentration; increased risk of digoxin toxicity	Monitor for signs and symptoms of digoxin toxicity, check digoxin concentration, and reduce dosage of digoxin accordingly
	Dofetilide	Additive effects on QT prolongation	Increased risk of cardiotoxicity (QT prolongation, torsades de pointes, cardiac arrest)	Concurrent use of 2 class III antiarrhythmics is not recommended
	Dolasetron	Additive effects on QT prolongation	Increased risk of cardiotoxicity (QT prolongation, torsades de pointes, cardiac arrest	Cardiac function should be closely monitored

Drug	Mechanism	Result	Recommendation
Flecainide	Decreased flecainide metabolism; additive effects on QT prolongation	Increased flecainide plasma concentration; increased risk of flecainide toxicity (cardiac arrhythmias, neurologic effects, exacerbation of heart failure) Increased risk of cardiotoxicity (QT prolongation, torsades de pointes, cardiac arrest)	Monitor ECG and monitor for signs and symptoms of flecainide toxicity; check serum flecainide concentration and reduce dosage of flecainide accordingly
Fluoroquinolones	Additive effects on QT prolongation	Increased risk of cardiotoxicity (QT prolongation, torsades de pointes, cardiac arrest)	Monitor cardiac function closely; concurrent use of 2 or more drugs that prolong QT interval is generally not recommended
Grapefruit juice	Inhibition of CYP3A-mediated metabolism of amiodarone to N-DEA by grapefruit juice	Increased amiodarone plasma concentration and decreased metabolite (N-DEA) activity, which may lead to inconsistent clinical effects from amiodarone	Coadministration of amiodarone and grapefruit juice should be avoided
Phenytoin and fosphenytoin	Decreased phenytoin metabolism and increased amiodarone metabolism	Increased phenytoin plasma concentration; increased risk of phenytoin toxicity Decreased plasma amiodarone concentration and decreased amiodarone effectiveness	Monitor serum phenytoin concentrations and adjust dosage accordingly; assess amiodarone clinical responses
Lidocaine	Decreased lidocaine clearance	Increased lidocaine plasma concentration; increased risk of lidocaine toxicity	Monitor for signs and symptoms of lidocaine toxicity (neurotoxicity, cardiac arrhythmias, hypotension, seizures) and reduce lidocaine dose as needed

(continued on next page)

Table 3
(continued)

Primary Drugs	Interacting Drugs	Proposed Mechanism of Interaction	Possible Effects	Clinical Management
	Procainamide	Decreased procainamide clearance	May increase serum procainamide concentration and lead to procainamide toxicity	Monitor for signs of procainamide toxicity (QT prolongation, torsades de points), check procainamide levels, and reduce procainamide dose accordingly
	Quinidine	Additive cardiac toxicity; additive effects on QT prolongation	May increase serum quinidine concentration Increased risk of cardiotoxicity (QT prolongation, torsades de pointes, cardiac arrest)	Concurrent use of a class Ia and a class III antiarrhythmic agent is generally not recommended; if concurrent use is deemed necessary, quinidine dose should be reduced by one-third and the patient should be monitored for signs of arrhythmias
	Theophylline	Decreased theophylline metabolism	Increased theophylline plasma concentration; increased risk of theophylline toxicity (nausea, vomiting, palpitation, seizures)	Monitor for signs and symptoms of theophylline toxicity, check theophylline serum concentration, and adjust dose of theophylline as needed
	Warfarin	Decreased warfarin metabolism	Increased bleeding risk from warfarin	Monitor INR; adjust warfarin dose as needed
Dofetilide	Cimetidine	Cimetidine inhibits dofetilide renal tubular secretion and metabolism through CYP3A4	Increased dofetilide plasma concentration; increased risk of cardiac arrhythmia	Concurrent use of dofetilide and cimetidine is contraindicated; if antacid therapy is required, use omeprazole, ranitidine, or antacids containing aluminum and magnesium hydroxides

	Interacting agent	Mechanism	Effect	Recommendation
	Ketoconazole	Inhibition of CYP3A4-mediated dofetilide metabolism; inhibition of renal cation transport system; additive effects on QT prolongation	Increased dofetilide plasma concentration; increased risk of cardiac arrhythmia	Concurrent use of dofetilide and ketoconazole is contraindicated
	Megestrol	Inhibition of renal cation transport system; reduced elimination of dofetilide	Increased dofetilide plasma concentration; increased risk of cardiac arrhythmia	Concurrent use of dofetilide and megestrol is contraindicated
	Prochlorperazine	Inhibition of renal cation transport system; reduced elimination of dofetilide	Increased dofetilide plasma concentration; increased risk of cardiac arrhythmia	Concurrent use of dofetilide and prochlorperazine is contraindicated
	Trimethoprim (including cotrimoxazole)	Inhibition of renal cation transport system; reduced elimination of dofetilide Additive effects on QT prolongation	Increased dofetilide plasma concentration; increased risk of cardiac arrhythmia	Concurrent use of dofetilide and trimethoprim is contraindicated
	Verapamil	Increased oral absorption of dofetilide by verapamil	Increased dofetilide plasma concentration; increased risk of cardiac arrhythmia	Concurrent use of dofetilide and verapamil is contraindicated
Dronedarone	Potent CYP3A inhibitors (clarithromycin, itraconazole, ketoconazole, nefazodone ritonavir, telithromycin voriconazole)	Inhibition of CYP3A4-mediated dronedarone metabolism	Increased dronedarone plasma concentration; increased risk of cardiac arrhythmia	Concurrent use of dofetilide and potent CYP3A inhibitors is contraindicated
	CYP3A inducers (carbamazepine, phenobarbital, phenytoin, rifampin)	Increased dronedarone metabolism	Decreased plasma dronedarone concentration and decreased dronedarone effectiveness	Concurrent use of dronedarone and enzyme inducers may result in decreased dronedarone exposure and should be avoided

(continued on next page)

Table 3
(continued)

Primary Drugs	Interacting Drugs	Proposed Mechanism of Interaction	Possible Effects	Clinical Management
	Digoxin	Inhibition of P-glycoprotein transporter of digoxin by dronedarone; reduced digoxin clearance	Increased digoxin plasma concentration; increased risk of digoxin toxicity	Monitor for signs and symptoms of digoxin toxicity, check digoxin concentration, and reduce dosage of digoxin accordingly
	Grapefruit juice	Inhibition of CYP3A-mediated dronedarone metabolism	Increased dronedarone plasma concentration; increased risk of dronedarone toxicity	Coadministration of dronedarone and grapefruit juice should be avoided
	Metoprolol	Possible CYP2D6 inhibition of β-blocker metabolism by dronedarone	Increased bioavailability of metoprolol; increased risk of bradycardia	Monitor cardiac function (especially heart rate); adjust metoprolol dose as needed
Ibutilide	Dolasetron	Additive effects on QT prolongation	Increased risk of cardiotoxicity (QT prolongation, torsades de pointes, cardiac arrest	Cardiac function should be closely monitored
Sotalol	α-Adrenergic blockers (doxazosin, prazosin, terazosin)	Suppression of β-mediated compensatory increases in heart rate	Increased hypotensive effect	Monitor blood pressure closely; use lowest possible initial dose of α-adrenergic blocker
	Dihydropyridine calcium blockers	Additive cardiovascular effects	Increased hypotensive effects	Monitor blood pressure and cardiac function, especially in patients predisposed to heart failure
	Digoxin	Additive cardiac effects, possibly increased digoxin bioavailability	Increased bradycardic effects	Monitor ECG and serum digoxin concentrations; adjust dose accordingly

Interactions with β-Blockers

β-blockers (all)			
α-blockers (doxazosin, prazosin, terazosin)	Suppression of β-mediated compensatory increases in heart rate	Increased risk for first-dose hypotension	Initiate the α-blocker with a lower dose, preferably at bedtime; monitor patient for hypotension
Antidiabetics	Altered glucose metabolism and β-blockade	Prolonged hypoglycemia; masking of hypoglycemic effects	Monitor patient's blood glucose closely; educate patients on the recognition of signs of hypoglycemia and action to take when hypoglycemic
β₂-adrenergic agonists (albuterol, levalbuterol, terbutaline)	Pharmacologic antagonism	Decreased effectiveness of either β-blocker or the β₂ agonist	Consider use of a cardioselective β-blocker with caution
Calcium antagonists (diltiazem, verapamil)	Additive cardiovascular effects Diltiazem and verapamil may decrease the metabolism of propranolol	Increased risk of hypotension, bradycardia, AV conduction disturbances	Monitor cardiac function and blood pressure closely; adjust dosages as needed
Clonidine	Unopposed α effect after withdrawal of clonidine in patients who received a β-blocker and clonidine concurrently	Rebound hypertension after withdrawal of clonidine in patients who received a β-blocker and clonidine concurrently	Consider use of cardioselective β-blockers (eg, atenolol, metoprolol) or an α-β-blocker (eg, labetalol); consider withdrawal of β-blocker before clonidine withdrawal; monitor blood pressure closely
Digoxin	Additive cardiac effects	Potentiation of bradycardia and AV block	Monitor patient for bradycardia and AV conduction delay on ECG and adjust dosages as needed
Disopyramide	Additive negative inotropic effects	Bradycardia, decreased cardiac output	Monitor heart rate, signs and symptoms of reduced cardiac output

(continued on next page)

Table 3
(continued)

Primary Drugs	Interacting Drugs	Proposed Mechanism of Interaction	Possible Effects	Clinical Management
	Epinephrine	Enhanced pressor response to adrenaline caused by unopposed peripheral α-receptor effects Blocked β-effects of epinephrine	Hypertension, bradycardia, resistance to epinephrine in anaphylaxis	Avoid this combination or use adrenaline cautiously in patients on β-blockers; monitor blood pressure carefully
	NSAIDs (indomethacin, phenylbutazone)	Decreased production of vasodilating and renal prostaglandins	Attenuation of the antihypertensive effect of β-blockers with possible loss of blood pressure control	Monitor blood pressure regularly and adjust dose of β-blocker as needed; use NSAIDs for short durations to minimize risk of interaction
β-Blockers (metoprolol, propranolol)	Amiodarone, dronedarone	Additive cardiac effects; possible inhibition of β-blocker metabolism by amiodarone	Potential for bradycardia or arrhythmias on initiation of combination therapy	Initiate combination therapy in a controlled clinical environment; monitor heart rate and ECG
	Fluoxetine	Decreased metabolism of β-blockers	Potentiation of β-blocker effects	Monitor for signs and symptoms of β-blocker toxicity; consider switching to a renally eliminated β-blocker (eg, atenolol) or an SSRI that does not inhibit CYP2D6 (eg, citalopram, nefazodone)
	Lidocaine	Decreased hepatic clearance of lidocaine by lipid-soluble β-blockers	Enhanced lidocaine toxicity (anxiety, myocardial depression, cardiac arrest)	Use combination with caution; use lower doses of lidocaine
	Propafenone	Decreased metabolism of β-blockers	Potentiation of β-blocker effects	Monitor blood pressure and cardiac function; adjust dosage of β-blocker as needed

	Rifampin	Increased metabolism of β-blockers	Decreased β-blocker effectiveness	Monitor blood pressure and adjust dosages of β-blockers accordingly; consider use of atenolol or nadolol, which are not likely to be affected
β-Blocker (propranolol)	Chlorpromazine	Decreased chlorpromazine metabolism; decreased propranolol clearance	Chlorpromazine toxicity (sedation, extrapyramidal effects, delirium); increased propranolol effect	Monitor for an enhanced effect of either drug and reduce the dosage of 1 or both drugs if needed
	Haloperidol	Unknown	Increased risk of hypotension and cardiac arrest	Use concomitant therapy with caution; monitor for signs of hypotension
	Thioridazine	Inhibition of thioridazine metabolism	Increased risk of thioridazine toxicity and cardiotoxicity (QT prolongation, torsades de pointes, cardiac arrest)	Concurrent use of propranolol and thioridazine is contraindicated
	Flecainide	Additive cardiovascular effects, decreased flecainide metabolism, decreased propranolol metabolism	Additive negative inotropic effects	Monitor for signs and symptoms of reduced cardiac output; adjust dosages as needed
	Theophylline	Pharmacologic antagonism Theophylline clearance may also be decreased by propranolol	Attenuation of bronchodilatory effects of theophylline; more pronounced with noncardioselective β-blockers	Monitor theophylline serum concentration; use of cardioselective β-blockers is preferable

Interactions with Calcium Antagonists

Calcium antagonists (all)	Cimetidine	Decreased hepatic metabolism of calcium antagonists	Increased effects/toxicity of calcium antagonists	Monitor heart rate and blood pressure and adjust dosages as needed; consider using another H₂ antagonist such as ranitidine

(continued on next page)

Table 3
(continued)

Primary Drugs	Interacting Drugs	Proposed Mechanism of Interaction	Possible Effects	Clinical Management
	Cyclosporine	Decreased cyclosporine metabolism (interaction is more prominent with diltiazem and verapamil)	Increased risk of cyclosporine toxicity (renal dysfunction, neurotoxicity)	Monitor for signs and symptoms of cyclosporine toxicity; monitor circulating cyclosporine levels and adjust cyclosporine dosage as needed; alternative calcium antagonist with minimal impact on cyclosporine levels such as isradipine may be used
	Enzyme inducers (carbamazepine, phenytoin, phenobarbital)	Increased metabolism of calcium antagonists	Decreased effectiveness of calcium antagonists	Monitor patients for loss of calcium antagonist effects, including clinical signs or symptoms of hypertension or angina; adjust dose of calcium antagonist accordingly
	Enzyme inhibitors (fluconazole, itraconazole, ketoconazole)	Decreased hepatic metabolism of calcium antagonists	Increased effects/toxicity of calcium antagonists	Monitor heart rate and blood pressure and adjust dosages as needed
	Grapefruit juice	Decreased hepatic metabolism of calcium antagonists (Interaction is more prominent with certain dihydropyridines: felodipine, nicardipine, nimodipine, nisoldipine, and nitrendipine)	Increased effects/toxicity of calcium antagonists	Tell patients to avoid grapefruit juice if possible (drink orange juice instead); otherwise, monitor blood pressure and adjust dosages as needed to avoid hypotension

Calcium antagonists (diltiazem, verapamil)	Amiodarone	Additive cardiac effects; inhibitor of metabolism of either agent via CYP3A4	Bradycardia, AV block or sinus arrest	Monitor for bradycardia and signs and symptoms of reduced cardiac output; avoid concurrent use in patients with sick sinus syndrome or partial AV block
	β-blockers, digoxin	Additive cardiac effects	Potential for bradycardia or heart block	Monitor heart and PR interval; adjust dosages as needed
	Carbamazepine	Decreased carbamazepine metabolism	Carbamazepine toxicity (ataxia, nystagmus, headache, vomiting, seizures)	Avoid concurrent use; use dihydropyridine calcium antagonists such as nifedipine instead
	Digoxin	Decreased renal or extrarenal clearance of digoxin	Increased serum digoxin concentration and toxicity (nausea, vomiting, arrhythmias)	Monitor patients for signs and symptoms of digoxin toxicity, check digoxin levels, and adjust dosage as needed
	Quinidine	Additive cardiac effects; inhibition of quinidine metabolism	Increased quinidine concentration and toxicity (ventricular arrhythmias, hypotension, exacerbation of heart failure)	Monitor for signs and symptoms of quinidine toxicity, check quinidine concentrations, and adjust dosage of quinidine as needed; consider alternative calcium antagonists

(continued on next page)

Table 3
(continued)

Interactions with Digoxin

Primary Drugs	Interacting Drugs	Proposed Mechanism of Interaction	Possible Effects	Clinical Management
Digoxin	Alprazolam	Decreased renal clearance of digoxin	Increased digoxin plasma concentration; increased risk of digoxin toxicity (nausea, vomiting, arrhythmias)	Monitor for signs and symptoms of digoxin toxicity, check digoxin concentration, and reduce dosage of digoxin accordingly
	Amiodarone, dronedarone	Inhibition of *P*-glycoprotein; reduced digoxin clearance	Increased digoxin plasma concentration; increased risk of digoxin toxicity	Monitor for signs and symptoms of digoxin toxicity, check digoxin concentration, and reduce dosage of digoxin accordingly
	Antibiotics (erythromycin, tetracycline)	Decreased digoxin bioinactivation by bacteria flora	Increased digoxin plasma concentration; increased risk of digoxin toxicity	Monitor digoxin serum concentrations when antibiotic is added to or withdrawn from therapy
	β-blockers	Additive cardiac effects	Potentiation of bradycardia and AV block	Monitor patient for bradycardia and AV conduction delay on ECG and adjust dosages as needed
	Calcium, intravenous	Additive or synergistic cardiac effects	Arrhythmias and cardiovascular collapse	Administer intravenous calcium slowly over several hours; monitor patients closely; coadministration of oral calcium acetate and digoxin is not recommended because of the risk of hypercalcemia and subsequent arrhythmias

Calcium antagonists (diltiazem, verapamil)	Decreased renal or extrarenal clearance of digoxin	Increased serum digoxin concentration and toxicity	Monitor patients for signs and symptoms of digoxin toxicity, check digoxin levels and adjust dosage as needed
Cholestyramine, colestipol	Cholestyramine and colestipol bind to digoxin, reducing its absorption	Decreased digoxin concentration and possible effectiveness	Administer digoxin 2 h before or 4–6 h after cholestyramine or colestipol; monitor digoxin serum concentration and observe patient for changes in response to digoxin
Disopyramide, flecainide	Unknown	Increased plasma digoxin concentrations and increased risk of digoxin toxicity	Monitor for signs and symptoms of digoxin toxicity, check digoxin level, and decrease dose of digoxin as needed
Diuretics (loop diuretics, thiazide diuretics and other potassium or magnesium wasting drugs)	Potassium and magnesium loss	Increased risk of digoxin toxicity	Monitor electrolytes and provide replacements as needed; educate patient regarding the importance of maintaining adequate dietary potassium intake; alternatively, use potassium-sparing diuretics
Itraconazole	Decreased digoxin metabolism and clearance	Increased plasma digoxin concentrations and increased risk of digoxin toxicity	Monitor for signs and symptoms of digoxin toxicity, check digoxin level, and decrease dose of digoxin as needed
Neomycin	Decreased digoxin absorption	Decreased digoxin serum concentration	Monitor digoxin serum concentrations

(continued on next page)

Table 3
(*continued*)

Primary Drugs	Interacting Drugs	Proposed Mechanism of Interaction	Possible Effects	Clinical Management
	Propafenone	Decreased digoxin volume of distribution and decreased nonrenal clearance of digoxin	Increased digoxin plasma concentration; increased risk of digoxin toxicity	Monitor for signs and symptoms of digoxin toxicity, check digoxin concentration, and reduce dosage of digoxin accordingly
	Quinidine	Decreased renal and nonrenal clearance of digoxin	Increased plasma digoxin concentrations and increased risk of digoxin toxicity	Monitor for signs and symptoms of digoxin toxicity, check digoxin level, and decrease dose of digoxin as needed
	Rifampin	Increased digoxin hepatic metabolism	Decrease plasma digoxin concentration and possibly effectiveness	Monitor digoxin concentration and adjust dose accordingly
	Sotalol	Additive cardiac effects, possibly increased digoxin bioavailability	Increased bradycardic effects	Monitor electrocardiogram and serum digoxin concentrations; adjust dose accordingly
	Spironolactone	Inhibition of active tubular secretion of digoxin	Increased plasma digoxin concentrations and increased risk of digoxin toxicity	Monitor for signs and symptoms of digoxin toxicity; false increase of digoxin concentrations may occur with some testing methods

Abbreviations: INR, international normalized ratio; N-DEA, *N*-desethylamiodarone; NSAIDs, nonsteroidal antiinflammatory drugs; SSRI, selective serotonin reuptake inhibitor.

[a] All class III antiarrhythmic agents may interact with other drugs that prolongs QT intervals (ie, class I or class III antiarrhythmics, antibacterials, antidepressants, antifungals, antipsychotics) to cause additive effects on QT prolongation. Some of these interactions are not listed in this table.

Data from Cheng-Lai A, Nawarskas JJ, Frishman WH. Cardiovascular drug-drug interactions. In: Frishman WH, Sica DA, editors. Cardiovascular pharmacotherapeutics. 3rd edition. Minneapolis (MN): Cardiotext; 2011. p. 511–3.

SUMMARY

Although elderly patients older than 65 years make up only 14% of the population in the United States, they receive more than 30% of prescribed medications.[6] The anti-arrhythmic drugs are as effective in elderly patients as they are in younger patients, but elderly patients may have more adverse effects from the drugs because of age-related changes in drug pharmacokinetics, concomitant disease, and drug-drug interactions.[6] In using antiarrhythmic drugs in elderly patients, it is important to acquire a full history of medication use from the patient, including the use of herbal and other alternative treatments (eg, nutriceuticals such as magnesium). The physician should be aware of the physiologic mechanisms of action of the antiarrhythmic drugs, patients and their caregivers should be aware of proper drug use, and the treatment plan should be reviewed regularly with patients, especially with regard to changes of drug dose and the abrupt discontinuation of drug treatment.

REFERENCES

1. Schwartz JB, Zipes DP. Cardiovascular disease in the elderly. In: Bonow RO, Mann DL, Zipes DP, Libby P, editors. Braunwald's heart disease–a textbook of cardiovascular medicine. 9th edition. Philadelphia: Saunders; 2011. p. 1727–56.
2. Fleg JL, Lakatta EG. Normal aging of the cardiovascular system. In: Aronow WS, Fleg JL, Rich MW, editors. Cardiovascular disease in the elderly. 4th edition. New York: Informa; 2008. p. 1–43.
3. Aronow WS, Sorbera C. Supraventricular tachyarrhythmias in the elderly. In: Aronow WS, Fleg JL, Rich MW, editors. Cardiovascular disease in the elderly. 4th edition. New York: Informa; 2008. p. 577–603.
4. Frishman MD. Alpha- and beta-adrenergic blocking drugs. In: Frishman WH, Sica DA, editors. Cardiovascular pharmacotherapeutics. 3rd edition. Minneapolis (MN): Cardiotext; 2011. p. 57–85.
5. Aronow WS, Sorbera C. Ventricular arrhythmias in the elderly. In: Aronow WS, Fleg JL, Rich MW, editors. Cardiovascular disease in the elderly. 4th edition. New York: Informa; 2008. p. 605–25.
6. Frishman WH, Aronow WS, Cheng-Lai A. Cardiovascular drug therapy in the elderly. In: Aronow WS, Fleg JL, Rich MW, editors. Cardiovascular disease in the elderly. 4th edition. New York: Informa; 2008. p. 99–135.
7. Novak LP. Aging, total body potassium, fat-free mass and cell mass in males and females between the ages of 18 and 85 years. J Gerontol 1972;27:438–43.
8. Vestal RE, Norris AH, Tobin JD, et al. Antipyrine metabolism in man: influence of age, alcohol, caffeine, and smoking. Clin Pharmacol Ther 1975;18:425–32.
9. Cusack B, Kelly J, O'Malley K, et al. Digoxin in the elderly: pharmacokinetic consequences of old age. Clin Pharm 1979;2:722–6.
10. Abernethy DR, Kerzner L. Age effects on alpha-1 acid glycoprotein concentration and imipramine plasma protein binding. J Am Geriatr Soc 1984;32:705–8.
11. Holt DW, Hayler AM, Healey GF. Effect of age and plasma concentrations of albumin and alpha-1 acid glycoprotein on protein binding of disopyramide. Br J Clin Pharmacol 1983;16:344–5.
12. Schmucker DL. Aging and drug disposition: an update. Pharmacol Rev 1985;37: 133–48.
13. Hayes MJ, Langman MJ, Short AH. Changes in drug metabolism with increasing age. II. Phenytoin clearance and protein binding. Br J Clin Pharmacol 1975;2: 73–9.

14. Cheng-Lai A, Frishman WH. Appendices. In: Frishman WH, Sica DA, editors. Cardiovascular pharmacotherapeutics. 3rd edition. Minneapolis (MN): Cardiotext; 2011. p. 633–51.

15. Wynne HA, Cope LH, Mutch E, et al. The effect of age upon liver volume and apparent liver blood flow in healthy man. Hepatology 1989;9:297–301.

16. Rowe JW, Andres R, Tobin JD, et al. The effect of age on creatinine clearance in man: a cross-sectional and longitudinal study. J Gerontol 1976;31:155–63.

17. Bender AD. The effect of increasing age on the distribution of peripheral blood flow in man. J Am Geriatr Soc 1965;13:192–8.

18. Cockcroft DW, Gault MH. Prediction of creatinine clearance from serum creatinine. Nephron 1976;16:31–41.

19. Levey AS, Coresh J, Balk E, et al. National Kidney Foundation practice guidelines for chronic kidney disease: evaluation, classification, and stratification. Ann Intern Med 2003;39:137–47.

20. Zimetbaum P, Kowey PR, Michelson EL. Antiarrhythmic drugs. In: Frishman WH, Sica DA, editors. Cardiovascular pharmacotherapeutics. 3rd edition. Minneapolis (MN): Cardiotext; 2011. p. 227–56.

21. Teo KK, Yusuf S, Furberg CD. Effects of prophylactic antiarrhythmic drug therapy in acute myocardial infarction: an overview of results from randomized controlled trials. JAMA 1993;270:1589–95.

22. Danahy DT, Aronow WS. Propranolol and lidocaine: clinical use as antiarrhythmic agents. Postgrad Med 1977;61:113–7.

23. Fenster PE, Bressler R. Treating cardiovascular diseases in the elderly. Part 2: antiarrhythmics, diuretics and calcium channel blockers. Drug Ther 1984;14(3):209–16.

24. Ochs HR, Carstens G, Greenblatt DJ. Reduction of lidocaine clearance during continuous infusion and by coadministration of propranolol. N Engl J Med 1980;303:373–7.

25. Frishman WH, Furberg CD, Friedewald WT. β-Adrenergic blockade in survivors of acute myocardial infarction. N Engl J Med 1984;310:830–7.

26. Lichstein E, Morganroth J, Harrist R, et al, The BHAT Study Group. Effect of propranolol on ventricular arrhythmias: the beta blocker heart attack trial experience. Circulation 1983;67(Suppl I):I5–10.

27. Hansteen V. Beta blockade after myocardial infarction: the Norwegian propranolol study in high-risk patients. Circulation 1983;67(Suppl I):I57–60.

28. Aronow WS, Ahn C, Mercando AD, et al. Effect of propranolol versus no antiarrhythmic drug on sudden cardiac death, total cardiac death, and total death in patients ≥62 years of age with heart disease, complex ventricular arrhythmias, and left ventricular ejection fraction ≥40%. Am J Cardiol 1994;74:267–70.

29. Aronow WS, Ahn C, Mercando AD, et al. Decrease of mortality by propranolol in patients with heart disease and complex ventricular arrhythmias is more an antiischemic than an antiarrhythmic effect. Am J Cardiol 1994;74:613–5.

30. Norris RM, Barnaby PF, Brown MA, et al. Prevention of ventricular fibrillation during acute myocardial infarction by intravenous propranolol. Lancet 1984;2:883–6.

31. Stone PH, Gibson RS, Glasser SP, et al. Comparison of propranolol, diltiazem and nifedipine in the treatment of ambulatory ischemia in patients with stable angina: differential effects on ambulatory ischemia, exercise performance, and anginal symptoms. Circulation 1990;82:1962–72.

32. Hawkins CM, Richardson DW, Vokonas PS, The BHAT Research Group. Effect of propranolol in reducing mortality in older myocardial infarction patients: the beta blocker heart attack trial experience. Circulation 1983;67(Suppl I):I94–7.

33. Hallstrom AP, Cobb LA, Yu BH, et al. An antiarrhythmic drug experience in 941 patients resuscitated from an initial cardiac arrest between 1970 and 1985. Am J Cardiol 1991;68:1025–31.
34. Aronow WS, Ahn C, Mercando AD, et al. Circadian variation of sudden cardiac death or fatal myocardial infarction is abolished by propranolol in patients with heart disease and complex ventricular arrhythmias. Am J Cardiol 1994;74: 819–21.
35. Kennedy HL, Brooks MM, Barker AH, et al. Beta-blocker therapy in the Cardiac Arrhythmia Suppression Trial. Am J Cardiol 1994;74:674–80.
36. Aronow WS. Management of the older person with atrial fibrillation. J Gerontol A Biol Sci Med Sci 2002;57:M352–63.
37. Lang R, Klein HO, Weiss E, et al. Superiority of oral verapamil therapy to digoxin in treatment of chronic atrial fibrillation. Chest 1983;83:491–9.
38. Roth A, Harrison E, Mitani G, et al. Efficacy and safety of medium and high-dose diltiazem alone and in combination with digoxin for control of heart rate at rest and during exercise in patients with chronic atrial fibrillation. Circulation 1986; 73:316–24.
39. David D, DiSegni E, Klein HO, et al. Inefficacy of digitalis in the control of heart rate in patients with chronic atrial fibrillation: beneficial effect of an added beta-adrenergic blocking agent. Am J Cardiol 1979;44:1378–82.
40. Nicklas JM, McKenna WJ, Stewart RA, et al. Prospective, double-blind, placebo-controlled trial of low dose amiodarone in patients with severe heart failure and asymptomatic frequent ventricular ectopy. Am Heart J 1991;122:1016–21.
41. Hockings B, George T, Mahrous F, et al. Effectiveness of amiodarone on ventricular arrhythmias during and after acute myocardial infarction. Am J Cardiol 1987; 60:967–70.
42. Pfisterer M, Kiowski W, Burckhardt D, et al. Beneficial effect of amiodarone on cardiac mortality in patients with asymptomatic complex ventricular arrhythmias after acute myocardial infarction and preserved but not impaired left ventricular function. Am J Cardiol 1992;69:1399–402.
43. Julian DG, Camm AJ, Frangin G, et al. Randomized trial of effect of amiodarone on mortality in patients with left-ventricular dysfunction after recent myocardial infarction: EMIAT. Lancet 1997;349:667–74.
44. Cairns JA, Connolly SJ, Roberts R, et al. Randomised trial of outcome after myocardial infarction in patients with frequent or repetitive ventricular premature depolarisations: CAMIAT. Lancet 1997;349:675–82.
45. Doval HC, Nul DR, Grancelli HO, et al. Randomised trial of low dose amiodarone in severe congestive heart failure. Lancet 1994;344:493–8.
46. Singh SN, Fletcher RD, Fisher SG, et al. Amiodarone in patients with congestive heart failure and asymptomatic ventricular arrhythmias. N Engl J Med 1995;333: 77–82.
47. Bardy GH, Lee KL, Mark DB, et al. Amiodarone or an implantable cardioverter-defibrillator for congestive heart failure. N Engl J Med 2005;352:225–37.
48. Herre J, Sauve M, Malone P, et al. Long-term results of amiodarone therapy in patients with recurrent sustained ventricular tachycardia or ventricular fibrillation. J Am Coll Cardiol 1989;13:442–9.
49. Greene HL, for the CASCADE Investigators. The CASCADE study: randomized anti-arrhythmic drug therapy in survivors of cardiac arrest in Seattle. Am J Cardiol 1993;72:70F–4F.
50. Gold RL, Haffajee CI, Charos G, et al. Amiodarone for refractory atrial fibrillation. Am J Cardiol 1986;57:124–7.

51. Cavusoglu E, Frishman WH. Sotalol: a new beta-adrenergic blocker for ventricular arrhythmias. Prog Cardiovasc Dis 1995;37:423–40.

52. Pedersen HS, Elming H, Seibaek M, et al. Risk factors and predictors of torsade de pointes ventricular tachycardia in patients with left ventricular systolic dysfunction receiving dofetilide. Am J Cardiol 2007;100:876–80.

53. Køber L, Bloch Thomsen PE, Møller M, et al. Effect of dofetilide in patients with recent myocardial infarction and left ventricular dysfunction: a randomised trial. Lancet 2000;356:2052–8.

54. Schmiegelow MD, Pedersen OK, Køber L, et al. Incidence of atrial fibrillation in patients with either heart failure or acute myocardial infarction and left ventricular dysfunction: a cohort study. BMC Cardiovasc Disord 2001;11:19.

55. Naccarelli GV, Wolbrette DL, Khan M, et al. Old and new antiarrhythmic drugs for converting and maintaining sinus rhythm in atrial fibrillation: comparative efficacy and results of trials. Am J Cardiol 2003;91(6A):15D–26D.

56. Chatterjee S, Ghosh J, Lichstein E, et al. Meta-analysis of cardiovascular outcomes with dronedarone in patients with atrial fibrillation or heart failure. Am J Cardiol 2012;110(4):607–13.

57. Connolly SJ, Camm AJ, Halperin JL, et al, for the PALLAS Investigators. Dronedarone in high-risk permanent atrial fibrillation. N Engl J Med 2011;365:2268–76.

58. Nattel S. Dronedarone in atrial fibrillation - Jekyll and Hyde? (editorial). N Engl J Med 2011;365:2321–2.

59. Tian D, Frishman WH. Vernakalant. A new drug to treat patients with acute onset atrial fibrillation. Cardiol Rev 2011;19:41–4.

60. Fuccelletti F, Iacomini P, Botta G, et al. Efficacy and safety of vernakalant in recent-onset atrial fibrillation after the European Medicines Agency approval: systematic review and meta-analysis. J Clin Pharmacol 2011. [Epub ahead of print].

61. Frishman WH, Sica DA. Calcium channel blockers. In: Frishman WH, Sica DA, editors. Cardiovascular pharmacotherapeutics. 3rd edition. Minneapolis (MN): Cardiotext; 2011. p. 99–120.

62. Hunt SA, Abraham WT, Feldman AM, et al. ACC/AHA 2005 Guideline Update for the Diagnosis and Management of Chronic Heart Failure in the Adult: a report of the American College of Cardiology/American Heart Association Task Force on Practice Guidelines (Writing Committee to Update the 2001 Guidelines for the Evaluation and Management of Heart Failure). Developed in collaboration with the American College of Chest Physicians and the International Society for Heart and Lung Transplantation. Endorsed by the Heart Rhythm Society. Circulation 2005;112:1825–52.

63. LeJemtel TH, Klapholz M, Frishman WH. Inotropic agents. In: Frishman WH, Sica DA, editors. Cardiovascular pharmacotherapeutics. 3rd edition. Minneapolis (MN): Cardiotext; 2011. p. 189–203.

64. Aronow WS, Ahn C, Kronzon I. Comparison of incidences of congestive heart failure in older African-Americans, Hispanics, and whites. Am J Cardiol 1999;84:611–2.

65. Gottdiener JS, McClelland RL, Marshall R, et al. Outcome of congestive heart failure in elderly persons: influence of left ventricular systolic function. The Cardiovascular Health Study. Ann Intern Med 2002;137:631–9.

66. Aronow WS. Echocardiography should be performed in all elderly patients with congestive heart failure. J Am Geriatr Soc 1994;42:1300–2.

67. Fleg JL, Gottlieb SH, Lakatta EG. Is digoxin really important in treatment of compensated heart failure? A placebo-controlled crossover study in patients with sinus rhythm. Am J Med 1982;73:244–50.

68. Aronow WS, Starling L, Etienne F. Lack of efficacy of digoxin in treatment of compensated congestive heart failure with third heart sound and sinus rhythm in elderly patients receiving diuretic therapy. Am J Cardiol 1986;58:168–9.
69. Murgatroyd FD, Xie B, Gibson SM, et al. The effects of digoxin in patients with paroxysmal atrial fibrillation: analysis of Holter data from the CRAFT-I trial [abstract]. J Am Coll Cardiol 1993;21:203A.
70. Galun E, Flugelman MY, Glickson M, et al. Failure of long-term digitalization to prevent rapid ventricular response in patients with paroxysmal atrial fibrillation. Chest 1991;99:1038–40.
71. Aronow WS. Digoxin or angiotensin converting enzyme inhibitors for congestive heart failure in geriatric patients: which is the preferred treatment? Drugs Aging 1991;1:98–103.
72. Butler VP Jr, Odel JG, Rath E, et al. Digitalis-induced visual disturbances with therapeutic serum digitalis concentrations. Ann Intern Med 1995;123:676–80.
73. Meyer BR, Frishman WH. Cholinergic and anticholinergic drugs. In: Frishman WH, Sica DA, editors. Cardiovascular pharmacotherapeutics. 3rd edition. Minneapolis (MN): Cardiotext; 2011. p. 93–7.
74. Cheng-Lai A, Nawarskas JJ, Frishman WH. Cardiovascular drug-drug interactions. In: Frishman WH, Sica DA, editors. Cardiovascular pharmacotherapeutics. 3rd edition. Minneapolis (MN): Cardiotext; 2011. p. 493–518.

Atrial Fibrillation
Stroke Prevention in Older Adults

Gene R. Quinn, MD, MS[a], Margaret C. Fang, MD, MPH[b],*

KEYWORDS

- Atrial fibrillation • Stroke prevention • Anticoagulants • Bleeding risk

KEY POINTS

- Antithrombotic treatment of atrial fibrillation (AF), including paroxysmal AF, should be guided by stroke risk stratification tools.
- Bleeding risk stratification tools may help clinicians counsel patients about bleeding risk on anticoagulants and are most appropriate when applied to patients at low or intermediate stroke risk in which the net benefit of anticoagulation is less clear.
- Newer fixed-dose oral anticoagulants have emerged as viable alternatives to warfarin and choice of anticoagulant should depend on comorbidities (eg, renal function), side-effect profile, cost, and patient preference.
- Stroke prevention in atrial flutter should be managed using the same recommendations as those for AF.

INTRODUCTION

The prevalence of atrial fibrillation (AF), the most common clinically significant cardiac arrhythmia, is increasing as the population of the United States ages.[1–3] AF disproportionately affects the elderly and confers a significant stroke risk.[1] With appropriate preventive strategies, the negative consequences of AF can be dramatically reduced; yet there is widespread underuse of proven antithrombotic therapies, particularly among older patients.[4] This article reviews stroke prevention in AF, including risk stratification for stroke and advances in newer oral anticoagulants, with a focus on treatment of the elderly.

Note that the available literature suggests that stroke risk related to paroxysmal AF is similar to the risk with chronic AF, as well as atrial flutter.[5] Thus, the recommendations in this article addressing chronic AF should be applied to paroxysmal AF and atrial flutter except as specifically noted.

Disclosures: None.
[a] Department of Medicine, University of California San Francisco, Box 0320, San Francisco, CA 94143, USA; [b] Division of Hospital Medicine, University of California San Francisco, 533 Parnassus Avenue, Box 0131, San Francisco, CA 94143, USA
* Corresponding author.
E-mail address: mfang@medicine.ucsf.edu

Clin Geriatr Med 28 (2012) 617–634
http://dx.doi.org/10.1016/j.cger.2012.08.003   geriatric.theclinics.com
0749-0690/12/$ – see front matter © 2012 Elsevier Inc. All rights reserved.

Epidemiology of AF

AF disproportionately affects older adults. The overall prevalence of AF in the United States is about 1%, but it is considerably higher in older populations. When stratified by age, the prevalence in adults older than age 65 is approximately 5%, and in those older than age 85 it nears 10% (**Fig. 1**). It is estimated that there will be approximately 5.6 million people with AF in the United States by the year 2050 and recent reports have suggested even higher growth projections.[2,6] Most of this disease burden will likely be borne by the elderly.

Common risk factors for chronic AF include advancing age, hypertension, underlying heart disease, and hyperthyroidism.[7,8] There may also be contributory genetic and lifestyle factors.

The negative health consequences of AF stem largely from the risk of AF-related ischemic stroke. An estimated 15% of ischemic strokes in the United States are related to AF and a substantial proportion of patients with cryptogenic strokes (eg, without a history of clinical AF) are later found to have atrial tachyarrhythmias on cardiac monitoring.[9,10] AF-related strokes also tend to be more severe than other ischemic stroke types, leading to longer hospital stays, higher rates of disability, and increased mortality in comparison with patients without AF.[11–14] The public health impact of AF is thus considerable.

Nonvalvular AF confers an increased stroke risk of at least two, and perhaps up to seven, times that of patients without the disease.[1,15] Rheumatic AF confers an even greater stroke risk—approximately 17 times as high as that found in patients without the disease, and five times higher than in patients with nonvalvular AF.[1,15] The stroke risk attributable to AF varies by age. In the Framingham cohort study, subjects ages 50 to 59 had 1.5% of their stroke risk attributable to AF, whereas subjects ages 80 to 89 had 23.5% of their stroke risk attributable to AF. Overall mortality was doubled in subjects with AF as opposed to those in normal sinus rhythm.[1]

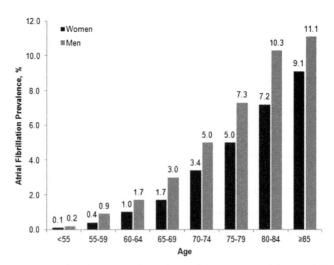

Fig. 1. The prevalence of AF by age and sex. (*Data from* Go AS, Hylek EM, Phillips KA, et al. Prevalence of diagnosed atrial fibrillation in adults: national implications for rhythm management and stroke prevention: the AnTicoagulation and Risk Factors in Atrial Fibrillation (ATRIA) Study. JAMA 2001;285(18):2370–5.)

STROKE PREVENTION IN AF

Chronic management of AF includes arrhythmia management and prevention of stroke. Stroke risk seems to be the same regardless of whether a rate control or a rhythm control strategy is adopted.[16] The cornerstone of stroke prevention in AF is the use of anticoagulants; however, patients do not derive the same degree of benefit equally. Estimating a given individual's risk of stroke is the first step in determining the appropriateness of antithrombotic therapy, as is weighing the comparative efficacy and safety of available antithrombotic options.[17] Stroke risk prevention strategies for chronic AF should be applied similarly to patients with paroxysmal AF, who seem to have a similar risk of thromboembolism.[18]

Although the benefits of anticoagulant treatment have been well established in the prevention of AF-related stroke, there are significantly less data for antithrombotic therapy in atrial flutter. There is an increased risk of ischemic stroke in patients with atrial flutter compared with patients with normal sinus rhythm.[19] Atrial flutter and AF often coexist, making the differentiation of the risk contribution from each disorder difficult. The 2006 American College of Cardiology, American Heart Association, and the European Society of Cardiology (ACC/AHA/ESC) guidelines make a class I recommendation for antithrombotic therapy in atrial flutter to mirror that in AF, but this is based on a low level of evidence.[5]

Risk Stratification for Stroke

The benefits of antithrombotic therapy in terms of stroke risk reduction need to be balanced by consideration of bleeding risk, difficulty of monitoring, and cost. Certain patients may be at such low stroke risk that the absolute benefits are too small to justify the use of an anticoagulant. To aid in deciding between recommending an anticoagulant, antiplatelet, or no antithrombotic therapy, risk stratification schemes have been developed to estimate the risk of stroke without anticoagulants.[7,20,21]

Out of the various available risk stratification schemes, the $CHADS_2$ score has been the most widely used and validated, although all risk schemes have only modest predictive ability. $CHADS_2$ is an acronym for five clinical factors: congestive heart failure, hypertension, age greater than or equal to 75 years, diabetes mellitus, and prior stroke (ischemic) or transient ischemic attack (TIA). The presence of each factor counts as one point, except for stroke or TIA, which count as two. Patients with a $CHADS_2$ score of 0 are considered low risk, those with a score of 1 are considered intermediate risk, and those with scores of greater than or equal to 2 are considered high risk (**Fig. 2**). These scores can also be translated into events per 100 person years and a number needed to treat (NNT) to prevent a thromboembolic event in 100 person years. The NNT to prevent stroke declines dramatically as the $CHADS_2$ score increases: to prevent 1 stroke, 417 people with a $CHADS_2$ score of 0 need to be treated with warfarin, compared to 125 people with a score of 1, and <50 people if the $CHADS_2$ score is 3 or higher. Patients with $CHADS_2$ score of 0 derive little absolute benefit from anticoagulation; patients with scores of 2 or higher have a baseline stroke risk that warrants anticoagulation if it can be tolerated.[22]

A more recently developed risk scheme, the CHA_2DS_2-VASc score, incorporated additional stroke risk factors (female sex, additional age strata, and vascular disease) in an attempt to improve on the performance of $CHADS_2$.[23] In general, $CHADS_2$ and CHA_2DS_2-VASc seem to perform similarly. By considering all women and patients ages 65 to 74 as being at intermediate stroke risk and, therefore, candidates for anticoagulation, CHA_2DS_2-VASc leads to a much larger percentage of patients being considered for anticoagulant therapy.[23,24] CHA_2DS_2-VASc was adopted by the ESC

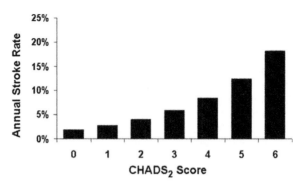

Fig. 2. Annual stroke rate by CHADS$_2$ score in a Medicare population. (*Data from* Gage BF, Waterman AD, Shannon W, et al. Validation of clinical classification schemes for predicting stroke: results from the National Registry of Atrial Fibrillation. JAMA 2001;285(22):2864–70.)

in its latest consensus statement, whereas the ninth edition of the American College of Chest Physicians (ACCP-9) Antithrombotic Guidelines is largely based on CHADS$_2$.[17,25] In general CHA$_2$DS$_2$-VASc seems most useful in providing additional risk stratification in patients with a low CHADS$_2$ risk (eg, a score of 0 or 1) to identify patients at an even lower risk for stroke (ie, CHA$_2$DS$_2$-VASc score = 0).[17]

Pharmacologic Treatments

Several anticoagulant and antiplatelet agents are currently available for use in preventing AF-related thromboembolism (**Table 1**). For decades, vitamin K antagonists were the only available oral anticoagulants. In recent years, the advent of orally available direct thrombin inhibitors and factor Xa inhibitors has expanded the therapeutic options for AF. The selection of therapy depends on the relative advantages and disadvantages of the medications for an individual patient (**Table 2**).

Vitamin K antagonists

Vitamin K antagonists, such as warfarin, have long been the mainstay of anticoagulant treatment of AF. They reduce stroke risk by approximately 68% and overall mortality by approximately 33%.[18,26–28] In addition, strokes that occur in patients treated at therapeutic levels of warfarin are less severe than among patients without anticoagulant treatment.[29]

The recommended target international normalized ratio (INR) range for AF is 2.0 to 3.0, which maximizes stroke prevention while minimizing bleeding risk (**Fig. 3**). This target INR range also seems to be the appropriate range for older patients and those with a prior history of stroke.[30]

Warfarin has several notable disadvantages. Drug-drug interactions are of particular concern, including commonly used antibiotics, amiodarone, and statins. Dietary intake of vitamin K can also alter warfarin's function and patients must be counseled to maintain a consistent diet. There are genetic variations in warfarin metabolism and activity that contribute to interindividual differences in dosing.[31]

Because of these factors, chronic warfarin therapy is associated with a considerable burden related to monitoring and dose adjustment. To accommodate the frequent monitoring needs, specialized anticoagulation clinics have been developed that are at least as effective at warfarin management as individual physician practices are, and may have lower rates of anticoagulation-related side effects and improved anticoagulation control.[32–34] Patients can also be taught to self-monitor and dose-adjust at

Table 1
Antithrombotic therapy options for AF

Agent	Dosing	Advantages	Disadvantages
Aspirin	81 mg or 325 mg Once daily	Ease of use Less bleeding complications compared with warfarin	Minimal efficacy in stroke prevention
Aspirin plus Clopidogrel	81 mg aspirin plus 75 mg clopidogrel daily	More effective than aspirin alone in stroke reduction	Less effective than warfarin in stroke prevention
Warfarin	Once daily Target INR 2.0–3.0	High efficacy in stroke risk reduction Reversible Can monitor anticoagulation levels	Requires frequent monitoring and dose adjustment Numerous drug-drug interactions Affected by dietary vitamin K
Dabigatran	150 mg twice daily for CrCl >30 mL/min 75 mg twice daily for CrCl 15–30 mL/min	No need for routine monitoring Fixed oral dosing	No way to monitor anticoagulant effect Not reversible Possible increase in myocardial infarction No long-term safety data Use with caution in patients with renal impairment
Rivaroxaban	20 mg once daily CrCl >50 mL/min 15 mg once daily CrCl 15–50 mL/min	No need for routine monitoring Fixed oral dosing (once daily)	No way to monitor anticoagulant effect Not reversible No long-term safety data Use with caution in patients with renal or hepatic impairment
Apixaban	5 mg twice daily	No need for routine monitoring Fixed oral dosing May have mortality benefit compared with warfarin	No way to monitor anticoagulant effect Not reversible Not yet FDA approved

home, a strategy that seems to be as effective as clinic-based monitoring in selected patients, and may result in slightly lower complication rates.[35,36]

Direct thrombin inhibitors
Dabigatran is the only oral direct thrombin inhibitor available since ximelagatran was withdrawn from the market due to excess hepatotoxicity.[37,38] It represents the first

Table 2
ACCP-9 guidelines on antithrombotic therapy for AF

	Recommendation	Comments
$CHADS_2 = 0$[a]	No antithrombotic therapy Or, if antithrombotic therapy is used, aspirin 75–325 mg daily	Aspirin provides low net clinical benefit in patients with low stroke risk
$CHADS_2 = 1$[a]	Anticoagulant therapy (preferred) Or antiplatelet therapy	Consider patient-specific bleeding risk Presence of additional stroke risk factors (female gender, age 65–74, or vascular disease) may help influence decision between anticoagulant and antiplatelet therapy
$CHADS_2 \geq 2$[a]	Anticoagulant therapy preferred	Dabigatran 150 mg twice daily preferred over vitamin K antagonist therapy if no contraindication to dabigatran

Additional Recommendations
- Patients with an indication for oral anticoagulant therapy, but who are deemed inappropriate for reasons other than bleeding risk, are recommended for combination therapy with aspirin and clopidogrel
- In those patients with an indication for oral anticoagulant therapy, but who are deemed inappropriate because of bleeding risk, are recommended aspirin
- Treat paroxysmal AF according to the same guidelines as permanent or persistent AF

Anticoagulation for Cardioversion of AF
- In patients with AF for >48 h or of unknown duration, $\geq$3 wk of therapeutic anticoagulation is recommended before cardioversion; alternatively, transesophageal echocardiography (TEE) to exclude thrombus may be performed, with maintenance of full anticoagulation from the time of TEE to cardioversion
- In patients with documented AF $\leq$48 h, initiate anticoagulation and proceed to electrical or pharmacologic cardioversion
- In patients undergoing urgent cardioversion, start parental anticoagulation before cardioversion if possible, but do not delay emergency intervention
- Therapeutic anticoagulation for at least 4 wk after cardioversion with decisions about long-term anticoagulation based on stroke risk stratification

[a] $CHADS_2$ stroke risk score: 1 point for congestive heart failure, hypertension, age $\geq$75, diabetes mellitus; 2 points for stroke or transient ischemic attack.
From You JJ, Singer DE, Howard PA, et al. Antithrombotic therapy for atrial fibrillation: Antithrombotic Therapy and Prevention of Thrombosis, 9th ed: American College of Chest Physicians Evidence-Based Clinical Practice Guidelines. Chest 2012;141(Suppl 2):e531S–75S; with permission.

oral anticoagulant in the United States since warfarin. Advantages over warfarin are fixed, twice daily dosing without the need for coagulation monitoring (**Table 1**).

The efficacy of dabigatran for stroke prevention was established by the Randomized Evaluation of Long-Term Anticoagulation Therapy (RE-LY) trial. Subjects were randomized to dabigatran at one of two doses (150 mg or 110 mg twice daily) or warfarin therapy. Dabigatran at the lower dose of 110 mg was noninferior to warfarin in preventing stroke with a significantly lower rate of major bleeding. The higher dose of dabigatran at 150 mg had a similar rate of major bleeding to warfarin, less intracranial hemorrhage risk, and a lower rate of ischemic stroke.[39]

Dabigatran is currently approved in the United States for use in AF at two doses: 150 mg twice a day and a reduced dose of 75 mg twice a day for patients with renal disease. Advantages of dabigatran are that it reaches efficacy within 2 to 3 hours after

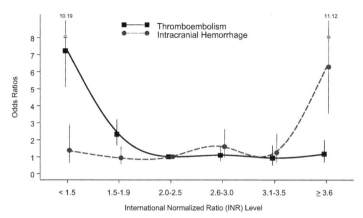

Fig. 3. The risk of thromboembolism and intracranial hemorrhage at different levels of international normalized ratio (INR). (*Data from* Singer DE, Chang Y, Fang MC, et al. Should patient characteristics influence target anticoagulation intensity for stroke prevention in nonvalvular atrial fibrillation?: the ATRIA study. Circ Cardiovasc Qual Outcomes 2009;2(4):297–304.)

an oral dose, does not need to be adjusted or monitored, and may have improved stroke protection in comparison with warfarin coupled with less intracranial hemorrhage. Because it is renally cleared, dabigatran should be avoided in individuals with severe renal disease and used with caution in patients with mild-to-moderate renal disease. There is no widely available way to monitor anticoagulation levels or effectively reverse anticoagulation in patients who are bleeding. Dabigatran may affect the partial thromboplastin time (PTT) level in patients, but degree of PTT elevation does not correlate with anticoagulant activity.

Fewer long-term safety data are available for dabigatran than for warfarin. Severe bleeding events have been reported in dabigatran users, many of whom were elderly, and there is significant concern with use of dabigatran in patients greater than 75 years old.[40] Moreover, a recent meta-analysis showed a significant increase in myocardial infarction in patients treated with dabigatran.[41]

Despite these disadvantages, because of the similar efficacy in preventing ischemic stroke and lower rates of intracranial hemorrhage, the ACCP-9 guidelines suggests that dabigatran at 150 mg twice per day be used instead of adjusted dose vitamin K antagonists in patients who require anticoagulation and are similar to the patients included in the RE-LY trial.[17]

Despite its higher cost, cost-effectiveness analyses comparing dabigatran to warfarin highlight the potential advantages of decreased stroke risk and intracranial hemorrhage. Most studies indicate that dabigatran is likely to be cost-effective, especially in patients at high stroke risk and higher bleeding risk. The cost-effectiveness is reduced in patients with lower stroke risk and lower bleeding risk.[42,43]

Oral factor Xa agents

Oral factor Xa agents, such as rivaroxaban and apixaban, directly inhibit factor Xa, the enzyme that converts prothrombin into active thrombin, an anticoagulant activity that is also shared with low-molecular-weight heparins, such as enoxaparin. These agents also do not require coagulation monitoring or dose adjustment (see **Table 1**).

Rivaroxaban is approved in the United States for use in nonvalvular AF based on the results of the Rivaroxaban Once Daily Oral Direct Factor Xa Inhibition Compared with

Vitamin K Antagonism for Prevention of Stroke and Embolism Trial in AF (ROCKET AF) trial, which demonstrated noninferiority to warfarin in stroke prevention with a similar overall bleeding risk and lower risks of fatal and intracranial bleeding. Rivaroxaban is dosed once daily at 20 mg per day for patients with normal renal function, or 15 mg per day for those with creatinine clearances of 15–50 mL/min. It should be used with caution in patients with creatinine clearances lower than 30 mL/min, and it is contra-indicated if the creatinine clearance is less than 15 mL/min. It is also unsuitable for patients with significant hepatic dysfunction.[44]

There are little long-term safety data for rivaroxaban. Rivaroxaban may affect the prothrombin time/INR, but INR levels do not correlate with degree of anticoagulation. There is no demonstrated way to reverse its anticoagulant effect, although early inves-tigation suggests that prothrombin complex concentrates might be of use.[45]

Apixaban is another oral factor Xa inhibitor that has been investigated for use in AF. The Apixaban for Reduction in Stroke and Other Thromboembolic Events in Atrial Fibrillation (ARISTOTLE) trial found apixaban to be superior to warfarin in preventing stroke and systemic embolism, noninferior in preventing ischemic or unknown-type strokes, and to have a lower rate of major bleeding and hemorrhagic stroke. This trial also found an overall mortality benefit after a median 1.8 years of follow-up, with borderline statistical significance ($P = .047$).[46]

The second major trial for apixaban in AF was the Apixaban vs Acetylsalicylic Acid to Prevent Stroke in Atrial Fibrillation Patients Who Have Failed or Are Unsuitable for Vitamin K Antagonist Treatment (AVERROES) trial, which compared apixaban with aspirin in subjects at risk for stroke but deemed not to be candidates for vitamin K antagonists. Apixaban decreased the rates of stroke compared with use of aspirin without significantly increasing major bleeding or intracranial hemorrhage.[47]

In the ARISTOTLE and AVERROES trials, subjects with serum creatinine levels greater than 2.5 mg/dL were excluded. Most subjects were dosed at 5 mg twice daily. A decreased dose of 2.5 mg twice daily was given to subjects with two or more of the following three factors: age 80 years or older, weight 60kg or less, or a serum creat-inine level of 1.5 to 2.5 mg/dL.

Other factor Xa inhibitors are currently in development, including edoxaban and betrixaban, but efficacy data are not yet available.[48,49]

Antiplatelet agents

Though not as effective as warfarin, antiplatelet agents have some efficacy in stroke reduction. Aspirin confers an approximately 20% reduction in stroke risk, with a concomitant increase in bleeding risk, and an unclear net benefit when balancing the two.[28,50,51] In the ACCP-9 guidelines, this balance between a small stroke risk reduction and an increase in bleeding risk led to the recommendation that patients with a CHADS$_2$ score of 0 take no antithrombotic medication.[17]

The optimal dosage of aspirin is unclear. A dosage of either 81 mg or 325 mg may be appropriate, and with the lack of evidence indicating superior efficacy with higher aspirin doses, a lower dose may be preferred to minimize side-effects.

Aspirin in combination with full-dose warfarin is often used in patients with indica-tions for warfarin therapy who also have separate indications for aspirin treatment, such as coronary artery disease. Select patients with certain conditions, such as acute coronary syndromes or placement of an intracoronary stent, may require therapy with a combination of antiplatelet agents and warfarin. The ACCP-9 guidelines recommend that patients with AF requiring anticoagulation and concomitant stable coronary disease be treated with vitamin K antagonists alone without the addition of aspirin, reflecting the lack of evidence supporting the efficacy of combination therapy in that population. In patients who have undergone placement of a coronary stent, patients with a CHADS$_2$ score of 2 or greater should be treated with triple therapy (aspirin, clopidogrel, and adjusted dose vitamin K antagonist) for a period of 1 month after bare metal stent placement, or 3 to 6 months after drug-eluting stent placement. After that initial period, vitamin K antagonist therapy along with a single antiplatelet agent is recommended until 12 months after stent placement, at which time the recommendation is to return to vitamin K antagonist alone. In patients with a CHADS$_2$ score of 0 or 1, dual antiplatelet therapy (aspirin and clopidogrel) is sufficient for the first 12 months after stent placement, after which patients should be treated as if they had stable coronary artery disease. Finally, in patients experiencing acute coronary syndromes who do not undergo intracoronary stent placement, those with a CHADS$_2$ score of 1 or greater should receive a vitamin K antagonist plus a single antiplatelet agent for the first 12 months and those with a CHADS$_2$ score of 0 should receive dual antiplatelet therapy for the same duration. After 12 months, recommendations mirror patients with stable coronary artery disease.[17]

Dual antiplatelet therapy in AF with aspirin plus clopidogrel has been studied in the Atrial Fibrillation Clopidogrel Trial with Irbesartan for Prevention of Vascular Events (ACTIVE) studies.[52,53] In the ACTIVE W trial, warfarin was superior to the combination of aspirin plus clopidogrel for stroke prevention, the rates of myocardial infarction were lower with warfarin, and the rates of major bleeding were similar in the two groups. Thus, aspirin plus clopidogrel should not be used in place of anticoagulants in patients who can take anticoagulant therapy.[52]

The ACTIVE A trial was conducted with subjects deemed ineligible for warfarin therapy and dual antiplatelet therapy was superior to aspirin alone, though with an increased rate of major bleeding. The increased bleeding rate and the benefits in stroke prevention were almost equal so that the net clinical benefit was minimal.[53] Furthermore, subgroup analysis showed that the benefits of adding clopidogrel to aspirin were limited to those subjects who were less than 75 years of age.[53]

The role of dual antiplatelet therapy in AF is probably limited owing to the availability of the newer fixed-dose oral anticoagulants; aspirin plus clopidogrel may be used as an alternative for stroke prevention in patients who would normally require oral anticoagulants but are deemed inappropriate for reasons other than bleeding risk.

Stroke Prevention Around Cardioversion

Patients with AF or flutter who are experiencing symptomatic arrhythmia, hemodynamic compromise, or their first episode of arrhythmia are often treated with either direct current or pharmacologic cardioversion. The time of cardioversion from AF or flutter to sinus rhythm is associated with an increased risk of stroke, presumably due to embolization of left atrial thrombus that either is preexisting at the time of cardioversion, or develops shortly thereafter.[54]

Patients in AF for fewer than 48 hours with hemodynamic compromise should be cardioverted without delay. For patients who have been in AF or flutter for more than 48 hours, two strategies for stroke reduction before cardioversion are recommended (**Table 2**). The first strategy is empiric treatment with at least 3 weeks of therapeutic anticoagulation before cardioversion. Alternatively, patients may undergo transesophageal echocardiography before cardioversion to exclude left atrial thrombus. If no thrombus is detected, patients can be cardioverted immediately after therapeutic anticoagulation is applied. However, if left atrial thrombus is detected, patients must be treated with anticoagulation for at least 3 weeks before cardioversion is attempted.[5,17]

In patients with AF or flutter for longer than 48 hours before cardioversion, anticoagulation should continue for at least 4 weeks. If the patient has evidence for recurrent AF at follow-up, anticoagulation should be continued based on stroke risk stratification as in other patients with AF.[5,17]

Procedures to Restore Sinus Rhythm

Procedures aimed at stopping AF and restoring sinus rhythm do not obviate the need for anticoagulation. Until there is strong evidence demonstrating reduced stroke risk with restoration of sinus rhythm, antithrombotic treatment should be applied based on baseline stroke risk factors as in patients with chronic AF.

Radiofrequency catheter ablation

Percutaneous radiofrequency catheter ablation can serve to eliminate or reduce AF burden, usually by isolating the pulmonary veins where AF often originates.[55] These procedures are indicated for otherwise healthy patients with symptomatic arrhythmia that limits quality of life and has not responded to conventional rhythm control strategies. Catheter ablation has not been demonstrated to reduce stroke risk, possibly because most patients relapse into AF within 5 years.[56]

Cox maze procedure

The Cox maze surgical procedure serves to create pathways of myocardium that can channel atrial depolarization to decrease microreentrant circuits. It is performed by cardiothoracic surgeons at experienced referral centers and requires cardiopulmonary bypass. Success rates for ablation of AF are greater than 90% with modern techniques, and there is evidence that a successful Cox maze procedure reduces stroke risk.[57] However, because most patients had another indication for long-term anticoagulation, it is not clear that patients may stop anticoagulant therapy after the Cox maze procedure.

Left atrial appendage procedures

Most thrombi in the left atria that lead to embolism arise from the left atrial appendage (LAA). Procedures have been developed to isolate, remove, or occlude this anatomic area with the goal of decreasing rates of ischemic stroke in patients with AF.[5]

Surgical ligation or amputation of the LAA can be performed in patients undergoing cardiothoracic surgery for another indication. Many patients undergoing either mitral valve replacement or Cox maze procedure have ligation performed concurrently.[58] These procedures likely decrease the rates of embolic stroke; however, most patients are concurrently treated with anticoagulation and there is no evidence that anticoagulation can be discontinued in these patients.

Percutaneous approaches to LAA occlusion are undergoing ongoing research. Studies of one such device, the percutaneous left atrial appendage transcatheter occlusion (PLAATO) device (Appriva Medical Inc, Sunnyvale, CA), have been discontinued because of an increase in adverse events.[59] The WATCHMAN device (Atritech Inc, Plymouth, Minnesota) is still being investigated and has not received approval in the United States. Preliminary reports showed a low rate of stroke even off anticoagulants.[60] However, more evidence is needed before percutaneous LAA occlusion can be considered a viable alternative to anticoagulation.

SPECIAL CONSIDERATIONS IN THE ELDERLY

Older patients are disproportionately affected by AF.[1,2] Not only is AF more prevalent in the elderly, but stroke risk also increases with age.[7,61] Older patients are also at greater risk from bleeding complications from anticoagulants, and may have more difficulty with the frequent dose-adjustments and monitoring required by vitamin K antagonists.[62-64] These factors make antithrombotic decision making and management in older patients with AF particularly challenging.

Net Clinical Benefit of Anticoagulation in the Elderly

The Birmingham Atrial Fibrillation Treatment of the Aged (BAFTA) trial quantified the benefit of warfarin therapy in patients greater than age 75 (mean age 81.5), randomizing patients to either aspirin or adjusted-dose warfarin. Warfarin was considerably more effective than aspirin, with a relative risk of 0.46 for any stroke, and the risk of bleeding was not statistically different between aspirin and warfarin.[65] The BAFTA trial confirmed the efficacy and relative safety of warfarin in an elderly population.

Although bleeding complications of anticoagulant therapy are more common in the elderly, the overall net clinical benefit favors anticoagulation in most older patients.[66] Intracranial hemorrhage is the complication that rivals ischemic stroke in terms of morbidity and mortality, whereas extracranial bleeding events are usually much less consequential than stroke.[29,67] In fact, the net clinical benefit of warfarin becomes progressively greater as patients age and accumulate additional stroke risk factors (**Fig. 4**).[66] The benefits of anticoagulation in older patients are reflected in the CHA_2DS_2-VASc scoring system, which suggests anticoagulation for patients ages 65 to 74 and recommends anticoagulation for all patients older than 75.[23]

Estimating Bleeding Risk on Anticoagulants

Older patients have a higher risk of anticoagulant-associated hemorrhage.[64] Although all bleeding events are more common with older age, intracranial hemorrhage is the most feared complication. Among patients with warfarin-related hemorrhage, 90% of deaths and most disability are caused by intracranial hemorrhage.[67] Risk factors for the development of intracranial hemorrhage include hypertension, increasing age, and prior stroke, but these factors also elevate ischemic stroke risk.[17] Patients with prior lobar intracranial hemorrhage are at particular risk of rebleeding and, thus, should generally not be rechallenged with anticoagulants.[68] The newer oral anticoagulants were associated with lower intracranial hemorrhage risk than warfarin in clinical trials, which, if borne out in clinical practice, would constitute a significant advantage over warfarin.

Several clinical factors in addition to older age have been linked to anticoagulant-associated bleeding risk.[69-72] Based on these factors, several bleeding risk prediction models have been developed to help clinicians estimate the risk on anticoagulants. One commonly cited score is the Outpatient Bleeding Risk Index, which assigns one point to age greater than 65, history of stroke, history of gastrointestinal bleeding, and one point if one or more of the following are present: recent myocardial infarction, hematocrit less than 30%, serum creatinine greater than 1.5 mg/dL, or diabetes mellitus.[69] Additional risk factors for hemorrhage were incorporated into the HEMORR2HAGES (Hepatic or Renal Disease, Ethanol abuse, Malignancy, Older age [≥75 years], Reduced platelet count or function including aspirin use, Rebleeding risk (history of prior bleeding), Hypertension, Anemia, Genetic factors, Excessive fall Risk, and Stroke) risk index.[70] The HAS-BLED (Hypertension, Abnormal renal and liver function, Stroke, Bleeding history, Labile INR, Elderly [age >65], and Drugs and alcohol use) score is another risk scheme that has been validated in various populations.[71] The ATRIA Bleeding Risk Score relies on five clinical variables (anemia, renal disease, age ≥75 years, prior bleeding, and hypertension). Using these variables, most patients could be classified into a low bleeding risk category, with hemorrhage rates of less than 1% per year while

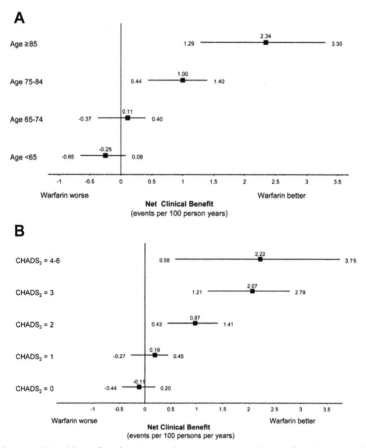

Fig. 4. The net clinical benefit of anticoagulant treatment with warfarin by age (*A*) and by CHADS₂ stroke risk score (*B*). Net clinical benefit calculated based on ischemic strokes prevented by warfarin minus the intracranial hemorrhage induced. (*Data from* Singer DE, Chang Y, Fang MC, et al. The net clinical benefit of warfarin anticoagulation in atrial fibrillation. Ann Intern Med 2009;151(5):297–305.)

taking warfarin. In contrast, patients with the highest risk score had hemorrhage rates of nearly 18% per year (**Fig. 5**).[72] In general, bleeding risk tools are probably most useful for patients at a low or intermediate risk for stroke, in whom the net clinical benefit of warfarin is less clear and the risk of bleeding becomes more influential.

A limitation of all bleeding risk schemes is that they do not distinguish between intracranial and extracranial bleeding events. In part because of the rarity of intracranial hemorrhage, clinically useful risk stratification schemes for intracranial hemorrhage do not yet exist.

Fall Risk and Anticoagulation

Perceived risk of falls in elderly patients often deters administration of anticoagulation for fear of intracranial hemorrhage.[73–75] The actual risk of fall-related hemorrhage is difficult to determine because high fall-risk patients are less likely to be included in

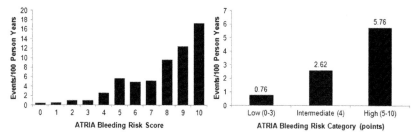

Fig. 5. Major bleeding events per 100 person years by ATRIA bleeding score (continuous score and three category score). ATRIA bleeding risk calculated by total points based on anemia (3 points), renal disease (3 points), age ≥75 (2 points), prior bleeding (1 point), and hypertension (1 point). (*Data from* Fang MC, Go AS, Chang Y, et al. A new risk scheme to predict warfarin-associated hemorrhage: the ATRIA (Anticoagulation and Risk Factors in Atrial Fibrillation) Study. J Am Coll Cardiol 2011;58(4):395–401.)

clinical studies of anticoagulation. However, the risk of fall-induced hemorrhage is likely outweighed by the benefits of anticoagulation for many older patients, with estimates that a person would need to fall an average of 300 times per year to outweigh the benefits gained in stroke prevention from anticoagulant therapy.[73,74,76] In one study of patients with AF, patients with high fall risk had almost twice the risk of intracranial hemorrhage, but the net benefit in high fall-risk patients still favored warfarin because of the large reduction in ischemic stroke rates.[77]

Warfarin Control

Chronic warfarin therapy requires ongoing monitoring and dose adjustments. Elderly patients are usually more sensitive to treatment with vitamin K antagonists and require lower doses of warfarin, often with maintenance doses of less than or equal to 5 mg daily.[62–64] In addition, polypharmacy is common in older patients, making drug-drug interactions more likely. Initiation of warfarin in the elderly generally requires lower doses than in younger patients.[62] Frequent medication review and close monitoring of INR around times of medication changes, acute illnesses, or hospitalization is recommended.

The newer oral anticoagulants have advantages over warfarin in terms of fewer drug-drug interactions and fixed daily dosing without requiring routine INR monitoring. These characteristics make direct thrombin inhibitors and factor Xa inhibitors more appealing with patients who have difficulty maintaining a stable INR or who decline frequent INR monitoring. However, because of the shorter half-life of these medications, adherence is important, with missed doses resulting in a quicker lack of anticoagulant effect. There are also no reliable coagulation tests that can determine whether patients are therapeutic or not, unlike INR testing for patients on warfarin. Severe bleeding events, particularly an increased risk of gastrointestinal hemorrhage, have been reported in dabigatran users, many of whom were elderly or who had renal dysfunction, thus demonstrating the need for long-term safety data related to the use of these agents in the elderly.[40] Now that there are multiple options for stroke prevention in AF, the final choice of antithrombotic therapy should be individualized and depend on safety, potential for drug-drug interactions, adherence, ability to monitor therapy, and costs.

SUMMARY

AF is a common condition that accounts for a large proportion of the ischemic stroke burden in the elderly. Although bleeding risk is elevated in older patients, the net clinical benefit favors anticoagulation for most older adults. The development of newer fixed-dose oral anticoagulants represents a promising alternative to conventional warfarin therapy and these agents may be associated with lower risk of intracranial hemorrhage. Use of newer agents may be appropriate for patients who have difficulty in maintaining stable INRs on warfarin or who prefer to forgo the regular monitoring required by warfarin. However, patients should be counseled about the need for adherence, the lack of ability to test for therapeutic efficacy, and the lack of proven options to reverse anticoagulant effect.

Recommendations include

1. Antithrombotic treatment of AF, including paroxysmal AF, should be guided by stroke risk stratification tools.
2. Bleeding risk stratification tools may help clinicians counsel patients about bleeding risk on anticoagulants and are most appropriate when applied to patients at low or intermediate stroke risk in whom the net benefit of anticoagulation is less clear.
3. Newer fixed-dose oral anticoagulants have emerged as viable alternatives to warfarin and choice of anticoagulant should depend on comorbidities (eg, renal function), side-effect profile, cost, and patient preference.
4. Stroke prevention in atrial flutter should be managed using the same recommendations as for AF.

REFERENCES

1. Wolf PA, Abbott RD, Kannel WB. Atrial fibrillation as an independent risk factor for stroke: the Framingham Study. Stroke 1991;22(8):983–8.
2. Go AS, Hylek EM, Phillips KA, et al. Prevalence of diagnosed atrial fibrillation in adults: national implications for rhythm management and stroke prevention: the AnTicoagulation and Risk Factors in Atrial Fibrillation (ATRIA) Study. JAMA 2001;285(18):2370–5.
3. Heeringa J, van der Kuip DA, Hofman A, et al. Prevalence, incidence and lifetime risk of atrial fibrillation: the Rotterdam study. Eur Heart J 2006;27(8):949–53.
4. Brass LM, Krumholz HM, Scinto JM, et al. Warfarin use among patients with atrial fibrillation. Stroke 1997;28(12):2382–9.
5. Fuster V, Ryden LE, Cannom DS, et al. ACC/AHA/ESC 2006 Guidelines for the Management of Patients with Atrial Fibrillation: a report of the American College of Cardiology/American Heart Association Task Force on Practice Guidelines and the European Society of Cardiology Committee for Practice Guidelines (Writing Committee to Revise the 2001 Guidelines for the Management of Patients With Atrial Fibrillation): developed in collaboration with the European Heart Rhythm Association and the Heart Rhythm Society. Circulation 2006;114(7):e257–354.
6. Naccarelli GV, Varker H, Lin J, et al. Increasing prevalence of atrial fibrillation and flutter in the United States. Am J Cardiol 2009;104(11):1534–9.
7. Fang MC, Go AS, Chang Y, et al. Comparison of risk stratification schemes to predict thromboembolism in people with nonvalvular atrial fibrillation. J Am Coll Cardiol 2008;51(8):810–5.
8. Benjamin EJ, Levy D, Vaziri SM, et al. Independent risk factors for atrial fibrillation in a population-based cohort. The Framingham Heart Study. JAMA 1994;271(11):840–4.
9. Elijovich L, Josephson SA, Fung GL, et al. Intermittent atrial fibrillation may account for a large proportion of otherwise cryptogenic stroke: a study of 30-day cardiac event monitors. J Stroke Cerebrovasc Dis 2009;18(3):185–9.

10. Healey JS, Connolly SJ, Gold MR, et al. Subclinical atrial fibrillation and the risk of stroke. N Engl J Med 2012;366(2):120–9.
11. Ivan CS, Seshadri S, Beiser A, et al. Dementia after stroke: the Framingham Study. Stroke 2004;35(6):1264–8.
12. Lamassa M, Di Carlo A, Pracucci G, et al. Characteristics, outcome, and care of stroke associated with atrial fibrillation in Europe: data from a multicenter multinational hospital-based registry (The European Community Stroke Project). Stroke 2001;32(2):392–8.
13. Lin HJ, Wolf PA, Kelly-Hayes M, et al. Stroke severity in atrial fibrillation. The Framingham Study. Stroke 1996;27(10):1760–4.
14. Jorgensen HS, Nakayama H, Reith J, et al. Acute stroke with atrial fibrillation. The Copenhagen Stroke Study. Stroke 1996;27(10):1765–9.
15. Wolf PA, Dawber TR, Thomas HE Jr, et al. Epidemiologic assessment of chronic atrial fibrillation and risk of stroke: the Framingham study. Neurology 1978;28(10): 973–7.
16. Wyse DG, Waldo AL, DiMarco JP, et al. A comparison of rate control and rhythm control in patients with atrial fibrillation. N Engl J Med 2002;347(23):1825–33.
17. You JJ, Singer DE, Howard PA, et al. Antithrombotic therapy for atrial fibrillation: Antithrombotic Therapy and Prevention of Thrombosis, 9th ed: American College of Chest Physicians Evidence-Based Clinical Practice Guidelines. Chest 2012; 141(Suppl 2):e531S–75S.
18. van Walraven C, Hart RG, Singer DE, et al. Oral anticoagulants vs aspirin in nonvalvular atrial fibrillation: an individual patient meta-analysis. JAMA 2002;288(19): 2441–8.
19. Halligan SC, Gersh BJ, Brown RD Jr, et al. The natural history of lone atrial flutter. Ann Intern Med 2004;140(4):265–8.
20. Gage BF, van Walraven C, Pearce L, et al. Selecting patients with atrial fibrillation for anticoagulation: stroke risk stratification in patients taking aspirin. Circulation 2004;110(16):2287–92.
21. Van Staa TP, Setakis E, Di Tanna GL, et al. A comparison of risk stratification schemes for stroke in 79,884 atrial fibrillation patients in general practice. J Thromb Haemost 2011;9(1):39–48.
22. Gage BF, Waterman AD, Shannon W, et al. Validation of clinical classification schemes for predicting stroke: results from the National Registry of Atrial Fibrillation. JAMA 2001;285(22):2864–70.
23. Lip GY, Nieuwlaat R, Pisters R, et al. Refining clinical risk stratification for predicting stroke and thromboembolism in atrial fibrillation using a novel risk factor-based approach: the euro heart survey on atrial fibrillation. Chest 2010;137(2):263–72.
24. Chao TF, Lin YJ, Tsao HM, et al. CHADS(2) and CHA(2)DS(2)-VASc scores in the prediction of clinical outcomes in patients with atrial fibrillation after catheter ablation. J Am Coll Cardiol 2011;58(23):2380–5.
25. European Heart Rhythm Association, European Association for Cardio-Thoracic Surgery, Camm AJ, et al. Guidelines for the management of atrial fibrillation: the Task Force for the Management of Atrial Fibrillation of the European Society of Cardiology (ESC). Eur Heart J 2010;31(19):2369–429.
26. Ezekowitz MD, Bridgers SL, James KE, et al. Warfarin in the prevention of stroke associated with nonrheumatic atrial fibrillation. Veterans Affairs Stroke Prevention in Nonrheumatic Atrial Fibrillation Investigators. N Engl J Med 1992;327(20): 1406–12.
27. Warfarin versus aspirin for prevention of thromboembolism in atrial fibrillation: Stroke Prevention in Atrial Fibrillation II Study. Lancet 1994;343(8899):687–91.

632 Quinn & Fang

28. Hart RG, Pearce LA, Aguilar MI. Meta-analysis: antithrombotic therapy to prevent stroke in patients who have nonvalvular atrial fibrillation. Ann Intern Med 2007; 146(12):857–67.
29. Fang MC, Go AS, Chang Y, et al. Thirty-day mortality after ischemic stroke and intracranial hemorrhage in patients with atrial fibrillation on and off anticoagulants. Stroke 2012;43(7):1795–9.
30. Singer DE, Chang Y, Fang MC, et al. Should patient characteristics influence target anticoagulation intensity for stroke prevention in nonvalvular atrial fibrillation?: the ATRIA study. Circ Cardiovasc Qual Outcomes 2009;2(4):297–304.
31. International Warfarin Pharmacogenetics Consortium, Klein TE, Altman RB, et al. Estimation of the warfarin dose with clinical and pharmacogenetic data. N Engl J Med 2009;360(8):753–64.
32. Chiquette E, Amato MG, Bussey HI. Comparison of an anticoagulation clinic with usual medical care: anticoagulation control, patient outcomes, and health care costs. Arch Intern Med 1998;158(15):1641–7.
33. Wilson SJ, Wells PS, Kovacs MJ, et al. Comparing the quality of oral anticoagulant management by anticoagulation clinics and by family physicians: a randomized controlled trial. CMAJ 2003;169(4):293–8.
34. Aziz F, Corder M, Wolffe J, et al. Anticoagulation monitoring by an anticoagulation service is more cost-effective than routine physician care. J Vasc Surg 2011; 54(5):1404–7.
35. Menendez-Jandula B, Souto JC, Oliver A, et al. Comparing self-management of oral anticoagulant therapy with clinic management: a randomized trial. Ann Intern Med 2005;142(1):1–10.
36. Matchar DB, Jacobson A, Dolor R, et al. Effect of home testing of international normalized ratio on clinical events. N Engl J Med 2010;363(17):1608–20.
37. Albers GW, Diener HC, Frison L, et al. Ximelagatran vs warfarin for stroke prevention in patients with nonvalvular atrial fibrillation: a randomized trial. JAMA 2005; 293(6):690–8.
38. Albers GW, Diener HC, Frison L, et al. Trials and tribulations of noninferiority: the ximelagatran experience. J Am Coll Cardiol 2006;48(5):1058 [author reply: 1059].
39. Connolly SJ, Ezekowitz MD, Yusuf S, et al. Dabigatran versus warfarin in patients with atrial fibrillation. N Engl J Med 2009;361(12):1139–51.
40. Legrand M, Mateo J, Aribaud A, et al. The use of dabigatran in elderly patients. Arch Intern Med 2011;171(14):1285–6.
41. Uchino K, Hernandez AV. Dabigatran association with higher risk of acute coronary events: meta-analysis of noninferiority randomized controlled trials. Arch Intern Med 2012;172(5):397–402.
42. Shah SV, Gage BF. Cost-effectiveness of dabigatran for stroke prophylaxis in atrial fibrillation. Circulation 2011;123(22):2562–70.
43. Kamel H, Johnston SC, Easton JD, et al. Cost-effectiveness of dabigatran compared with warfarin for stroke prevention in patients with atrial fibrillation and prior stroke or transient ischemic attack. Stroke 2012;43(3):881–3.
44. Patel MR, Mahaffey KW, Garg J, et al. Rivaroxaban versus warfarin in nonvalvular atrial fibrillation. N Engl J Med 2011;365(10):883–91.
45. Eerenberg ES, Kamphuisen PW, Sijpkens MK, et al. Reversal of rivaroxaban and dabigatran by prothrombin complex concentrate: a randomized, placebo-controlled, crossover study in healthy subjects. Circulation 2011;124(14): 1573–9.
46. Granger CB, Alexander JH, McMurray JJ, et al. Apixaban versus warfarin in patients with atrial fibrillation. N Engl J Med 2011;365(11):981–92.

47. Connolly SJ, Eikelboom J, Joyner C, et al. Apixaban in patients with atrial fibrillation. N Engl J Med 2011;364(9):806–17.
48. Ruff CT, Giugliano RP, Antman EM, et al. Evaluation of the novel factor Xa inhibitor edoxaban compared with warfarin in patients with atrial fibrillation: design and rationale for the Effective aNticoaGulation with factor xA next GEneration in Atrial Fibrillation-Thrombolysis In Myocardial Infarction study 48 (ENGAGE AF-TIMI 48). Am Heart J 2010;160(4):635–41.
49. Turpie AG, Bauer KA, Davidson BL, et al. A randomized evaluation of betrixaban, an oral factor Xa inhibitor, for prevention of thromboembolic events after total knee replacement (EXPERT). Thromb Haemost 2009;101(1):68–76.
50. Flaker GC, Gruber M, Connolly SJ, et al. Risks and benefits of combining aspirin with anticoagulant therapy in patients with atrial fibrillation: an exploratory analysis of stroke prevention using an oral thrombin inhibitor in atrial fibrillation (SPORTIF) trials. Am Heart J 2006;152(5):967–73.
51. Gage BF, Cardinalli AB, Albers GW, et al. Cost-effectiveness of warfarin and aspirin for prophylaxis of stroke in patients with nonvalvular atrial fibrillation. JAMA 1995;274(23):1839–45.
52. ACTIVE Writing Group of the ACTIVE Investigators, Connolly S, Pogue J, Hart R, et al. Clopidogrel plus aspirin versus oral anticoagulation for atrial fibrillation in the Atrial fibrillation Clopidogrel Trial with Irbesartan for prevention of Vascular Events (ACTIVE W): a randomised controlled trial. Lancet 2006;367(9526): 1903–12.
53. ACTIVE Investigators, Connolly SJ, Pogue J, Hart RG, et al. Effect of clopidogrel added to aspirin in patients with atrial fibrillation. N Engl J Med 2009;360(20): 2066–78.
54. Gentile F, Elhendy A, Khandheria BK, et al. Safety of electrical cardioversion in patients with atrial fibrillation. Mayo Clin Proc 2002;77(9):897–904.
55. Wazni O, Wilkoff B, Saliba W. Catheter ablation for atrial fibrillation. N Engl J Med 2011;365(24):2296–304.
56. Weerasooriya R, Khairy P, Litalien J, et al. Catheter ablation for atrial fibrillation: are results maintained at 5 years of follow-up? J Am Coll Cardiol 2011;57(2): 160–6.
57. Cox JL, Ad N, Palazzo T. Impact of the maze procedure on the stroke rate in patients with atrial fibrillation. J Thorac Cardiovasc Surg 1999;118(5):833–40.
58. Garcia-Fernandez MA, Perez-David E, Quiles J, et al. Role of left atrial appendage obliteration in stroke reduction in patients with mitral valve prosthesis: a transesophageal echocardiographic study. J Am Coll Cardiol 2003;42(7): 1253–8.
59. Ostermayer SH, Reisman M, Kramer PH, et al. Percutaneous left atrial appendage transcatheter occlusion (PLAATO system) to prevent stroke in high-risk patients with non-rheumatic atrial fibrillation: results from the international multi-center feasibility trials. J Am Coll Cardiol 2005;46(1):9–14.
60. Holmes DR, Reddy VY, Turi ZG, et al. Percutaneous closure of the left atrial appendage versus warfarin therapy for prevention of stroke in patients with atrial fibrillation: a randomised non-inferiority trial. Lancet 2009;374(9689):534–42.
61. Hobbs FD, Roalfe AK, Lip GY, et al. Performance of stroke risk scores in older people with atrial fibrillation not taking warfarin: comparative cohort study from BAFTA trial. BMJ 2011;342:d3653.
62. Garcia D, Regan S, Crowther M, et al. Warfarin maintenance dosing patterns in clinical practice: implications for safer anticoagulation in the elderly population. Chest 2005;127(6):2049–56.

63. Copland M, Walker ID, Tait RC. Oral anticoagulation and hemorrhagic complications in an elderly population with atrial fibrillation. Arch Intern Med 2001;161(17): 2125–8.
64. Perez-Gomez F, Iriarte JA, Zumalde J, et al. Antithrombotic therapy in elderly patients with atrial fibrillation: effects and bleeding complications: a stratified analysis of the NASPEAF randomized trial. Eur Heart J 2007;28(8):996–1003.
65. Mant J, Hobbs FD, Fletcher K, et al. Warfarin versus aspirin for stroke prevention in an elderly community population with atrial fibrillation (the Birmingham Atrial Fibrillation Treatment of the Aged Study, BAFTA): a randomised controlled trial. Lancet 2007;370(9586):493–503.
66. Singer DE, Chang Y, Fang MC, et al. The net clinical benefit of warfarin anticoagulation in atrial fibrillation. Ann Intern Med 2009;151(5):297–305.
67. Fang MC, Go AS, Chang Y, et al. Death and disability from warfarin-associated intracranial and extracranial hemorrhages. Am J Med 2007;120(8):700–5.
68. Eckman MH, Rosand J, Knudsen KA, et al. Can patients be anticoagulated after intracerebral hemorrhage? A decision analysis. Stroke 2003;34(7):1710–6.
69. Beyth RJ, Quinn LM, Landefeld CS. Prospective evaluation of an index for predicting the risk of major bleeding in outpatients treated with warfarin. Am J Med 1998; 105(2):91–9.
70. Gage BF, Yan Y, Milligan PE, et al. Clinical classification schemes for predicting hemorrhage: results from the National Registry of Atrial Fibrillation (NRAF). Am Heart J 2006;151(3):713–9.
71. Lip GY, Frison L, Halperin JL, et al. Comparative validation of a novel risk score for predicting bleeding risk in anticoagulated patients with atrial fibrillation: the HAS-BLED (Hypertension, Abnormal Renal/Liver Function, Stroke, Bleeding History or Predisposition, Labile INR, Elderly, Drugs/Alcohol Concomitantly) score. J Am Coll Cardiol 2011;57(2):173–80.
72. Fang MC, Go AS, Chang Y, et al. A new risk scheme to predict warfarin-associated hemorrhage: the ATRIA (Anticoagulation and Risk Factors in Atrial Fibrillation) Study. J Am Coll Cardiol 2011;58(4):395–401.
73. Man-Son-Hing M, Laupacis A. Anticoagulant-related bleeding in older persons with atrial fibrillation: physicians' fears often unfounded. Arch Intern Med 2003; 163(13):1580–6.
74. Man-Son-Hing M, Nichol G, Lau A, et al. Choosing antithrombotic therapy for elderly patients with atrial fibrillation who are at risk for falls. Arch Intern Med 1999;159(7):677–85.
75. Pugh D, Pugh J, Mead GE. Attitudes of physicians regarding anticoagulation for atrial fibrillation: a systematic review. Age Ageing 2011;40(6):675–83.
76. Sellers MB, Newby LK. Atrial fibrillation, anticoagulation, fall risk, and outcomes in elderly patients. Am Heart J 2011;161(2):241–6.
77. Gage BF, Birman-Deych E, Kerzner R, et al. Incidence of intracranial hemorrhage in patients with atrial fibrillation who are prone to fall. Am J Med 2005;118(6): 612–7.

Atrial Fibrillation and Atrial Flutter: Medical Management

Jane Chen, MD, FHRS

KEYWORDS

- Atrial fibrillation • Atrial flutter • Antiarrhythmic drugs • Elderly

KEY POINTS

- Atrial fibrillation and atrial flutter are common arrhythmias in the elderly.
- Rate control can be achieved with β-blockers, calcium channel blockers, and digoxin, and lenient rate control (resting heart rates of <110 bpm) seems to be an acceptable alternative to strict rate control.
- Antiarrhythmic agents are chosen based on the side effect profile, and dose adjustments are often required for age and renal function.
- Polypharmacy in the elderly is common, and drug interactions must be carefully taken into account when adjusting doses.
- Rate control and rhythm control strategies are associated with equivalent mortality and quality of life outcomes; therefore, in asymptomatic or minimally symptomatic patients, rate control is a reasonable therapeutic strategy.

INTRODUCTION

Atrial fibrillation (AF) and atrial flutter (AFL) are common cardiac rhythm disturbances that incur significant morbidity and mortality.[1,2] They are primarily disorders associated with aging. In a study of long-term care residents whose average age was 84 years, the prevalence of AF was 11% in women and 14% in men.[3] Currently, it is estimated that 3 million people in the United States have AF. This number is projected to double by the year 2050, with 50% of affected individuals older than the age of 80.[1] Age-related changes in the heart, including diastolic dysfunction and atrial remodeling, and increased incidence of hypertension and diabetes may account for the strength of association between age and AF. AF accounts for more cardiovascular hospitalizations than heart failure, atherosclerotic heart disease, or stroke.[4] In a retrospective study of Medicare patients 65 years and older, more than half of the patients diagnosed with AF were hospitalized within the first year of diagnosis, with a readmission rate of 43.7% over a mean of 24 months.[5]

Cardiovascular Division, Washington University School of Medicine, 660 South Euclid Avenue, Campus Box 8086, St. Louis, MO 63110, USA
E-mail address: janechen@dom.wustl.edu

Clin Geriatr Med 28 (2012) 635–647
http://dx.doi.org/10.1016/j.cger.2012.08.002
0749-0690/12/$ – see front matter © 2012 Elsevier Inc. All rights reserved.

geriatric.theclinics.com

The management of AF and AFL is multifaceted. Prevention of thromboembolism and stroke, control of heart rate, and the restoration of sinus rhythm are three major areas of therapy that should be addressed for each patient. Numerous methods are available to achieve each goal, and each method has a risk-benefit ratio that must be considered on an individual basis. Comorbidities, potential for drug intolerance, drug interactions caused by polypharmacy, and higher risk for procedural complications are among the factors that make management of AF and AFL challenging in older patients (**Box 1**). Prevention of thromboembolism and invasive methods of therapy are addressed elsewhere in this issue. This article reviews the most recent data on the medical management of AF and AFL in the elderly, including an in-depth evaluation of pharmacologic agents available for rate and rhythm management of AF and AFL, and a discussion of rate versus rhythm control.

RELATIONSHIP BETWEEN AF AND AFL

The pathophysiologic relationship between AF and AFL is not completely clear. AF is generally recognized as a result of chaotic atrial rhythm involving multiple microreentrant circuits within the atria, whereas AFL is a more organized, macroreentrant rhythm. The most common type of AFL has negative flutter waves ("saw-tooth pattern") in the inferior leads on the 12-lead electrocardiogram (ECG), and involves a reentrant circuit with a critical area of slow conduction in the isthmus bordered by the tricuspid valve, inferior vena cava, and coronary sinus (isthmus-dependent AFL).

AF was first observed to spontaneously organize into AFL in 1924.[6] It has also been noted that some antiarrhythmic drugs can convert AF to AFL.[7] Isthmus-dependent AFL is amenable to radiofrequency ablation, with long-term success rates approaching 80%.[8] For patients in whom AF is observed to convert to AFL with antiarrhythmic drugs, a hybrid approach, with ablation of AFL and continuation of antiarrhythmic drugs, has been advocated to control AF. Unfortunately, long-term follow-up demonstrates AF recurrences in 90% of patients.[9] In one study of patients with no documented AF before AFL ablation, the incidence of AF was 50% at a mean follow-up of 30 months.[10]

Box 1
Information required for drug choice and dosing in the elderly
Age
Gender
Body weight
Body mass index
Creatinine clearance
Hepatic function
Ejection fraction
Heart failure functional status
Comedications, including prescription, over-the-counter, and herbal preparations
Intake of grapefruit or grapefruit juice
Baseline electrocardiogram measurements of QRS and QT interval

Because of the close relationship between AF and AFL, although they are distinctly different arrhythmias, similar management strategies are applied to both. In general, the two main approaches to medical management of AF and AFL are rate control (ie, controlling the ventricular response rate) and rhythm control (ie, attempting to maintain sinus rhythm). As discussed elsewhere in this issue, most older adults require long-term anticoagulation, regardless of the choice of rate or rhythm control.

RATE CONTROL

Effective control of ventricular rate during AF and AFL is a primary goal in acute and chronic phases of management. Rate control is crucial for the relief of symptoms and the prevention of tachycardia-mediated cardiomyopathy. Guidelines suggest targeting a resting heart rate of 60 to 80 beats per minute, and a peak rate with exercise of 90 to 115 beats per minute.[1]

β-Blockers

β-Blockers are highly effective in controlling ventricular rates in AF in the acute and chronic settings. β-Blockers are not effective in the conversion of AF to sinus rhythm. The onset of action with intravenous β-blockers for rate control is usually within minutes. Because of their antisympathetic actions, oral β-blockers are the most effective drugs in controlling ventricular rates during exertion. β-Blockers also have the advantage of reducing mortality in patients with coronary artery disease.[11] β-Blockers given before cardiac surgery have been shown to decrease the incidence of postoperative AF.[12] For acute rate control, metoprolol and atenolol may be given as intravenous boluses, and esmolol may be administered as a continuous infusion. In addition to metoprolol and atenolol, propranolol, timolol, nadolol, bisoprolol, nebivolol, and carvedilol are available in the United States and may be used to maintain effective heart rate control. β-Blockers are contraindicated in patients with significant bradycardia (heart rate <40–45 bpm), atrioventricular (AV) nodal block, hypotension, bronchospasm, or decompensated heart failure. Additional side effects may include decreased exercise tolerance, fatigue, low mood, sleep disturbances, and sexual dysfunction.

Elderly patients with sinoatrial dysfunction are particularly prone to development of bradyarrhythmias when receiving β-blockers. Compared with younger men, a greater reduction in exercise heart rate at a given atenolol concentration has been reported in elderly men. Decreased number of β-adrenoreceptors and blunted β-adrenoreceptor responsiveness have been implicated as possible mechanisms.[13] A genetic polymorphism of the β_1-adrenergic receptor ADRB1 has been associated with favorable response to all rate-controlling agents. The presence of the polymorphism is postulated to have synergic effects to calcium channel blockers and digoxin. Carriers of the genetic variant seem to require lower doses of medication for rate control compared with noncarriers.[14]

Calcium Channel Blockers

Like β-blockers, the nonhydropyridine calcium channel blockers verapamil and diltiazem act directly on the AV node to slow conduction. They are not effective in converting AF to sinus rhythm. Intravenous verapamil and diltiazem have a rapid onset of action and are effective in acutely controlling the ventricular rate. Verapamil is more negatively inotropic than diltiazem, and it is also more likely to cause hypotension. Long-term use of these agents should be avoided in patients with decreased left ventricular systolic function. Diltiazem, 0.25 mg/kg, may be given intravenously every

5 to 10 minutes for acute rate control. If needed, this may be followed by a continuous infusion of 5 to 15 mg/h, titrated to achieve the desired heart rate. Verapamil may be given intravenously in 2.5- to 5-mg boluses. Oral maintenance doses for diltiazem and verapamil range from 120 to 360 mg daily in divided doses or as long-acting formulations. Major side effects include hypotension, bradycardia, heart block, and heart failure exacerbations. Constipation is a common side effect in older adults, especially with verapamil. Lower-extremity edema is also common, and may be erroneously attributed to worsening heart failure.

Digoxin

Neither intravenous nor oral digoxin facilitates conversion to sinus rhythm.[15] Digoxin is used primarily to control the ventricular response rate. However, because effective rate control with intravenous digoxin may take 12 hours or longer,[16] there is little role for intravenous digoxin in the acute setting. Digoxin slows ventricular rate by enhancing vagal tone, and the effect is easily overcome by sympathetic activity. Therefore, digoxin is generally not effective in the postoperative setting or in very active patients.

As monotherapy, digoxin is potentially useful in elderly and sedentary patients in whom hypotension, severe heart failure, or other conditions preclude the use of β-blockers or calcium channel blockers. Digoxin is most effective when used in combination with other drugs. In a clinical trial comparing digoxin, diltiazem, atenolol, and the combination of diltiazem or atenolol with digoxin, digoxin plus atenolol, 50 mg daily, provided the most effective rate control.[17]

The usual maintenance dose of digoxin is 0.125 to 0.375 mg per day. Decreased volume of distribution and glomerular filtration predispose elderly patients to an increased risk for digoxin toxicity, which may manifest as heart block, bradycardia, or ventricular arrhythmias. In elderly patients with reduced creatinine clearance (CrCl), it is generally recommended that a daily dose of 0.125 mg per day is sufficient. Because the cardiac effects of digoxin are potentiated by hypokalemia, hypomagnesia, and hypercalcemia, serum levels of these electrolytes should be maintained within the normal range. In addition, many medications increase the plasma concentration of digoxin, so careful scrutiny for potential drug interactions is extremely important to avoid toxicity (**Table 1**).

RHYTHM CONTROL

Restoration and maintenance of sinus rhythm is frequently necessary for symptomatic relief. Conversion of AF and AFL to sinus rhythm is best achieved with electrical cardioversion, and maintenance of sinus rhythm typically requires the use of antiarrhythmic drugs. Rhythm control becomes more difficult with prolonged duration in AF, depressed systolic function, severe diastolic dysfunction, and larger atrial size.

In patients with AF and rapid ventricular rate who are hemodynamically unstable, immediate electrical cardioversion is indicated. In stable patients, electrical cardioversion may be electively performed with low risk of thromboembolic events if the duration of AF is less than 48 hours, or if patients are on warfarin with therapeutic INRs for at least 3 consecutive weeks. If the duration is unknown, if patients are not on long-term anticoagulation, or if subtherapeutic INRs have recently been documented, a transesophageal echocardiogram is recommended to rule out the presence of left atrial thrombus before cardioversion. Anticoagulation with warfarin must be continued for a minimum of 1 month after cardioversion because of continuing risk of thrombus formation from atrial stunning after cardioversion. In patients with risk factors for

Table 1 Potential major drug interactions		
Drug	Plasma Concentration Increased By	Plasma Concentration Decreased By
Digoxin	Amiodarone Quinidine Propafenone Diltiazem Verapamil Erythromycin Itraconazole Dronedarone	
Metoprolol	CYP2D6 inhibitors: Quinidine Propafenone Amiodarone Paroxetine Dronedarone	
Dofetilide	Inhibition of renal tubular secretion: Hydrochlorothiazide Cimetidine Ketoconazole Trmethoprim Increased hepatic blood flow (increased absorption): Verapamil	CYP3A4 inducers: Carbamazepine Phenytoin Rifampin St John's Wort
Disopyramide Diltiazem Dronedarone	Cyp3A4 inhibitors: Itraconazole Ketoconazole Clarithromycin Grape fruit juice	CYP3A4 inducers: Carbamazepine Phenytoin Rifampin St John's Wort

stroke, warfarin should be continued indefinitely.[18] Elective cardioversion with the new anticoagulants, rivaroxiban and dabigatran, has not been well studied. However, continuous use of dabigatran for a minimum of 3 weeks before cardioversion does not seem to be associated with increased risk of stroke compared with warfarin.[19] Electrical conversion of AFL usually requires lower energy than AF. Occasionally, AFL can be terminated through rapid atrial pacing, which may be delivered by the atrial lead in patients with dual-chamber pacemakers or defibrillators.

Some antiarrhythmic agents may convert AF or AFL to sinus rhythm. Regardless of the method of conversion, whether electrical, pacing, or pharmacologic, appropriate anticoagulation status must be ascertained before initiation of therapy.

ANTIARRHYTHMIC DRUGS
Challenges in the Elderly

Administration of oral antiarrhythmic agents in elderly patients is frequently complicated by comorbidity, diminished drug clearance, compliance issues, and polypharmacy leading to drug interactions. Aging is usually associated with increases in total body fat and decreases in lean body mass and total body water. These changes can affect the volume of distribution of lipophilic and hydrophilic drugs, and may necessitate a reduction in dosages. Therapeutic drug monitoring of antiarrhythmic drugs has some role in the treatment of elderly patients. Measuring the plasma concentrations of these drugs may help to clarify whether dosage adjustments are possible when pharmacotherapy fails. However, monitoring plasma concentrations does not minimize the necessity of ECG monitoring for evaluation of QRS and QT intervals. Furthermore, significant signs of clinical toxicity can occur even at plasma levels that are at the lower end of the accepted therapeutic range.[20]

Vaughn-Williams Classification

The Vaughn-Williams Classification was introduced in 1970 and is one of the most widely used classification schemes for antiarrhythmic agents. This scheme classifies a drug based on the primary mechanism of its antiarrhythmic effect. It should be noted, however, that many antiarrhythmic drugs have multiple mechanisms of action. Class II (β-blockers) and intravenous (calcium channel blockers) are used for rate control and have been discussed previously. Class I and III drugs are used for rhythm control, and are discussed next.

Vaughn-Williams Class IA

Class IA antiarrhythmic drugs (quinidine, procainamide, and disopyramide) are sodium and potassium channel blockers that increase action potential duration and QT interval. They are not as commonly used nowadays as they were in the past, because they are only moderately effective and are associated with significant side effects. Because they can prolong the QT interval, the most serious side effect from these agents is torsades de pointes ventricular tachycardia (VT). Quinidine may be given as quinidine sulfate at 200 to 400 mg every 6 hours or as quinidine gluconate at 324 to 648 mg every 8 to 12 hours. It is frequently associated with nausea or diarrhea, and it has also been associated with increased mortality, presumably because of proarrhythmia.[21] The efficacy of intravenous procainamide for chemical conversion of recent-onset AF to sinus rhythm is unproved.[22] Procainamide is given orally at 1 to 6 grams per day in divided doses. Prolonged use of procainamide may be associated with a systemic lupus-like syndrome. Disopyramide, given 100 to 300 mg every 6 to 8 hours, has anticholinergic effects that may be useful for AF that is triggered by increased vagal tone. However, the anticholinergic actions may exacerbate glaucoma or urinary dysfunction in the elderly. Disopyramide also has potent negative inotropic action that precludes its use in patients with severe left ventricular dysfunction and chronic heart failure.

Vaughn-Williams Class IB

Class IB agents, such as mexiletine and lidocaine, have no effect on atrial tissues and are not used for treatment of AF or AFL.

Vaughn-Williams Class IC

Class IC drugs (flecainide and propafenone) are predominantly sodium channel blockers. They prolong the action potential duration to a significantly greater extent than they prolong the QT interval. As a result, cardiac toxicity manifests predominantly as widened QRS intervals. This effect is more pronounced at faster heart rates, and is more prominent with flecainide than with propafenone. Once maintenance dose has been achieved, an exercise stress test is recommended to monitor for QRS widening at higher heart rates. Flecainide and propafenone may convert AF to AFL. The slower flutter waves may then be conducted through the AV node with a 1:1 relationship, resulting in a rapid ventricular rate. Therefore, it is important to use AV nodal blocking agents concomitantly with class IC drugs. Propafenone also has β-blocking properties, and may exacerbate bradycardia.

Although these agents are effective in maintaining sinus rhythm, their safety profile has been in question since the publication of the Cardiac Arrhythmia Suppression Trial.[23] This study showed increased mortality in patients who were prophylactically treated with flecainide or encainide for suppression of premature ventricular complexes after uncomplicated myocardial infarctions. Whether flecainide or propafenone increases mortality in patients treated for atrial arrhythmias is unknown. However, the results of the Cardiac Arrhythmia Suppression Trial study have been generalized to patients with coronary artery disease or any structural heart disease, and class IC agents are not recommended in these populations (including most elderly patients). In patients with normal hearts, however, these drugs offer few side effects and have an excellent safety profile. The main side effects are sinus node depression and bradycardia.

Flecainide is given at 50 to 200 mg orally twice a day; many elderly patients only require 50 mg twice a day. The starting dose of propafenone is 150 mg every 8 to 12 hours. Metabolism of flecainide and propafenone are dependent on the activity of the CYP2D6 isoenzyme. Approximately 5% to 10% of the white population has mutations of this isoenzyme, making them "poor metabolizers" of the drugs, requiring a reduction in dose.[24]

Vaughn-Williams Class III

Class III drugs (sotalol, dofetilide, and ibutilide) are predominantly potassium channel blockers, with a tendency to cause QT prolongation. Torsade de pointes VT is a significant potential side effect from these agents. Sotalol is a racemic mixture with β-blocking (l-sotalol) and class III antiarrhythmic (d-sotalol) properties. Oral dosing is usually 80 to 160 mg twice a day. D-sotalol alone has been shown to increase mortality in postinfarction patients,[25] and is not clinically available. Sotalol is renally excreted, and the risk of QT prolongation and torsade de pointes VT is higher in patients with decreased CrCl. These issues are of particular importance in elderly women, in whom longer QT intervals may be noted at baseline. Sotalol is contraindicated in patients with CrCl less than 40 mL/min and should be administered once daily in patients with CrCl of 40 to 60 mL/min. Initiation of sotalol, especially in elderly patients, should ideally be in the hospital setting for monitoring of QT intervals and creatinine. Sotalol may exacerbate chronic heart failure, and it is not recommended in patients with acute heart failure exacerbations.

The main advantages of dofetilide over sotalol are its safety profile in patients with severe left ventricular dysfunction or chronic heart failure and lower likelihood to cause significant bradycardia.[26,27] Initiation of dofetilide requires hospitalization with continuous telemetry monitoring for a minimum of six doses. Dofetilide dosing does not need to be adjusted for age, but is dependent on the baseline QT interval and CrCl. A baseline corrected QT (QTc) interval of more than 440 milliseconds, or more than 500 milliseconds with a bundle branch block or paced rhythm, precludes the use of dofetilide, as does a CrCl of less than 20 mL/min. Initial dose of dofetilide is 500 μg twice a day if the CrCl is more than 60 mL/min, 250 μg twice a day if the CrCl is 40 to 60 mL/min, and 125 μg twice a day if the CrCl is 20 to 40 mL/min. A 12-lead ECG must be obtained 1 to 2 hours after each dose and the QT interval carefully measured. If the QTc is more than 500 milliseconds after one dose, the subsequent dose must be reduced by half. If the subsequent ECG shows QTc more than 500 milliseconds, then the drug must be discontinued.[28]

Ibutilide is currently the only intravenous drug approved for chemical conversion of AF. It is more effective when used in AF of short duration (<7 days), and more effective in AFL than AF.[22] Ibutilide is associated with QT prolongation and a 4% to 8% risk of torsade de pointes VT, especially in the first 2 to 4 hours after administration of the drug. The risk for VT is higher in patients with cardiomyopathy and chronic heart failure. Ibutilide is given as intravenous bolus at a dose of 1 mg over 10 minutes or until conversion, whichever occurs first. It should only be given under carefully monitoring by personnel familiar with the drug, and an external defibrillator should be readily available in case of torsades de pointes VT. Patients must be monitored on telemetry for at least 4 hours after being given the drug. Ibutilide is not available in oral form for maintenance of sinus rhythm.

Amiodarone

Amiodarone is a complex drug that blocks sodium, potassium, calcium, and β-receptors. Intravenous amiodarone may facilitate conversion to sinus rhythm, although usually only after 48 hours of treatment.[29] Oral amiodarone can also convert a small proportion of patients with AF to sinus rhythm.[30] Prophylactic amiodarone given for a minimum of 7 days before cardiac surgery has been shown to reduce postoperative AF, thereby shortening hospital stay and reducing hospitalization costs.[31] Amiodarone may be used safely in patients with a history of myocardial infarction or left ventricular dysfunction. A loading dose of amiodarone is usually required to achieve steady-state blood levels. For oral therapy, the usual starting dose is 400 mg three times a day, with subsequent dosage reductions over a period of several weeks to a maintenance dose of 200 mg per day. Maintenance doses as low as 50 to 100 mg per day may be sufficient in the elderly. Amiodarone is a highly lipophilic drug for which fat is a major site of distribution.[32] In elderly patients with high body fat, a larger loading dose may be required.

Short-term use of amiodarone is usually well tolerated, but side effects are common during long-term administration. Major side effects include thyroid dysfunction, liver function abnormalities, pulmonary toxicity, photosensitivity, skin discoloration, bradycardia, and neurologic dysfunction, all of which are usually reversible with early detection and discontinuation of the drug. Before initiation of amiodarone, baseline thyroid function tests, liver function tests, chest radiograph, and pulmonary function tests should be obtained. Laboratory tests should be followed every 6 months. Chest films and pulmonary function tests are usually followed every 1 to 2 years, or whenever patients develop symptoms of shortness of breath. Amiodarone-induced bradycardia is more common in older patients, especially those with prior myocardial infarctions or sinus node dysfunction, and may require pacemaker implantation.[33] Although prolongation of the QT interval may occur, torsades de pointes VT is less common with amiodarone than with other antiarrhythmic drugs. Amiodarone is excreted through the skin, and has an elimination half-life of 1 to 2 months. In elderly patients with higher total body fat, clearance from the circulation may take even longer.

Dronedarone

Dronedarone is a relatively new antiarrhythmic drug that is pharmacologically related to amiodarone but lacks the iodine moiety that is associated with thyroid and pulmonary side effects.[34] Dronedarone is given at a set dose of 400 mg twice a day. Initial studies in patients with a mean age of 63 years and paroxysmal AF showed that dronedarone was better at maintaining sinus rhythm and ventricular rate control than placebo.[35] In direct comparison with amiodarone, dronedarone was associated with more AF recurrence, although amiodarone was associated with more side effects and higher rate of drug discontinuation.[36] Dronedarone has been shown to reduce the incidence of hospitalization for cardiovascular causes and death compared with placebo.[37] The reduction in cardiovascular events led to the hypothesis that the benefits of dronedarone may extend beyond rhythm control. This hypothesis was tested in the PALLAS trial, which showed that administration of dronedarone in patients with permanent AF was in fact associated with an increase in the rates of heart failure hospitalization, stroke, and death.[38] This trial is particularly relevant to elderly patients because patients 75 years or older constituted more than 50% of the study population. Elderly patients with asymptomatic permanent AF should not be treated with dronedarone for rate control. Dronedarone is also contraindicated in patients with severe left ventricular systolic dysfunction or recent heart failure exacerbation, because it has been shown to increase total mortality in such patients.[39]

Choice of Antiarrhythmic Drugs

The first step in choosing an antiarrhythmic agent for a patient with AF is to determine the presence or absence of structural heart disease. In patients without structural heart, flecainide or propafenone, along with an AV nodal blocking agent, are an excellent first choice. Disopyramide may be used in patients without known glaucoma or urinary retention if AF is triggered by high vagal tone. In patients with structural heart disease, including significant left ventricular hypertrophy, in conjunction with normal baseline QT interval and renal function, sotalol is an appropriate first-choice agent. In patients with active heart failure or baseline bradycardia, dofetilide is a reasonable alternative. In elderly patients, presence of heart disease and decreased renal function frequently preclude the use of many of the previously mentioned agents. As a result, amiodarone is commonly used in older patients. Dronedarone is a reasonable alternative to amiodarone in patients with paroxysmal AF in the absence of heart failure, although its efficacy seems to be inferior to amiodarone.

RATE VERSUS RHYTHM CONTROL

Elderly patients were not well represented in major trials evaluating the comparative effectiveness of rate versus rhythm control strategies. The mean age of patients in these trials was less than 70 years. The largest trial, AFFIRM, was an international study that randomized asymptomatic patients to rate versus rhythm control.[40] There was no difference in the primary outcome of overall mortality between these two groups. The PIAF trial[41] studied symptomatic patients with persistent AF. During follow-up, quality of life improved for rate and rhythm control groups, but there was no difference between groups. The AF-CHF trial studied the effects of rate or rhythm control in patients with left ventricular ejection fractions of 35% or less, and found that even in this high-risk population, there was no difference between groups in the primary endpoint of time to death from cardiovascular causes.[42] The results of other major studies are shown in **Table 2**, with no significant differences in major composite endpoints of death, thromboembolic events, or major bleeding between rate and rhythm control. The RACE II trial importantly showed that patients treated with "lenient" rate control, defined as a resting heart rate of less than 110 bpm, have the same quality of life scores as patients treated with "strict" rate control, defined as a resting heart rate of less than 80 bpm and exercise heart rates of less than 110 bpm.[43] The results of these trials suggest that for most patients with minimal symptoms, rate control is an acceptable therapeutic option, and does not increase mortality or major cardiovascular events. Additionally, lenient rate control is a very reasonable therapeutic approach in elderly patients.

Table 2
Major studies of rate versus rhythm control

Study	# Rhythm Control	# Rate Control	Mean Age (y)	% Women	Mean Follow-up	% SR in Rhythm Control Group at Follow-up	Primary Endpoint	Result
AFFIRM[40] (2002)	2033	2027	69	40	3.5 y	73	Overall mortality	No difference
RACE[44] (2002)	266	256	68	37	2.3 ± 0.6 y	39	Composite[a]	No difference
PIAF[41] (2003)	127	127	61	28	1 y	56	Quality of life	No difference
STAF[45] (2003)	100	100	65	40	19.6 ± 8.9 mo	23	Composite[a]	No difference
HOT CAFE[46] (2004)	104	101	60	35	1.7 ± 0.4 y	63.5	Composite[a]	No difference
AF CHF[42] (2008)	682	694	66	20	37 ± 19 mo	73	Time to death from CV causes	No difference

Abbreviations: AF CHF, Atrial Fibrillation and Congestive Heart Failure; AFFIRM, Atrial Fibrillation Follow-Up Investigation of Rhythm Management; CV, cardiovascular; HOT CAFÉ, How To Treat Chronic Atrial Fibrillation; PIAF, Pharmacologic Intervention in Atrial Fibrillation; RACE, Rate Control versus Electrical Cardioversion; SR, sinus rhythm; STAF, Strategies of Treatment of Atrial Fibrillation.
[a] Composite endpoints = death, thromboembolic events, major bleeding.

SUMMARY

AF and AFL are common arrhythmias in elderly patients. Medical management of AF in the elderly is particularly challenging, and every decision regarding the management of AF has an associated risk. An understanding of potential drug interactions, vigilance in assessing comorbidities, and knowledge of drug side effects are important factors in determining appropriate drugs and dosages for each individual patient.

REFERENCES

1. Fang MC, Chen J, Rich MW. Atrial fibrillation in the elderly. Am J Med 2007;120: 481–7.
2. Wolf PA, Abbott RD, Kannel WB. Atrial fibrillation as an independent risk factor for stroke: the Framingham study. Stroke 1991;22:983–8.
3. Moore KL, Boscardin WJ, Steinman MA, et al. Age and sex variation in prevalence of chronic medical conditions in older residents of U.S. nursing homes. J Am Geriatr Soc 2012;60:756–64.
4. Roger VL, Go AS, Lloyd-Jones DM, et al. Heart disease and stroke statistics - 2011 update: a report from the American Heart Association. Circulation 2011; 123:e18–209.
5. Naccarelli GV, Johnston SS, Dalal M, et al. Rates and implications for hospitalization of patients ≥65 years of age with atrial fibrillation/flutter. Am J Cardiol 2012; 109:543–9.
6. Garrey WE. Auricular Fibrillation. Physiol Rev 1924;4:215–50.
7. Nabar A, Rodriguez LM, Timmermans C, et al. Class IC antiarrhythmic drug induced atrial flutter: electrocardiographic and electrophysiological findings and their importance for long term outcome after right atrial isthmus ablation. Heart 2001;85:424–9.
8. Walters TE, Kistler PM, Kalman JM. Radiofrequency ablation for atrial tachycardia and atrial flutter. Heart Lung Circ 2012;21:386–94.
9. Anastasio N, Frankel DS, Deyell MW, et al. Nearly uniform failure of atrial flutter ablation and continuation of antiarrhythmic agents (hybrid therapy) for the long-term control of atrial fibrillation. J Interv Card Electrophysiol 2012. http://dx.doi.org/10.1007/s10840-012-9679-0.
10. Chinitz JS, Gerstenfeld EP, Marchlinski FE, et al. Atrial fibrillation is common after ablation of isolated atrial flutter during long-term follow-up. Heart Rhythm 2007;4: 1029–33.
11. Hjalmarson A, Elmfeldt D, Herlitz J, et al. Effect on mortality of metoprolol in acute myocardial infarction. A double-blind randomised trial. Lancet 1981;2:823–7.
12. Connolly SJ, Cybulsky I, Lamy A, et al. Double-blind, placebo-controlled, randomized trial of prophylactic metoprolol for reduction of hospital length of stay after heart surgery: the beta-Blocker Length Of Stay (BLOS) study. Am Heart J 2003;145:226–32.
13. Priebe HJ. The aged cardiovascular risk patient. Br J Anaesth 2000;85:763–78.
14. Parvez B, Chopra N, Rowan S, et al. A common β1-adrenergic receptor polymorphism predicts favorable response to rate-control therapy in atrial fibrillation. J Am Coll Cardiol 2012;59:49–56.
15. Intravenous digoxin in acute atrial fibrillation: results of a randomized, placebo-controlled multicentre trial in 239 patients. Eur Heart J 1997;18:649–54.
16. Roberts SA, Diaz C, Nolan PE, et al. Effectiveness and cost of digoxin treatment for atrial fibrillation and flutter. Am J Cardiol 1993;72:567–73.

17. Farshi R, Kistner D, Sarma JS, et al. Ventricular rate control in chronic atrial fibrillation during daily activity and programmed exercise: a crossover open-label study of five drug regimens. J Am Coll Cardiol 1999;33:304–10.

18. Fuster V, RYden LE, Cannom DS, et al. ACC/AHA/ESC 2006 Guidelines for the management of patients with atrial fibrillation. Circulation 2006;114:e257–354.

19. Nagarakanti R, Ezekowitz MD, Oldgren J, et al. Dabigatran versus warfarin in patients with atrial fibrillation: an analysis of patients undergoing cardioversion. Circulation 2011;123:131–6.

20. Campbell TJ, Williams KM. Therapeutic drug monitoring: antiarrhythmic drugs. Br J Clin Pharmacol 1998;46:307–19.

21. Coplen SE, Antman EM, Berlin JA, et al. Efficacy and safety of quinidine therapy for maintenance of sinus rhythm after cardioversion. A meta-analysis of randomized control trials. Circulation 1991;82:1106–16.

22. Volgman AS, Carberry PA, Stambler B, et al. Conversion efficacy and safety of intravenous ibutilide compared with intravenous procainamide in patients with atrial flutter or fibrillation. J Am Coll Cardiol 1998;31:1414–9.

23. Echt DS, Liebson PR, Mitchell LB, et al. The cardiac arrhythmia suppression trial. N Engl J Med 1991;324:781–8.

24. Chou WH, Yan FX, Robbins-Weilert DK, et al. Comparison of two CYP2D6 genotyping methods and assessment of genotype-phenotype relationships. Clin Chem 2003;49:542–51.

25. Waldo AL, Camm AJ, deRuyter H, et al. Effect of d-sotalol on mortality in patients with left ventricular dysfunction after recent and remote myocardial infarction. The SWORD Investigators. Survival With Oral d-Sotalol. Lancet 1996;348:7–12.

26. Torp-Pedersen C, Moller M, Block-Thomsen PE, et al. The Danish investigations of arrhythmia and mortality on dofetilide study group: dofetilide in patients with congestive heart failure and left ventricular dysfunction. N Engl J Med 1999; 341:857–65.

27. Pedersen OD, Bagger H, Keller N, et al. Efficacy of dofetilide in the treatment of atrial fibrillation-flutter in patients with reduced left ventricular function. A Danish Investigations of Arrhythmia and Mortality ON Dofetilide (DIAMOND) substudy. Circulation 2001;104:292–6.

28. Roukoz H, Waliba S. Dofetilide: a new class III antiarrhythmic agent. Expert Rev Cardiovasc Ther 2007;5:9–19.

29. Cotter G, Blatt A, Kaluski E, et al. Conversion of recent onset paroxysmal atrial fibrillation to normal sinus rhythm: the effect of no treatment and high-dose amiodarone. A randomized, placebo-controlled study. Eur Heart J 1999;20: 1833–42.

30. Kochiadakis GE, Igoumenidis NE, Parthenakis FI, et al. Amiodarone versus propafenone for conversion of chronic atrial fibrillation: results of a randomized, controlled study. J Am Coll Cardiol 1999;33:966–71.

31. Daoud EG, Strickberger SA, Man KC, et al. Preoperative amiodarone as prophylaxis against atrial fibrillation after heart surgery. N Engl J Med 1997;337:1785–91.

32. Fukuchi H, Nakashima M, Araki R, et al. Effect of obesity on serum amiodarone concentration in Japanese patients: population pharmacokinetic investigation by multiple trough screen analysis. J Clin Pharm Ther 2009;34:329–36.

33. Essebag V, Hadjis T, Platt RW, et al. Amiodarone and the risk of bradyarrhythmia requiring permanent pacemaker in elderly patients with atrial fibrillation and prior myocardial infarction. J Am Coll Cardiol 2003;41:249–54.

34. Cheng JW. New and emerging antiarrhythmic and anticoagulant agents for atrial fibrillation. Am J Health Syst Pharm 2010;67(Suppl 5):S26–34.

35. Singh BN, Connolly SJ, Crijns HJ, et al. Dronedarone for maintenance of sinus rhythm in atrial fibrillation or flutter. N Engl J Med 2007;357:987–99.
36. Le Heuzey JY, De Ferrari GM, Radzik D, et al. A short-term, randomized, double-blind, parallel-group study to evaluate the efficacy and safety of dronedarone versus amiodarone in patients with persistent atrial fibrillation: the DIONYSOS study. J Cardiovasc Electrophysiol 2010;21:597–605.
37. Hohnloser SH, Crijns HJ, van Eickels M, et al. Effect of dronedarone on cardiovascular events in atrial fibrillation. N Engl J Med 2009;360:668–78.
38. Connelly SJ, Camm AJ, Halperin JL, et al. Dronedarone in high-risk permanent atrial fibrillation. N Engl J Med 2011;365:2268–76.
39. Lober L, Torp-Pedersen C, McMurray JJ, et al. Increased mortality after dronedarone therapy for severe heart failure. N Engl J Med 2008;358:2678–87.
40. Wyse DG, Waldo AL, DiMarco JP, et al. A comparison of rate control and rhythm control in patients with atrial fibrillation. N Engl J Med 2002;347:1825–33.
41. Grönefeld GC, Lilienthal J, Kuck KH, et al. Impact of rate versus rhythm control on quality of life in patients with persistent atrial fibrillation. Eur Heart J 2003;24: 1430–6.
42. Roy D, Talajic M, Nattel S, et al. Rhythm control versus rate control for atrial fibrillation and heart failure. N Engl J Med 2008;358:2667–77.
43. Groenveld HF, Crijns HJ, Van den Berg MP, et al. The effect of rate control on quality of life in patients with permanent atrial fibrillation. Data from the RACE II (Rate Control Efficacy in Permanent Atrial Fibrillation II) study. J Am Coll Cardiol 2011;58:1795–803.
44. Van Gelder IC, Hagens VE, Bosker HA, et al. A comparison of rate control and rhythm control in patients with recurrent persistent atrial fibrillation. N Engl J Med 2002;347:1834–40.
45. Carlsson J, Miketic S, Windeler J, et al. Randomized trial of rate-control versus rhythm control in persistent atrial fibrillation. The Strategies of Treatment of Atrial Fibrillation (STAF) study. J Am Coll Cardiol 2003;41:1690–6.
46. Opolski G, Torbicki A, Kosior DA, et al. Rate control vs rhythm control in patients with nonvalvular persistent atrial fibrillation: the results of the Polish How to Treat Chronic Atrial Fibrillation (HOT CAFE) study. Chest 2004;126:476–86.

Atrial Fibrillation and Atrial Flutter: Nonpharmacologic Therapy

David L. Johnson, MS, PAC[a], John D. Day, MD[a], John R. Doty, MD[b], T. Jared Bunch, MD[a],*

KEYWORDS

- Atrial fibrillation • Atrial flutter • Catheter ablation • Rhythm control

KEY POINTS

- As elderly patients present significant challenges for long-term pharmacologic management, nonpharmacologic approaches will continue to be a vital option for clinicians to improve the quality of life and function of these patients.
- For rhythm control, observational studies of catheter ablation suggest similar long-term efficacy and safety rates in elderly and very elderly populations in comparison with younger groups.
- Minimally invasive surgical approaches have distinct advantages in certain populations, but require further study in the elderly to define and understand the potential benefits and risks in comparison with younger patients.

Atrial fibrillation (AF) is the most common cardiac arrhythmia encountered clinically, and affects more than 2 million people in the United States alone.[1] With advances in medicine, patients are living longer with diseases such as cardiovascular disease. Enhanced longevity with cardiovascular disease is one of the suspected mechanisms behind the increase in the prevalence of AF (0.1% <55 years to 9.0% >80 years).[2] Statistics have shown that the median age of patients with AF is 75 years, and 70% of the AF patients are 65 to 85 years old.[2,3] Unfortunately for health care providers, the number of individuals who have AF is only going to increase. It is expected that in the next 20 to 30 years, as the Western population ages, the number of people with AF will double or triple.[2,4]

AF management in the elderly can present unique challenges. These challenges stem from concurrent cardiovascular diseases and physiologic changes secondary to age, which make these patients more susceptible to drug toxicities and interactions.[5] In addition, elderly patients are frequently using numerous medications to improve their health and longevity, resulting in a myriad of potential drug-to-drug

[a] Intermountain Heart Institute, Department of Cardiology, Intermountain Medical Center, Murray, UT, USA; [b] Intermountain Heart Institute, Department of Cardiovascular Surgery, Murray, UT, USA
* Corresponding author. Intermountain Medical Center, Eccles Outpatient Care Center, 5169 Cottonwood Street, Suite 510, Murray, UT.
E-mail address: Thomas.bunch@imail.org

Clin Geriatr Med 28 (2012) 649–663
http://dx.doi.org/10.1016/j.cger.2012.07.004
0749-0690/12/$ – see front matter © 2012 Elsevier Inc. All rights reserved.

geriatric.theclinics.com

interactions that can minimize medication effects and potentially expose patients to harm.[5] Such challenges underlie need to explore and refine all treatment strategies in the elderly, particularly those not based on long-term medication dependency.

Across all age strata, but particularly in the elderly, the optimal timing of a treatment approach, as well as the approach in general for AF, continues to evolve. Often a patient's age and objective frailty come into the decision-making process, particularly in decisions involving invasive and noninvasive options. Furthermore, the extent of an invasive procedure may also have been minimized in the elderly to avoid a perceived risk of higher complications. The challenge with a therapy-decision construct of avoiding more aggressive or invasive procedures in the elderly is that it typically is not based on evidence or potential benefit, but more on anticipated or perceived risk. At a minimum, a careful age-based review of the true benefits and risks of invasive procedures is essential in understanding their place and relevance in the care of an aging population.

In the treatment of AF, 3 primary concepts are essential: (1) to minimize risk of thromboembolism, (2) to reduce cardiovascular morbidity such as heart failure, and (3) to improve quality of life and symptoms. To this extent this review discusses the nonpharmacologic treatment options for AF in the elderly, in particular atrioventricular (AV) node ablation and pacemaker implantation, catheter ablation, and surgical Maze procedures.

When choosing a treatment strategy, the ability of the strategy to reduce symptoms and cardiovascular morbidity must be weighed against the relative risk and burden imposed by the approach. There is significant variability in response, and treatment approaches must be considered dynamically as disease processes advance and evolve.

RATE CONTROL

In most patients, rate-control medications become the first line of approach. The relative use of these agents increases as the AF disease progresses from paroxysmal to persistent/long-standing persistent, and with advancing age.[6]

Rate control is a preferable option in many patients based on the results of the AFFIRM and RACE trials, which not only showed equivalence in outcomes compared with those treated with rhythm options, but actually revealed trends toward benefit with rate control.[7,8] A meta-analysis of 5 rate-control trials confirmed a trend toward a reduction in total mortality with rate control in comparison with rhythm control (13.0% vs 14.6%, odds ratio 0.87, 95% confidence interval [CI] 0.74–1.02).[9] This outcome was not totally unexpected, as the AFFIRM study accounted for 77% of the patients. Unfortunately, the very elderly are often underrepresented in these clinical trials. Nonetheless, rate-control strategies are often chosen in the elderly, owing to the potential of proarrhythmia from rhythm-control drugs and more advanced AF subtypes.[10]

Radiofrequency (RF) ablation of the AV node and/or the His bundle is the most common form of nonpharmacologic rate control. Because of the invasive nature of the procedure and the requirement for permanent pacemaker implantation, this treatment is reserved for patients in whom pharmacologic rate-control therapy is either unsuccessful or not tolerated.[11,12] In looking at these patients in aggregate, patients reported an enhanced quality of life after AV node ablation.[13–16] In addition to improvement in quality-of-life scores, patients with AV node ablation report fewer physician visits, hospital admissions, and heart-failure episodes, and a general improvement in ejection fraction.[13,16] Unlike the aggregate data from the rhythm versus rate-control studies, there does not appear to be a clear mortality advantage in AV node ablation and pacemaker implantation. In a study of 350 patients, 3-year survival rates after AV node ablation and pacemaker implantation and that with pharmacologic therapy for rate control were similar, and the same as the expected survival in the general population.[14]

The majority of patients do well after AV node ablation with standard right ventricular pacing. However, right ventricular pacing causes electrical and mechanical dyssynchrony, which in some patients can impair left ventricular function, increase mortality, and reduce function.[17] In patients who experience such a cardiovascular decline, adding an additional lead to pace the left ventricle (cardiac resynchronization therapy) can improve the outcome and largely reverse the negative impact of right ventricular pacing alone.[18,19] Although there are no trials that specifically look for a potential benefit or detriment to this strategy in the elderly, when patients are followed long term the risk of heart failure after AV node ablation with standard right ventricular pacing becomes significant, and advanced age appears to increase the risk. For example, in a study of 213 patients with follow-up on average of 6 years, 13% developed new heart failure. The 2 risk factors for new or aggravated heart failure were a low ejection fraction and age.[20] From the cardiac resynchronization trials one can expect elderly patients to respond to biventricular pacing, similar to younger patients. In a substudy of MADIT CRT (Multicenter Automatic Defibrillator Implantation Trial—Cardiac Resynchronization Therapy), patients were stratified into 3 age-based groups: patients younger than 60 years (n = 548), age 60 to 74 years (n = 941) and older than 75 years (n = 331). The 3 age cohorts with cardiac resynchronization therapy showed a significant reduction in left ventricular end-systolic volume and end-diastolic volume, left atrial volume, and an increase in left ventricular ejection fraction at 1 year in comparison with the baseline echocardiogram.[21]

RHYTHM CONTROL
Catheter-Based Radiofrequency Ablation

RF catheter ablation has been shown to be effective in eliminating or significantly reducing AF. In a recent worldwide survey that comprised a wide variety of select patients, 10,488 of 16,309 (64%) patients after catheter ablation for AF had no clinical AF (ie, asymptomatic) without the need of an antiarrhythmic drug at their last follow-up. Another 2047 (13%) were without clinical AF with the use of a previously ineffective antiarrhythmic drug. AF subtype influenced outcomes in this analysis, with success rates free of antiarrhythmic drugs in patients with paroxysmal AF of 69%, persistent AF of 59%, and long-lasting persistent AF of 60%. Major complications were reported in 741 patients (4.5%). These complications included: 25 (0.15%) procedure-related deaths, 37 (0.23%) strokes, 115 (0.71%) transient ischemic attacks, 213 (1.3%) episodes of tamponade. and 48 (0.29%) patients who received intervention for severe pulmonary vein stenosis.[22]

Fortunately, as RF ablation has become more commonplace in the management of AF, its use has been expanded to broader groups. As such, one can glean a broad understanding of the efficacy and safety of the therapeutic approach. Inclusive in this expansion to new patient populations of RF ablation for AF is the use of therapy in elderly and very elderly populations. **Table 1** shows the outcomes and complications in 3 studies that examined the use of catheter ablation for AF in octogenarians. In aggregate, the success rates from 1 to 2 years ranged between 69% and 78%, with the lower success rates found as the follow-up times increased. Total complications were relatively rare, occurring in 9 of 175 patients included in these studies (incidence: 5.1%). As already mentioned, this complication rate is similar to that reported in the worldwide survey and, more importantly, the complication rates were similar to those in the younger comparative cohorts from each reporting center.[23–25]

These data are similar to those collected in a slightly younger population of patients 75 years or older (average: 77 ± 6 years). In this study of 174 consecutive patients,[26]

Table 1
Outcomes after catheter ablation for symptomatic AF in patients older than 80 years

Study	Patients >80 y	Outcome	Complications	Comparison with Younger Patients
Bunch et al,[23] 2010	35 of 752	1-y survival free of AF without drugs: 78%	Tamponade (1), deep venous thrombosis (1), urinary tract infection (1)	No difference in success rates or complications (>80, <80 y)
Santangeli et al,[24] 2012	103 of 2754	Survival free of AF without drugs (18 ± 6 mo): 69%	Pericardial effusion (1), minor bleeding (3)	No difference in success rates or complications (>80, <80 y)
Tan et al,[25] 2010	37 of 377	Survival free of AF without drugs (mean 18 mo): 70%	Retroperitoneal bleed (1), deep venous thrombosis (1), large hematoma (1)	No difference in success rates or complications between 3 age cohorts (>80, 79–70, 69–60 y)

127 (73%) maintained sinus rhythm after a single procedure over a mean follow-up 20 ± 14 months. Major acute complications included 1 stroke and 1 hemothorax.

These data in elderly patients were largely collected from high-volume centers and may not fully approximate those obtained in low-volume centers and/or with low-volume operators. Furthermore, elderly patients may experience unique complications that are not necessarily collected during routine follow-up care after an ablation. For example, the authors found that hospital stay was longer in older patients (2.9 ± 7.7 vs 2.1 ± 1.1 days, P = .001). The primary reason for the extra day of hospitalization was for fluid management and heart failure. Also noted was a nonsignificant trend toward a higher risk (hazard ratio 3.62, P = .13) of urinary tract infections in the older group.[23] To truly understand the risk and benefits of catheter ablation in the elderly, additional end points such as recovery from anesthesia, the influence of polypharmacy, rehabilitation, and functional status need to be collected prospectively and reported. It is likely that multiple variables lead to a higher risk of rehospitalization at 30 days that was age-dependent in 4156 patients who underwent their first ablation and were included in the California State Inpatient Database (**Fig. 1**).[27]

Given the challenges with fluid retention, longer hospital stays, and higher admission rates in the elderly, the question naturally arises as to whether the ablation approach should be altered to minimize periprocedural morbidity (**Fig. 2**). Although reducing the extent of ablation decreases catheter manipulation and intravenous/catheter-based fluid administration, it may also negatively affect elderly patients who often present with more coexistent heart disease and more advanced subtypes of AF. Modification of ablation strategy coupled with more advanced AF disease may underlie why Tan and colleagues[25] found a greater need for repeat procedures and long-term requirement of antiarrhythmic medications in older patients than in younger patients.

The authors previously examined the question of age-based risk relative to the aggressiveness of the ablation performed.[28] To understand this risk, 2 catheter ablation approaches were compared: wide-area circumferential ablation (WACA) and a more aggressive approach of WACA plus additional linear lines in the left atrium

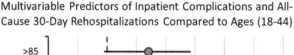

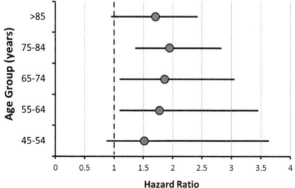

Fig. 1. Multivariate adjusted odds ratios for inpatient complications and 30-day rehospitalization based on age-separated strata. In general, there was a trend toward increasing risk with advancing age. (*Adapted from* Shah RU, Freeman JV, Shilane D, et al. Procedural complications, rehospitalizations, and repeat procedures after catheter ablation for atrial fibrillation. J Am Coll Cardiol 2012;59(2):143–9.)

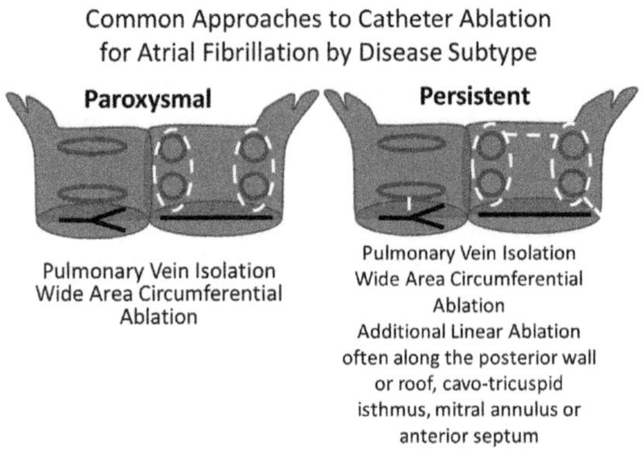

Common Approaches to Catheter Ablation
for Atrial Fibrillation by Disease Subtype

Paroxysmal

Persistent

Pulmonary Vein Isolation
Wide Area Circumferential
Ablation

Pulmonary Vein Isolation
Wide Area Circumferential
Ablation
Additional Linear Ablation
often along the posterior wall
or roof, cavo-tricuspid
isthmus, mitral annulus or
anterior septum

Fig. 2. Common catheter-ablation approaches for paroxysmal versus persistent/long-standing persistent atrial fibrillation (AF). In patients with paroxysmal AF, typically pulmonary vein isolation is performed in isolation using a wide-area circumferential approach. In patients with more advanced AF subtypes, additional linear ablation in the right and left atrium is often required.

(WACA-L). The results were then compared based on procedure type between 3 age categories; younger than 50, 50 to 75, older than 75 years. As suspected, patients with paroxysmal AF only were more likely to receive a WACA than a WACA-L (88.1% vs 47.7%, P<.0001). WACA-L patients were more likely to have congestive heart failure (40.9% vs 19.4%, P<.0001). Across all age groups, the 1-year survival rates free of AF were 82.9% (WACA) and 81.8% (WACA-L) (P = .52). There was no difference in 1-year survival free of AF rates based on ablative procedure type across all age groups (**Fig. 3**). However, the largest age-based difference based on procedure type was seen in the oldest group studied, where the WACA-L patients actually did better and had rates very similar to the younger groups. At a minimum, these single-center study data suggest that age alone should not be used to determine ablation strategy, but rather the extent of coexistent disease and AF subtype.[28] As important in this study was that when comparing WACA-L with WACA, no association was found to suggest an increased risk of periprocedural or long-term complications.

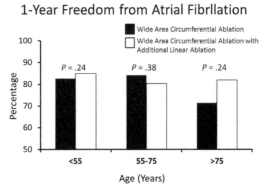

Fig. 3. Success rates of 1-year freedom from AF based on age and ablation strategy. Overall success rates were similar across all age groups and treatment approaches. There was a trend toward better outcomes in the elderly group when a more aggressive AF strategy was used.

All these studies in aggregate suggest that significant periprocedural complications, such as stroke, heart failure, and mortality, are not increased in elderly patients undergoing ablation in comparison with younger counterparts during the follow-up periods. An interesting and important finding reported by Santangeli and colleagues[24] was that they were able to discontinue warfarin anticoagulation in 49 of 71 (69%) octogenarian patients, this despite 66% of this population having a CHADS$_2$ score of at least 2. The primary reason cited by the investigators for continuing warfarin was left atrial appendage isolation during the procedure in 22 patients. Despite this strategy, the investigators did not observe any cerebral ischemic events in the older cohort. These data are vital in understanding the dynamic treatment of elderly patients after ablation over time, as they may encounter increased comorbidities and/or fall risks that increase their risk of significant bleeding on long-term anticoagulation.

In summary, there are accumulating data suggesting that catheter-based AF ablation among elderly patients confers similar clinical benefit to that among younger patients.

However, these data in the elderly are limited to retrospective subgroup analyses in small numbers of elderly patients, and as such should be interpreted with a degree of caution until larger prospective trials become available.

Unique Challenges in the Elderly

There are unique challenges in performing ablation in the elderly. For example, osteoporosis is a common disease stemming from low bone mass with microarchitectural disruption, resulting in skeletal fragility and fracture risk. This process can result in marked chest-wall deformities, and often leads to a unilateral cephalization of the pulmonary veins (**Fig. 4**). Cephalad-oriented pulmonary veins can present a challenge in isolation of pulmonary veins because a transseptal ablation approach orients the tools to a lateral position. Also, cephalad-oriented veins can approximate the esophagus, which further impairs an operator's ability to fully isolate them. In addition, chest-wall deformities can lead to difficulties in recovery of respiratory function in patients who undergo general anesthesia, and can place patients at risk for poor secretion clearance and pneumonia.

Similarly, esophageal disorders are more common in the elderly. In particular, disorders such as esophageal dilatation from dysmotility and a hiatal hernia can expose large regions of the esophagus to thermal injury during posterior left atrial ablation (**Fig. 5**). In a large meta-analysis, the risk of a hiatal hernia increased significantly in patients older than 50 years (odds ratio 2.17, 95% CI 1.35–3.51, $P = .001$).[29] Furthermore, multiple aspects of gastroesophageal reflex disease and esophageal dysmotility are more common with aging.[30]

Surgical Approaches for Atrial Fibrillation

Predating catheter-based approaches were surgical therapies for AF. Early work in catheter ablation was patterned after the proven surgical approaches. The standard surgical approach was developed in 1990 and the final iteration is known as the Cox Maze III operation.[31–33] This operation and its variations aim to surgically create a "maze" of functional myocardium within the atrium, which allows for propagation of atrial depolarization but reduces the likelihood of wave fronts responsible for microreentry. These procedures have evolved to minimize the chronotropic intolerance and atrial transport, and reduce procedural times. Although most postsurgical studies have limited cardiac monitoring follow-up, one series reported 197 patients with an actuarial freedom from AF rate of 89.3% at 10 years.[34]

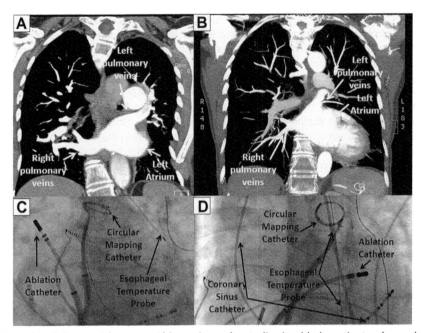

Fig. 4. (*A, B*) Computed tomographic angiography studies in elderly patients who underwent catheter ablation. In both patients, skeletal abnormalities from degenerative joint disease and osteoporosis result in anatomic variation of the atrial and pulmonary vein positions with a cephalad orientation of the left-sided pulmonary veins. (*C*) Left anterior oblique fluoroscopic image demonstrating a cephalad pulmonary vein that was ultimately isolated electrically. (*D*) Left anterior oblique fluoroscopy image with a cephalad left superior pulmonary vein whose course was immediately parallel to the esophagus, which prohibited the ability to perform radiofrequency ablation along the posterior aspect of that vein.

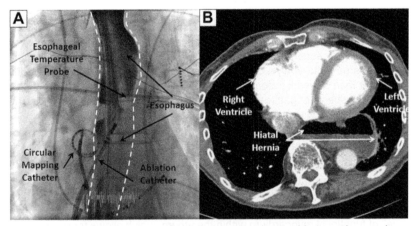

Fig. 5. (*A*) Barium esophagram performed during catheter ablation. The esophagus is moderately dilated (projected course marked by the white lines) along the complete aspect of the posterior left atrium. (*B*) Computed tomography study (axial image) reveals a massive hiatal hernia that spanned completely along the posterior left atrium, and which severely affected the ablation procedure because of inability to perform radiofrequency ablation along the posterior wall.

The standard Maze procedure requires multiple atrial incisions that are sewn back together to create linear scars, and has therefore not been widely adopted. Various modifications have been developed that primarily use RF or cryoablation to create the lesion set. These modified Maze procedures are more rapid and less technically demanding. The use of alternative energy sources also allows for minimally invasive approaches that do not require sternotomy.[35–38] Success rates of short-term arrhythmia control with minimally invasive surgical ablation vary widely, but are generally lie between those of catheter-based procedures and standard "cut-and-sew" Maze operations.[39,40]

Although endocardial catheter-based approaches offer advantages regarding recovery and invasiveness, there are several potential advantages with minimally invasive surgical ablation that are applicable to an elderly population. Such advantages include removal or ligation of the left atrial appendage, a reduced risk of phrenic nerve and esophageal injury, and a lower risk of intracardiac thrombus formation and subsequent thromboembolism. In addition, the surgical approach allows for direct identification and elimination of epicardial sources of arrhythmogenesis, such as autonomic ganglia.

Similar to catheter-based approaches, there are small observational studies describing surgical ablation outcomes in elderly and very elderly patients in comparison with their younger counterparts. In one study, 28 octogenarians who underwent a concomitant Maze procedure at the time of another cardiac surgery were compared with 172 younger patients.[41] In the octogenarian group, the postoperative rates of renal failure (17.8% vs 7.0%, $P = .05$) and sepsis (10.7% vs 2.3%, $P = .025$) were higher and the hospital stay longer (20 ± 24 vs 14 ± 31 days, $P = .004$). Over a follow-up of 12 ± 6 months, recurrence of AF was similar between the older and younger groups (11.8% vs 26.3%, $P = .187$). No strokes were recorded in either group. Mortality was higher in the octogenarians than in the younger group (16.7% vs 6.1%, $P = .065$). Although these event rates are higher than those for catheter-based ablation, the subjects were sicker patients who underwent cardiac surgery with a concomitant Maze procedure. As with other studies of complex cardiac surgery, the addition of surgical ablation to other cardiac operations can substantially increase the risk profile for an elderly patient.

At present, there are no age-based comparative data with minimally invasive surgical ablative procedures. In a systematic review of such procedures with a focus on outcomes and patient selection, the mean age of patients in published reports of the minimally invasive Maze procedure is 61 ± 2.9 years. This mean age is similar to catheter-based outcomes data, particularly as reports have expanded to older populations. The aggregate procedural complication rate is 7.7% after a minimally invasive surgical ablation, which is slightly higher than that for catheter ablation. However, serious complications such as stroke, tamponade, and atrioesophageal fistula are all lower in comparison with catheter ablation.[42]

Nonpharmacologic Stroke Prevention

Age, in particular older than 75 years, is in the CHADS$_2$ rule as a major risk factor of stroke in patients with AF. At the same time, age is a consistent reason reported by physicians that deters use of warfarin in elderly patients with AF. Physician surveys have consistently cited patient age as a deterrent to the use of warfarin in AF.[43] Although age is a blanket concern, it reflects a complex clinical scenario that includes fragility, falls, poor compliance, cognitive decline, polypharmacy, prior bleed, and comorbid diseases that affect drug metabolism and clearance.[44,45] However, these fears of age-based risk of bleed are not unfounded. Multiple bleeding-risk scores include age as a clinical variable associated with risk. For example, the HAS-BLED score contains hypertension, liver or renal failure, stroke, bleeding, labile international normalized ratios, elderly, and drugs/alcohol as risk factors.[46] Similarly, the HEMOR-R2HAGES risk index contains 11 variables to determine risk, of which one is an age older than 75.[46]

There are new and exciting nonpharmacologic approaches to prevent thromboembolism in patients with AF. These approaches are particularly important to consider in elderly patients who have a higher risks of anticoagulation-related adverse events. Surgical ligation of the left atrial appendage remains an important advantage to surgical approaches to AF. Recently, this approach has become available through a transcutaneous approach. With this system (**Fig. 6**), a standard percutaneous epicardial access is performed. Magnet-based guide wires are advanced into the left atrium and appendage, through a transseptal approach, and also through the epicardium. These magnets adhere to each other. Over the endocardial wire a balloon is inflated in the left atrial appendage. Over the epicardial wire, a lariat-shaped surgical ligation is advanced over the balloon and then synched down. Both the endocardial and epicardial systems are then removed, leaving in place the suture that occludes the appendage.

There are many catheter-based endocardial systems. Highlighted here is the one with the most comprehensive data to date. The Watchman device (Atritech, Minneapolis, MN) (see **Fig. 6**) involves an expandable system deployed in the left atrial appendage via a transseptal catheter. The implanted device has a self-expanding nitinol frame that secures it in the appendage. In the PROTECT AF trial of more than 700 patients with nonvalvular AF, randomly assigned in a 2:1 ratio to either the device or to long-term warfarin, the device was shown not to be inferior to warfarin. The composite primary efficacy end point was stroke, cardiovascular death, and systemic embolism. This event rate was similar in the Watchman group and the warfarin group (3.0 vs 4.9 events per 100 patient-years). However, the primary safety end point, which was a composite of major bleeding, pericardial effusion, procedure-related stroke, and device embolization, was more common in the Watchman group than in the warfarin group (7.4 vs 4.4 events per 100 patient-years).[47] The majority of the adverse

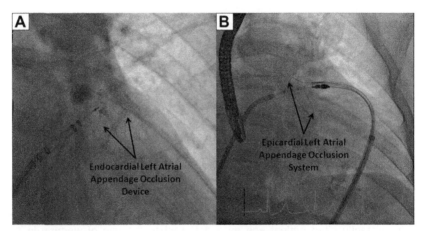

Fig. 6. (A) Endocardial placement of a left atrial appendage closure device (Watchman Device). There is a small amount of residual contrast noted above the device, which is on the tip of the occluded appendage. (B) A transseptally placed endocardial wire is magnetically attached to an epicardially placed wire. Over the epicardial wire a lariat-shaped suture is advanced over the appendage; this will ultimately be synched down to occlude the appendage.

events were related to pericardial effusions, a complication that improved dramatically with procedural experience.[48] As the use of these devices expands to sicker populations, clinicians will be able to glean an understanding of their utility in the elderly and very elderly populations. It is possible that nonpharmacologic approaches to stroke prevention may ultimately create a new paradigm for AF care in all patients, especially the elderly.

Patient Selection for Ablation

Although this review reports that nonpharmacologic therapies in the elderly have similar safety and efficacy rates as those achieved in younger patient groups, these outcomes need to be viewed in the context that the elderly cohorts were likely a "select" group. In other words, these patients were deemed candidates for a nonpharmacologic approach by a heart rhythm specialist as well as the referring cardiologist or primary care physician. Also, the outcomes were achieved in centers that perform a high volume of procedures, a characteristic that influences both efficacy and safety. With regard to AF, these were elderly patients who could receive general anesthesia, high doses of periprocedural anticoagulation, and cardiac stimulants such as isoproterenol and/or cardiac inotropes. Although typical atrial flutter is less invasive and requires access to the right atrium only, it still requires the need of anesthesia, anticoagulation, and, if a complete electrophysiology study is performed, exposure to cardiac stimulants.

The recent Heart Rhythm Society/European Heart Rhythm Association/European Cardiac Arrhythmia Society Expert consensus statement on catheter and surgical ablation of AF recommended an approach for patient selection based on baseline characteristics. These considerations include a patient's age, the left atrial size, especially the extent of left atrial enlargement, and the duration of AF. In particular, the expert consensus said that in the very elderly there is a higher risk of cardiac perforation and myocardial infarction.[49] There is a clear risk of perforation with age in patients who undergo placement of a permanent pacemaker, which is often performed at the time of AV node ablation.[50] There has not been a clear association between age and risk of perforation during catheter ablation, although this remains a pervasive hypothetical risk. Certainly the risk of periprocedural myocardial infarction is related to the coexistence of cardiovascular comorbidities, which increase with age. These comorbidities need to be considered in all patients who undergo procedures whereby general anesthesia and/or the need of cardiac stimulants are required.

The authors advocate that the very elderly are considered potential candidates for catheter ablation if they can undergo general anesthesia, receive high doses of anticoagulation and cardiac stimulants and/or inotropic agents, and be referred to center and operator that has high-volume experience in managing these types of patients. In patients who are not good candidates based on these criteria, other options can be considered: an ablation of right atrial flutter if this is dominant rhythm and then use of an antiarrhythmic drug for the AF; AV node ablation and pacemaker placement; or long-term antiarrhythmic drug therapy or rate-control therapy. If the risks and benefits are unclear, a referral can be made to discuss the risks and benefits of each option with an experienced heart rhythm specialist, with a subsequent conference call between this individual and the referring physician to formulate the best plan.

SUMMARY

The elderly population is growing and living longer with cardiac disease. These population-based trends provide a fertile environment for an ever-growing incidence of AF. As elderly patients present significant challenges for long-term pharmacologic management, nonpharmacologic approaches will continue to be a vital option for clinicians to improve the quality of life and function of these patients. For rhythm control, observational studies of catheter ablation suggest similar long-term efficacy and safety rates in elderly and very elderly populations as for younger groups. Minimally invasive surgical approaches have distinct advantages in certain populations, but require further study in the elderly to define and understand the potential benefits and risks in comparison with younger patients. Further research in prospective clinical trials, adequately powered to assess age-related differences, is needed to confirm the findings of observational studies in elderly patients who have undergone nonpharmacologic rhythm-control procedures.

REFERENCES

1. Lloyd-Jones D, Adams R, Carnethon M, et al. Heart disease and stroke statistics—2009 update: a report from the American Heart Association Statistics Committee and Stroke Statistics Subcommittee. Circulation 2009;119(3):e21–181.
2. Go AS, Hylek EM, Phillips KA, et al. Prevalence of diagnosed atrial fibrillation in adults: national implications for rhythm management and stroke prevention: the AnTicoagulation and Risk Factors in Atrial Fibrillation (ATRIA) Study. JAMA 2001;285(18):2370–5.
3. Feinberg WM, Blackshear JL, Laupacis A, et al. Prevalence, age distribution, and gender of patients with atrial fibrillation. Analysis and implications. Arch Intern Med 1995;155(5):469–73.
4. Miyasaka Y, Barnes ME, Gersh BJ, et al. Secular trends in incidence of atrial fibrillation in Olmsted County, Minnesota, 1980 to 2000, and implications on the projections for future prevalence. Circulation 2006;114(2):119–25.
5. Chatap G, Giraud K, Vincent JP. Atrial fibrillation in the elderly: facts and management. Drugs Aging 2002;19(11):819–46.
6. McNamara RL, Tamariz LJ, Segal JB, et al. Management of atrial fibrillation: review of the evidence for the role of pharmacologic therapy, electrical cardioversion, and echocardiography. Ann Intern Med 2003;139(12):1018–33.
7. Van Gelder IC, Hagens VE, Bosker HA, et al. A comparison of rate control and rhythm control in patients with recurrent persistent atrial fibrillation. N Engl J Med 2002;347(23):1834–40.
8. Wyse DG, Waldo AL, DiMarco JP, et al. A comparison of rate control and rhythm control in patients with atrial fibrillation. N Engl J Med 2002;347(23):1825–33.
9. de Denus S, Sanoski CA, Carlsson J, et al. Rate vs rhythm control in patients with atrial fibrillation: a meta-analysis. Arch Intern Med 2005;165(3):258–62.
10. Camm AJ, Kirchhof P, Lip GY, et al. Guidelines for the management of atrial fibrillation: the Task Force for the Management of Atrial Fibrillation of the European Society of Cardiology (ESC). Eur Heart J 2010;31(19):2369–429.
11. Curtis AB, Kutalek SP, Prior M, et al. Prevalence and characteristics of escape rhythms after radiofrequency ablation of the atrioventricular junction: results from the registry for AV junction ablation and pacing in atrial fibrillation. Ablate and Pace Trial Investigators. Am Heart J 2000;139(1 Pt 1):122–5.
12. Rosenquvist M, Lee MA, Moulinier L, et al. Long-term follow-up of patients after transcatheter direct current ablation of the atrioventricular junction. J Am Coll Cardiol 1990;16(6):1467–74.
13. Fitzpatrick AP, Kourouyan HD, Siu A, et al. Quality of life and outcomes after radiofrequency His-bundle catheter ablation and permanent pacemaker

implantation: impact of treatment in paroxysmal and established atrial fibrillation. Am Heart J 1996;131(3):499–507.

14. Ozcan C, Jahangir A, Friedman PA, et al. Long-term survival after ablation of the atrioventricular node and implantation of a permanent pacemaker in patients with atrial fibrillation. N Engl J Med 2001;344(14):1043–51.

15. Weerasooriya R, Davis M, Powell A, et al. The Australian Intervention Randomized Control of Rate in Atrial Fibrillation Trial (AIRCRAFT). J Am Coll Cardiol 2003; 41(10):1697–702.

16. Wood MA, Brown-Mahoney C, Kay GN, et al. Clinical outcomes after ablation and pacing therapy for atrial fibrillation: a meta-analysis. Circulation 2000;101(10):1138–44.

17. Szili-Torok T, Kimman GP, Theuns D, et al. Deterioration of left ventricular function following atrio-ventricular node ablation and right ventricular apical pacing in patients with permanent atrial fibrillation. Europace 2002;4(1):61–5.

18. Orlov MV, Gardin JM, Slawsky M, et al. Biventricular pacing improves cardiac function and prevents further left atrial remodeling in patients with symptomatic atrial fibrillation after atrioventricular node ablation. Am Heart J 2010;159(2): 264–70.

19. Valls-Bertault V, Fatemi M, Gilard M, et al. Assessment of upgrading to biventricular pacing in patients with right ventricular pacing and congestive heart failure after atrioventricular junctional ablation for chronic atrial fibrillation. Europace 2004;6(5):438–43.

20. Poci D, Backman L, Karlsson T, et al. New or aggravated heart failure during long-term right ventricular pacing after AV junctional catheter ablation. Pacing Clin Electrophysiol 2009;32(2):209–16.

21. Penn J, Goldenberg I, Moss AJ, et al. Improved outcome with preventive cardiac resynchronization therapy in the elderly: a MADIT-CRT substudy. J Cardiovasc Electrophysiol 2011;22(8):892–7.

22. Cappato R, Calkins H, Chen SA, et al. Updated worldwide survey on the methods, efficacy, and safety of catheter ablation for human atrial fibrillation. Circ Arrhythm Electrophysiol 2010;3(1):32–8.

23. Bunch TJ, Weiss JP, Crandall BG, et al. Long-term clinical efficacy and risk of catheter ablation for atrial fibrillation in octogenarians. Pacing Clin Electrophysiol 2010;33(2):146–52.

24. Santangeli P, Biase LD, Mohanty P, et al. Catheter Ablation of Atrial Fibrillation in Octogenarians: safety and outcomes. J Cardiovasc Electrophysiol 2012;23(7): 687–93.

25. Tan HW, Wang XH, Shi HF, et al. Efficacy, safety and outcome of catheter ablation for atrial fibrillation in octogenarians. Int J Cardiol 2010;145(1):147–8.

26. Corrado A, Patel D, Riedlbauchova L, et al. Efficacy, safety, and outcome of atrial fibrillation ablation in septuagenarians. J Cardiovasc Electrophysiol 2008;19(8): 807–11.

27. Shah RU, Freeman JV, Shilane D, et al. Procedural complications, rehospitalizations, and repeat procedures after catheter ablation for atrial fibrillation. J Am Coll Cardiol 2012;59(2):143–9.

28. Lim T, Day JD, Weiss JP, et al. More Aggressive Left Atrial Ablation in Elderly Patients does not Increase Procedural Complications and Favorably Impacts Outcomes. J Innovations Card Rhythm Manag 2011;2:206–11.

29. Menon S, Trudgill N. Risk factors in the aetiology of hiatus hernia: a meta-analysis. Eur J Gastroenterol Hepatol 2011;23(2):133–8.

30. Greenwald DA. Aging, the gastrointestinal tract, and risk of acid-related disease. Am J Med 2004;117(Suppl 5A):8S–13S.

31. Cox JL, Boineau JP, Schuessler RB, et al. Five-year experience with the maze procedure for atrial fibrillation. Ann Thorac Surg 1993;56(4):814–23 [discussion: 23–4].

32. Cox JL, Canavan TE, Schuessler RB, et al. The surgical treatment of atrial fibrillation. II. Intraoperative electrophysiologic mapping and description of the electrophysiologic basis of atrial flutter and atrial fibrillation. J Thorac Cardiovasc Surg 1991;101(3):406–26.

33. Cox JL, Jaquiss RD, Schuessler RB, et al. Modification of the maze procedure for atrial flutter and atrial fibrillation. II. Surgical technique of the maze III procedure. J Thorac Cardiovasc Surg 1995;110(2):485–95.

34. Gaynor SL, Schuessler RB, Bailey MS, et al. Surgical treatment of atrial fibrillation: predictors of late recurrence. J Thorac Cardiovasc Surg 2005;129(1):104–11.

35. Gaita F, Riccardi R, Caponi D, et al. Linear cryoablation of the left atrium versus pulmonary vein cryoisolation in patients with permanent atrial fibrillation and valvular heart disease: correlation of electroanatomic mapping and long-term clinical results. Circulation 2005;111(2):136–42.

36. Kottkamp H, Hindricks G, Autschbach R, et al. Specific linear left atrial lesions in atrial fibrillation: intraoperative radiofrequency ablation using minimally invasive surgical techniques. J Am Coll Cardiol 2002;40(3):475–80.

37. Melby SJ, Zierer A, Bailey MS, et al. A new era in the surgical treatment of atrial fibrillation: the impact of ablation technology and lesion set on procedural efficacy. Ann Surg 2006;244(4):583–92.

38. Sie HT, Beukema WP, Elvan A, et al. Long-term results of irrigated radiofrequency modified maze procedure in 200 patients with concomitant cardiac surgery: six years experience. Ann Thorac Surg 2004;77(2):512–6.

39. Doty JR, Doty DB, Jones KW, et al. Comparison of standard Maze III and radiofrequency Maze operations for treatment of atrial fibrillation. J Thorac Cardiovasc Surg 2007;133(4):1037–44.

40. Stulak JM, Dearani JA, Sundt TM 3rd, et al. Ablation of atrial fibrillation: comparison of catheter-based techniques and the Cox-Maze III operation. Ann Thorac Surg 2001;91(6):1882–8.

41. Grubitzsch H, Beholz S, Dohmen PM, et al. Concomitant ablation of atrial fibrillation in octogenarians: an observational study. J Cardiothorac Surg 2008;3:21.

42. Han FT, Kasirajan V, Wood MA, et al. Minimally invasive surgical atrial fibrillation ablation: patient selection and results. Heart Rhythm 2009;6(Suppl 12):S71–6.

43. McCrory DC, Matchar DB, Samsa G, et al. Physician attitudes about anticoagulation for nonvalvular atrial fibrillation in the elderly. Arch Intern Med 1995;155(3):277–81.

44. Kutner M, Nixon G, Silverstone F. Physicians' attitudes toward oral anticoagulants and antiplatelet agents for stroke prevention in elderly patients with atrial fibrillation. Arch Intern Med 1991;151(10):1950–3.

45. Man-Son-Hing M, Laupacis A. Anticoagulant-related bleeding in older persons with atrial fibrillation: physicians' fears often unfounded. Arch Intern Med 2003;163(13):1580–6.

46. Olesen JB, Lip GY, Hansen PR, et al. Bleeding risk in 'real world' patients with atrial fibrillation: comparison of two established bleeding prediction schemes in a nationwide cohort. J Thrombi Haemost 2011;9(8):1460–7.

47. Holmes DR, Reddy VY, Turi ZG, et al. Percutaneous closure of the left atrial appendage versus warfarin therapy for prevention of stroke in patients with atrial fibrillation: a randomised non-inferiority trial. Lancet 2009;374(9689):534–42.

48. Reddy VY, Holmes D, Doshi SK, et al. Safety of percutaneous left atrial appendage closure: results from the Watchman Left Atrial Appendage System

for Embolic Protection in Patients with AF (PROTECT AF) clinical trial and the Continued Access Registry. Circulation 2011;123(4):417–24.

49. Calkins H, Kuck KH, Cappato R, et al. HRS/EHRA/ECAS expert consensus statement on catheter and surgical ablation of atrial fibrillation: recommendations for patient selection, procedural techniques, patient management and follow-up, definitions, endpoints, and research trial design: a report of the Heart Rhythm Society (HRS) Task Force on Catheter and Surgical Ablation of Atrial Fibrillation. Developed in partnership with the European Heart Rhythm Association (EHRA), a registered branch of the European Society of Cardiology (ESC) and the European Cardiac Arrhythmia Society (ECAS); and in collaboration with the American College of Cardiology (ACC), American Heart Association (AHA), the Asia Pacific Heart Rhythm Society (APHRS), and the Society of Thoracic Surgeons (STS). Endorsed by the governing bodies of the American College of Cardiology Foundation, the American Heart Association, the European Cardiac Arrhythmia Society, the European Heart Rhythm Association, the Society of Thoracic Surgeons, the Asia Pacific Heart Rhythm Society, and the Heart Rhythm Society. Heart Rhythm 2012;9(4):632–696.e21.

50. Mahapatra S, Bybee KA, Bunch TJ, et al. Incidence and predictors of cardiac perforation after permanent pacemaker placement. Heart Rhythm 2005;2(9): 907–11.

Ventricular Arrhythmias in the Elderly: Evaluation and Medical Management

Miguel A. Leal, MD*, Michael E. Field, MD, Richard L. Page, MD

KEYWORDS

- Elderly • Ventricular arrhythmias • Evaluation • Management
- Antiarrhythmic therapy • Implantable Cardioverter-Defibrillators (ICDs)

KEY POINTS

- Ventricular tachycardia (VT) is an abnormally fast heart rate (greater than 100 beats per minute) originating from either the right or the left ventricle, presenting as monomorphic (uniform morphology on a surface electrocardiogram) or polymorphic (several different morphologies without a specific pattern).
- *Torsades de pointes* is a specific form of polymorphic VT characterized by a gradual change in the amplitude and twisting of the QRS complexes around the isoelectric line, associated with a prolonged QT interval. The cause may be congenital or acquired. *Torsades* usually terminates spontaneously but frequently recurs and may degenerate into ventricular fibrillation.
- Ventricular fibrillation is an abnormally fast heart rate (usually more than 300 beats per minute) that is almost invariably associated with syncope and potentially sudden death when sustained and characterized by very rapid and disorganized contractions of the ventricular chambers to an extent whereby there is no meaningful cardiac output.
- The causes include myocardial ischemia, abnormal myocardial substrate (previous myocardial infarction; valvular heart disease; infiltrative disorders, such as cardiac amyloidosis, sarcoidosis, hemochromatosis, and so forth), hypoxia, electrolyte abnormalities, drug effect or toxicity, ion channel disorders, and idiopathic (in the absence of structural heart disease or other identified cause).
- The mechanisms include reentry around the anatomic (scar, fibrosis) or functional area of conduction block, abnormal automaticity, and triggered activity.
- Treatment: implantable cardioverter-defibrillator (ICD) placement is indicated in many cases, with or without concomitant antiarrhythmic drug therapy. Pharmacologic treatment may also constitute the main basis of therapy in the case of individuals for whom ICD implantation may not be deemed appropriate or necessary.

Department of Medicine, University of Wisconsin, School of Medicine & Public Health, 600 Highland Avenue, Madison, WI 53792, USA
* Corresponding author.
E-mail address: maleal@medicine.wisc.edu

Clin Geriatr Med 28 (2012) 665–677
http://dx.doi.org/10.1016/j.cger.2012.07.006
0749-0690/12/$ – see front matter Published by Elsevier Inc.

geriatric.theclinics.com

INTRODUCTION

Ventricular arrhythmias are the most common cause of sudden cardiac death (SCD).[1–3] Approximately 50% of deaths related to cardiovascular causes are sudden, and many of these deaths are caused by ventricular tachycardia (VT) and/or ventricular fibrillation (VF).

VT is a wide complex tachycardia (greater than 100 beats per minute) originating from the ventricles. VT can be either monomorphic (**Fig. 1**) or polymorphic (**Fig. 2**), depending on its appearance on surface electrocardiography.

The differential diagnosis for a wide complex tachycardia includes the following:

- Supraventricular tachycardia (SVT)
  - With rate-related bundle branch block (aberrant) conduction
  - With a preexisting bundle branch block pattern (**Fig. 3**)
  - Conducted via an accessory pathway (Wolff-Parkinson-White syndrome)
  - In the setting of a paced ventricular rhythm
- Metabolic disorders leading to secondary changes in the QRS complex morphology, such as hyperkalemia
- Artifact (The example given in **Fig. 4** was caused by resting tremor and resulted in misclassification as nonsustained VT by the telemetry system in a patient with normal sinus rhythm.)

VF (**Fig. 5**) is faster than VT and disorganized. It can occur either as the primary rhythm or after VT degenerates into VF. Because VF is never compatible with an adequate cardiac output, all patients develop hemodynamic instability and, unless the phenomenon self-terminates (a rare occurrence in true VF), it is lethal.

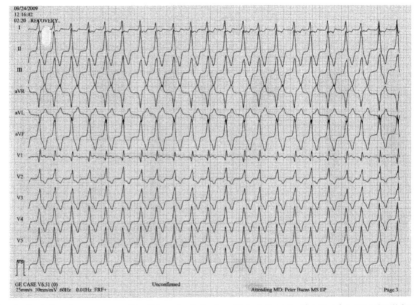

Fig. 1. Sustained monomorphic VT noted during the recovery phase of a treadmill-based exercise stress test.

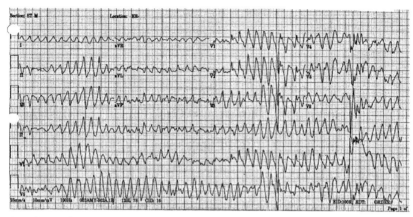

Fig. 2. Polymorphic VT with varying QRS complex morphologies.

EVALUATION

VTs typically present with palpitations, syncope, or cardiac arrest. In the elderly population, they may be manifested as intermittent confusion or unexplained falls. In some cases, they may also be asymptomatic.

The initial evaluation of patients presenting with ventricular arrhythmias, once stabilized, includes a full history and physical; 12-lead surface electrocardiogram (ECG); and comprehensive laboratory testing, including electrolytes, cardiac enzymes, thyroid function, and the evaluation of the cardiac structure (usually through transthoracic echocardiography). The goal of the evaluation is to identify potentially reversible causes and define the cardiac substrate. In addition, the laboratory analysis will

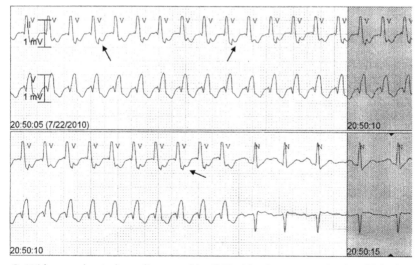

Fig. 3. Wide complex tachycardia caused by SVT with aberrant conduction (right bundle branch block pattern) mimicking VT. Note the retrograde P waves (*arrows*) at the terminal portion of the QRS complexes during SVT.

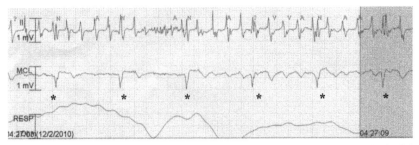

Fig. 4. Artifact caused by resting tremor in an elderly patient (affecting mainly the limb lead II and, less intensely, the precordial lead modified chest lead (MCL)), leading to the incorrect label of nonsustained VT by the telemetry system. The true QRS complexes (*asterisks*) are better identified in the precordial lead MCL, and the multiple deflections noted in lead II that do not correspond to true QRS complexes are secondary to artifact.

evaluate for renal or hepatic dysfunction that could alter clearance of antiarrhythmic drug agents.

Ventricular arrhythmias caused by secondary causes, such as ischemia; hypokalemia; hypomagnesemia; acidosis; and offending medications, such as QT prolonging drugs, should be excluded. Because ischemic heart disease is often the cause of ventricular arrhythmias, stress testing or coronary angiography may be warranted.

The extent and aggressiveness of the evaluation in the elderly population depends on several factors, including the severity of the episodes (asymptomatic vs symptomatic or hemodynamically significant) and the overall status of the patients (life expectancy, comorbidities, and quality of life). Careful evaluation of the primary data, including the 12-lead ECG and rhythm strips, should be undertaken to verify that the rhythm was indeed ventricular and not supraventricular in origin or simply an artifact. Occasionally, invasive electrophysiologic evaluation is required to distinguish between VT and SVT; such studies are generally well tolerated in the elderly.

In the case of patients who are asymptomatic with minimal to no structural heart disease and whose arrhythmias are nonsustained and always self-terminate, no further therapy may be warranted other than perhaps beta-blockers. On the other hand, patients with hemodynamically unstable or highly symptomatic episodes will require a thorough evaluation to rule out underlying causes, including coronary artery disease, and referral to a cardiac specialist.

In addition, special attention should be given to excluding recurrent arrhythmias caused by *torsades de pointes*, a form of polymorphic VT associated with prolonged QTc intervals. Several relatively common medications, including certain antibiotics,

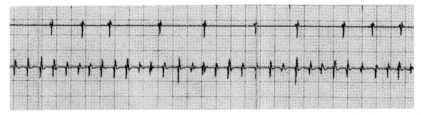

Fig. 5. Intracardiac electrograms obtained during interrogation of an ICD (implantable cardioverter-defibrillator), revealing one episode of VF. Note the atrioventricular (AV) dissociation (*top line, atrial-sensed events; bottom line, ventricular-sensed events*).

such as macrolides; some antidepressants and antipsychotic agents; and many other medications, may affect the cardiac ion channels in a way that prolongs the myocardial repolarization. The more prolonged the QTc interval becomes, the higher the risk of *torsades*.

PHARMACOLOGIC STRATEGIES

Drug therapy has an important but limited role in the treatment of ventricular arrhythmias.[4] As previously discussed, with the exception of beta-blockers, other antiarrhythmic drugs have not been shown to prevent SCD in the elderly. In general, antiarrhythmic drugs are used as adjunctive therapies for patients with or at risk for ventricular arrhythmias.[5] Because of the potential adverse effects, these agents must be used with caution. Elderly patients are at a higher risk of adverse effects of these drugs,[6] both caused by direct pharmacodynamic effects and also drug-drug interactions. The use of antiarrhythmic agents in this population must be selective, with a thorough understanding of drug interactions, elimination, and monitoring.

Beta-blockers

Beta-blockers are the most important class of drugs to treat patients with or at risk for ventricular arrhythmias. There is evidence that these drugs reduce mortality in patients with previous myocardial infarction and heart failure with left ventricular (LV) dysfunction.[7–11]

They represent a large category of drugs, including both selective and nonselective agents, with complex pharmacodynamic profiles (**Table 1**). Selective beta-blockers are associated with preferential or exclusive blockade of the beta-1 adrenergic

Table 1
Beta-blocker agents and their different pharmacologic properties and clinical indications

Class/Drug	HTN	Angina	Arrhythmias	Post-MI	Heart Failure	ISA	Alpha-Blockade
	Clinical Indications					Pharmacology	
Nonselective beta-blockers (β1 & β2)							
Carvedilol	X	—	—	—	X	—	X
Labetalol	X	X	—	—	—	X	X
Nadolol	X	X	X	X	—	—	—
Pindolol	X	X	—	—	—	X	—
Propranolol	X	X	X	X	—	—	—
Sotalol	—	—	X	—	—	—	—
Timolol	X	X	X	X	—	—	—
B1-selective							
Acebutolol	X	X	X	—	—	X	—
Atenolol	X	X	X	X	—	—	—
Bisoprolol	X	X	X	—	X	—	—
Esmolol	X	—	X	—	—	—	—
Metoprolol	X	X	X	X	X[a]	—	—

Abbreviations: HTN, hypertension; ISA, intrinsic sympathomimetic activity; MI, myocardial infarction.
[a] In patients with chronic LV systolic dysfunction, the long-acting form of metoprolol (succinate) is recommended.
Data from Refs.[9–11]

receptor and tend to cause less respiratory side effects. Nonselective beta-blockers can also block the beta-2 adrenergic receptor and, in some cases, the peripheral alpha-1 adrenergic receptors and are associated with lowering blood pressure through arteriolar vasodilatation in addition to other metabolic effects mediated by that pathway, such as improved sensitivity to insulin.

They are generally well tolerated, although their use may be limited by symptomatic bradycardia, reactive airway disease (asthma, chronic obstructive pulmonary disease), fatigue, and depression.

Some of these agents are renally cleared, and awareness of this property should allow more careful drug dosing and selection. Some commonly used beta-blockers with renal elimination include atenolol and nadolol. Safer choices in patients with renal insufficiency include metoprolol (either the short-acting formulation metoprolol tartrate or the long-acting salt metoprolol succinate) and carvedilol.

Class Ic Drugs (Flecainide and Propafenone)

Class Ic drugs (based on the Vaughan-Williams classification of antiarrhythmic drugs) are agents that inhibit the membrane-based sodium channel and decrease conduction velocity.

Although these agents were designed to suppress ventricular arrhythmias and in fact are quite effective in suppressing ventricular ectopy, they are contraindicated in patients with coronary artery disease and/or structural heart disease based on the Cardiac Arrhythmia Suppression Trial (CAST), which demonstrated a 3.6-fold risk of death.[12,13] Therefore, although recognized as commonly used agents to treat atrial arrhythmias in patients without structural heart disease, class Ic agents play a limited role in the treatment of ventricular tachycardia and should be avoided in patients with structural heart disease.

Calcium Channel Blockers

This class includes the 2 nondihydropyridine calcium channel blockers, diltiazem and verapamil. Both have negative chronotropic properties and are, therefore, contraindicated in patients with significant LV dysfunction of clinically overt heart failure states.

These drugs (especially verapamil) are particularly effective in the medical management of some types of idiopathic VT, such as fascicular VT (originating from the His-Purkinje system) or other forms of VT caused by triggered activity, such as VT arising from the right ventricular (RV) outflow tract (**Fig. 6**).

Sotalol

Sotalol is a class III antiarrhythmic drug with potassium channel-blocking effects as well as beta-blocking effects. Its use in ventricular arrhythmias is primarily limited to the prevention of recurrent VT in patients with implantable cardioverter-defibrillators (ICDs).[14] Sotalol is associated with QTc prolongation and torsades de pointes.

The risk of torsades caused by sotalol is higher in patients with bradycardia, hypokalemia or hypomagnesemia, and renal insufficiency (because it is renally cleared); therefore, caution must be taken with its use in elderly patients. It is recommended that all patients on sotalol receive routine monitoring of renal function and electrolytes as well as periodic surveillance ECGs to assess the duration of the QTc interval.

In addition, the care team must be mindful of the potential for interaction between sotalol and other QT-prolonging drugs, which may result in lethal proarrhythmic effects.[15] A complete list of QT-prolonging drugs can be obtained from the Web site www.qtdrugs.org. Furthermore, many commonly used prescription programs, such as Micromedex and Epocrates, are contemporary clinical tools that allow for

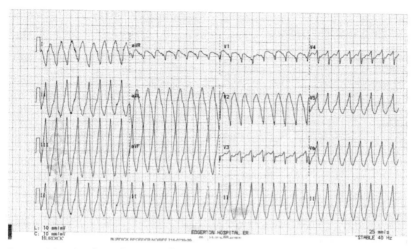

Fig. 6. VT originating from the RV outflow tract in a patient with no structural heart disease (idiopathic VT); this form of VT, characterized by a left bundle branch block pattern in lead V1 and inferior axis (broad monophasic R wave in the inferior leads), often is characterized by a good clinical response to oral verapamil.

an easy and clinically applicable way to evaluate the potential for drug-drug interactions and combined toxicity profiles.

Amiodarone

Amiodarone is an antiarrhythmic drug with complex antiarrhythmic properties, including the blockade of several ion channels (predominantly potassium and, to a less extent, sodium channels). Although it is generally classified as a class III agent, amiodarone rarely is associated with torsades de pointes. This drug has been used for many years to treat patients with both atrial and ventricular arrhythmias. The Food and Drug Administration has approved amiodarone for the management of life-threatening recurrent VF or hemodynamically unstable VT refractory to other antiarrhythmic agents or in patients intolerant of other agents used for these conditions.

Amiodarone has an important role in the acute cardiac life-support algorithm for resuscitation of patients with VT or VF.[16] Acute management of VT is beyond the scope of this review. Despite the fact that it rarely is the cause of torsades, amiodarone should not be used in patients who previously have demonstrated this arrhythmia.

Amiodarone has a limited role in the chronic treatment of VT. Although it is capable of suppressing VT, it has not been shown to provide a reduction in mortality. It is inferior to ICD therapy in the management of patients at risk for ventricular arrhythmias.[17] Its role in long-term therapy for VT is mainly confined to the prevention of recurrent ICD therapies, although it plays a limited role in the suppression of symptomatic ventricular arrhythmias in patients who are not candidates for ICDs who have inadequate suppression with beta-blocker therapy alone.[18,19]

Amiodarone is associated with a high incidence of adverse effects (**Table 2**). In general, there is a greater incidence with higher doses and longer duration of therapy. Commonly affected organ systems include the skin, thyroid, eye, lungs, liver, and the central nervous system (especially in the elderly).[20] The development of amiodarone-induced lung disease can be insidious, challenging to diagnose, and fatal. Early recognition and evaluation are essential.

Table 2
Adverse effects of amiodarone

Adverse Effect	Incidence (%)	Diagnosis	Treatment
Pulmonary toxicity	2–17	Cough or dyspnea; chest imaging, PFTs with DLCO	Stop amiodarone; possibly corticosteroids if severe
Thyroid	2–12	Hyperthyroidism	Corticosteroids, PTU, methimazole, possible thyroidectomy
	4–22	Hypothyroidism	Thyroid replacement
GI tract	30	Nausea, anorexia, constipation	Dose decrease or discontinuation
	15–30	Transaminase elevation	Consider discontinuation, other causes
Central Nervous System	3–30	Tremor, neuropathy, ataxia	May improve with dose decrease or discontinuation
Ocular	>90	Corneal microdeposits, halo vision, photophobia	Ophthalmology consult
	<1	Optic neuropathy	Discontinue drug, ophthalmology consult
Skin	25–75	Photosensitivity	Sun avoidance
	<10	Blue discoloration	Possibly decrease dose or no change
Heart	5	Bradycardia and AV block on ECG	Pacemaker placement in some cases
	<1	Proarrhythmia, including torsades	Discontinue drug

Abbreviations: AV, atrioventricular; DLCO, carbon monoxide diffusing capacity; GI, gastrointestinal; PFTs, pulmonary function tests; PTU, propylthiouracil.

Adapted from Goldschlager N, Epstein AE, Naccarelli GV, et al. A practical guide for clinicians who treat patients with amiodarone: 2007. Heart Rhythm 2007;4:1250.

Because of the potential for side effects, a systematic approach to surveillance is recommended (**Table 3**), and it should be clear which of the members of the care team is responsible for these follow-up studies.[20] Patient education may also be helpful in improving compliance with the follow-up.

NONPHARMACOLOGIC STRATEGIES

Several randomized controlled trials have demonstrated the superiority of ICD therapy over medical therapy in the prevention of SCD in patients with sustained VT/VF and cardiomyopathy.[21–26] ICDs are capable of treating ventricular arrhythmias by either antitachycardia pacing algorithms (**Fig. 7**) or cardioverter-defibrillator shocks (**Fig. 8**).

Indications for ICD therapy are detailed in published guideline documents[27] and summarized here:

Secondary Prevention

ICD implantation is recommended for the secondary prevention of VT/VF in the following clinical settings:

1. Patients with a prior episode of resuscitated VT/VF or sustained hemodynamically unstable VT in whom a completely reversible cause cannot be identified, excluding

Table 3
Suggested surveillance model for monitoring and early identification of amiodarone-induced end-organ toxicity

Test	Baseline	Every 6 mo	Every 12 mo
History & physical examination	Yes	Yes	Yes
Thyroid studies (TSH ± free T4)	Yes	Yes	Yes
Liver transaminases (AST, ALT)	Yes	Yes	Yes
Chest radiograph[a]	Yes	—	Yes
Pulmonary function tests (with DLCO)[a]	Yes	—	—
Eye examination	If visual impairment or symptoms	—	—
ECG	Yes	—	Yes

Abbreviations: ALT, alanine aminotransferase; AST, aspartate aminotransferase; DLCO, carbon monoxide diffusing capacity; TSH, thyroid-stimulating hormone.
[a] Repeat if symptoms.
Data from Goldschlager N, Epstein AE, Naccarelli GV, et al. A practical guide for clinicians who treat patients with amiodarone: 2007. Heart Rhythm 2007;4:1250.

patients who have VT/VF limited to the first 48 hours after an acute myocardial infarction.
2. Patients with episodes of spontaneous sustained VT in the presence of heart disease (valvular, ischemic, hypertrophic, dilated, or infiltrative cardiomyopathies) and other settings (eg, channelopathies).

Primary Prevention

Implantation of an ICD is recommended for the primary prevention of VT/VF in patients at risk of SCD caused by VT/VF who have optimal medical management (including the use of beta-blockers and angiotensin-converting enzyme inhibitors), including:

1. Patients with a prior myocardial infarction and LV ejection fraction of 30% or less

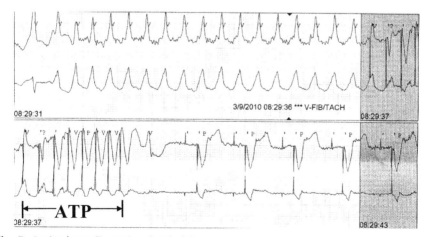

Fig. 7. Antitachycardia pacing (ATP) delivered by an ICD system successfully terminating rapid monomorphic VT (*top tracing*). Note the restoration of an atrioventricular paced rhythm following the burst ventricular pacing sequence. The ATP sequence in this case consisted of 8 ventricular paced events at a cycle length faster than the original VT.

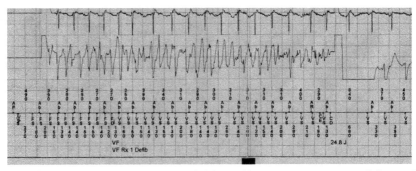

Fig. 8. Defibrillator shock (24.8 J discharge) delivered by an ICD system successfully treating VF. Note the atrioventricular (AV) dissociation pattern (*top line, atrial channel; midline, ventricular channel; bottom line, marker channel*). This recording is provided in the noninvasive interrogation of the ICD.

2. Patients with a cardiomyopathy, New York Heart Association functional class II to III, and LV ejection fraction of 35% or less (Patients with a nonischemic cardiomyopathy should receive optimal medical therapy for 3 months with documentation of persistent LV ejection fraction of 35% or less despite therapy.)
3. Recommendations are to defer primary prevention ICD placement until more than 40 days after medically managed myocardial infarctions or at least 3 months after coronary revascularization (either surgical or percutaneous).
4. Patients with a reasonable expectation of survival with good functional status for more than 1 year

In selected cases, such as reversible conditions that may lead to paroxysmal ventricular arrhythmias or until eligibility criteria for ICD implantation are met, patients can take advantage of the wearable vest-type defibrillator as an alternative for SCD prevention.

Elderly patients are underrepresented in trials involving ICD therapy. Trials have generally included patients with an average age of less than 65 years and relatively few comorbidities. In contrast, the average age of patients hospitalized for heart failure and reduced ejection fraction is 75 years old, with several comorbidities.

These discrepancies between the best available evidence and daily clinical practice must be taken into consideration when elderly patients are referred for ICD placement. It is certainly true that many elderly patients remain quite functional until their death and should receive similar treatment options as younger patients receive.

Catheter ablation of the arrhythmogenic ventricular substrate (**Fig. 9**) may be used early in the course of therapy in patients with focal idiopathic VT refractory to medical therapy (curative intent) or as suppressive therapy to minimize the occurrence of symptoms and ICD shocks in patients with advanced structural heart disease (palliative intent). Because of potential complications, such as cardiac perforation, tamponade, valvular damage, and stroke, catheter ablation is typically reserved for patients that have failed or cannot tolerate antiarrhythmic drug therapy.[28]

CLINICAL FOLLOW-UP

After treatment is instituted, patients with ventricular arrhythmias should have specific follow-up needs addressed by a multidisciplinary team of professionals, including a cardiologist (usually a clinical cardiac electrophysiologist), primary care physician, clinical pharmacist, and other specific services (eg, anticoagulation clinic), especially

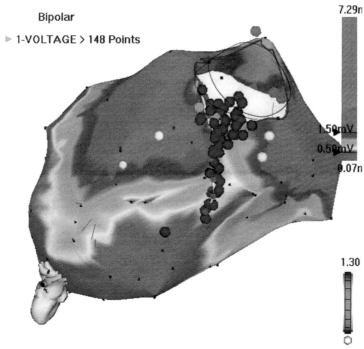

Bipolar

▶ 1-VOLTAGE > 148 Points

7.29n

1.50mV
0.50mV
0.07n

1.30

Fig. 9. Voltage map of the LV obtained during a catheter ablation procedure of a patient with previous history of inferior myocardial infarction. This view is a left posterior view of the LV endocardial surface. The areas in red indicate local voltage less than 0.5 mV, consistent with previous scar from infarction. Areas in purple indicate normal voltage and the graded colors in between represent intermediate voltage (scar border zone). The red dots indicate a line of radiofrequency lesions delivered to interrupt a critical isthmus, essential for the VT circuit.

if medical therapy with antiarrhythmic agents is maintained longitudinally. As described in the previous sections, every antiarrhythmic agent carries an intrinsic proarrhythmic risk given its specific mechanism of action and can be associated with adverse effects related to dosage issues or interactions with other medications.

It should also be noted that a careful and detailed medication reconciliation effort should be undertaken, especially in the elderly population, which is typically more vulnerable to polypharmacy and adverse reactions secondary to drug-drug interactions.[29]

The prognosis depends almost exclusively on the cause and mechanism of the ventricular arrhythmia, ranging from a normal life span with adequate treatment (such as observed in well-tolerated, idiopathic VT) to a significant decline in quality of life and survival, as seen in patients with severe LV systolic dysfunction and irreversible conditions, such as advanced cardiomyopathies that are refractory to conventional medical therapy.

SUMMARY

Ventricular arrhythmias, including VT and VF, constitute the major cause of SCD. They typically present with palpitations, syncope, or cardiac arrest. In the elderly population, their presentation may be intermittent confusion or unexplained falls. In some cases, they may also be asymptomatic. The primary management goals are to identify and treat the underlying cause and prevent recurrence.

Beta-blockers are commonly used to treat or prevent ventricular arrhythmias. Higher-risk patients often require an ICD. Aside from beta-blockers, the other antiarrhythmic drugs have not been shown to reduce mortality associated with ventricular arrhythmias and are primarily used as adjunctive therapy in patients with ICDs.

Antiarrhythmic drugs may be associated with a higher risk of adverse events in the elderly. In addition, the elderly population is vastly underrepresented in clinical trials and, therefore, the benefit of many treatment strategies, such as ICDs, is less clear. Management decisions must take into account patient and family preferences, comorbidities, and quality of life.

REFERENCES

1. Singh SN. Antiarrhythmic drug therapy of ventricular tachycardia in the elderly: lessons from clinical trials. Am J Geriatr Cardiol 1998;7(6):56–9.
2. Buxton AE. Patients with ventricular tachycardia. In: Akhtar M, Myerburg R, Ruskin J, editors. Sudden cardiac death: prevalence, mechanisms, and approach to diagnosis and management. Baltimore (MD): Williams & Wilkins; 1994. p. 465.
3. Larsen L, Markham J, Haffajee CI. Sudden death in idiopathic dilated cardiomyopathy: role of ventricular arrhythmias. Pacing Clin Electrophysiol 1993;16:1051.
4. Fozzard HA, Arnsdorf MF. Cardiac electrophysiology. In: Fozzard HA, Haber E, Jennings A, et al, editors. The heart and cardiovascular system. New York: Raven Press; 1991. p. 63.
5. Grant AO. Cardiac ion channels. Circ Arrythm Electrophysiol 2009;2:185.
6. Deneer VH, van Hemel NM. Is antiarrhythmic treatment in the elderly different? A review of the specific changes. Drugs Aging 2011;28(8):617–33.
7. Friedman LM, Byington RP, Capone RJ, et al. Effect of propranolol in patients with myocardial infarction and ventricular arrhythmia. J Am Coll Cardiol 1986;7:1.
8. Brophy JM, Joseph L, Rouleau JL. Beta-blockers in congestive heart failure. A Bayesian meta-analysis. Ann Intern Med 2001;134:550.
9. Foody JM, Farrell MH, Krumholz HM. Beta-Blocker therapy in heart failure: scientific review. JAMA 2002;287:883.
10. Sackner-Bernstein JD, Mancini DM. Rationale for treatment of patients with chronic heart failure with adrenergic blockade. JAMA 1995;274:1462.
11. Bristow MR. Beta-adrenergic receptor blockade in chronic heart failure. Circulation 2000;101:558.
12. Echt DS, Liebson PR, Mitchell LB, et al. Mortality and morbidity in patients receiving encainide, flecainide, or placebo. The Cardiac Arrhythmia Suppression Trial. N Engl J Med 1991;324:781.
13. Effect of the antiarrhythmic agent moricizine on survival after myocardial infarction. The Cardiac Arrhythmia Suppression Trial II Investigators. N Engl J Med 1992;327:227.
14. Connolly AJ, Dorian PD, Roberts RS, et al. Comparison of β-blockers, amiodarone plus β-blockers, or sotalol for prevention of shocks from implantable cardioverter defibrillators. The OPTIC study: a randomized trial. JAMA 2006;295(2):165–71.
15. Burkart F, Pfisterer M, Kiowski W, et al. Effect of antiarrhythmic therapy on mortality in survivors of myocardial infarction with asymptomatic complex ventricular arrhythmias: Basel Antiarrhythmic Study of Infarct Survival (BASIS). J Am Coll Cardiol 1990;16:1711.

16. Field JM, Hazinski MF, Sayre MR, et al. Part 1: executive summary: 2010 American Heart Association guidelines for cardiopulmonary resuscitation and emergency cardiovascular care. Circulation 2010;122:S640.
17. Bardy GH, Lee KL, Mark DB, et al. Amiodarone or an implantable cardioverter-defibrillator for congestive heart failure. N Engl J Med 2005;352:225.
18. Pfisterer M, Kiowski W, Burckhardt D, et al. Beneficial effect of amiodarone on cardiac mortality in patients with asymptomatic complex ventricular arrhythmias after acute myocardial infarction and preserved but not impaired left ventricular function. Am J Cardiol 1992;69:1399.
19. Cairns JA, Connolly SJ, Roberts R, et al. Randomised trial of outcome after myocardial infarction in patients with frequent or repetitive ventricular premature depolarisations: CAMIAT. Canadian Amiodarone Myocardial Infarction Arrhythmia Trial Investigators. Lancet 1997;349:675.
20. Goldschlager N, Epstein AE, Naccarelli GV, et al. A practical guide for clinicians who treat patients with amiodarone: 2007. Heart Rhythm 2007;4:1250.
21. Moss AJ, Hall WJ, Cannom DS, et al. Improved survival with an implanted defibrillator in patients with coronary disease at high risk for ventricular arrhythmia. Multicenter Automatic Defibrillator Implantation Trial Investigators. N Engl J Med 1996;335:1933.
22. Moss AJ, Fadl Y, Zareba W, et al. Survival benefit with an implanted defibrillator in relation to mortality risk in chronic coronary heart disease. Am J Cardiol 2001;88:516.
23. Senges JC, Becker R, Schreiner KD, et al. Variability of Holter electrocardiographic findings in patients fulfilling the noninvasive MADIT criteria. Multicenter Automatic Defibrillator Implantation Trial. Pacing Clin Electrophysiol 2002;25:183.
24. Every NR, Hlatky MA, McDonald KM, et al. Estimating the proportion of post-myocardial infarction patients who may benefit from prophylactic implantable defibrillator placement from analysis of the CAST registry. Cardiac Arrhythmia Suppression Trial. Am J Cardiol 1998;82:683.
25. Buxton AE, Fisher JD, Josephson ME, et al. Prevention of sudden death in patients with coronary artery disease: the Multicenter Unsustained Tachycardia Trial (MUSTT). Prog Cardiovasc Dis 1993;36:215.
26. Buxton AE, Lee KL, Fisher JD, et al. A randomized study of the prevention of sudden death in patients with coronary artery disease. Multicenter Unsustained Tachycardia Trial Investigators. N Engl J Med 1999;341:1882.
27. Epstein AE, DiMarco JP, Ellenbogen KA, et al. ACC/AHA/HRS 2008 guidelines for device-based therapy of cardiac rhythm abnormalities: a report of the American College of Cardiology/American Heart Association Task Force on Practice Guidelines (Writing Committee to Revise the ACC/AHA/NASPE 2002 Guideline Update for Implantation of Cardiac Pacemakers and Antiarrhythmia Devices): developed in collaboration with the American Association for Thoracic Surgery and Society of Thoracic Surgeons. Circulation 2008;117:e350.
28. Aliot EM, Stevenson WG, Almendral-Garrote JM, et al. EHRA/HRS expert consensus on catheter ablation of ventricular arrhythmias. Europace 2009;11:771–817.
29. Cho S, Lau SW, Tandon V, et al. Geriatric drug evaluation: where are we now and where should we be in the future? Arch Intern Med 2011;171:937.

Ventricular Arrhythmias
Device Therapy and Ablation

Jonathan P. Man, MD, Andrew E. Epstein, MD, FHRS*

KEYWORDS

- Ventricular arrhythmia • Catheter ablation • Device implantation therapy
- Heart failure

KEY POINTS

- Despite a growing elderly patient population, there are few randomized, well-controlled studies to guide decision making with respect to the treatment of ventricular arrhythmias with either device implantation or ablation.
- Using registries, subgroup analyses of existing trials and retrospective data may be misleading because of the lack of randomization, referral and inclusion bias, inhomogeneity, and small numbers.
- Although some data may be conflicting, there appears to be some degree of risk for treating the elderly; however, increased risk for these patients is in part a consequence of age itself and of comorbid conditions.
- In terms of benefit, however, although the data may be mixed, there are ample data suggesting that age should not contraindicate seemingly aggressive treatment when accepted indications for intervention exist.

INTRODUCTION

In the coming years there will be a demographic shift in the population of the United States, with a near doubling of people aged 65 years or older by 2050.[1] The elderly population (age $\geq$65 years) has been increasing over the last 30 years.[2–6] The proportion of people aged 65 or older was 13.0% in 2010[7] and it is projected to increase to 20.2% by 2050.[1] In terms of cardiovascular health, this increasing proportion of elderly people will increase the burden of cardiovascular disease in the American population.

Coronary heart disease (CHD) increases with age in both men and women.[2] **Fig. 1** shows the increasing rates of CHD as a function of age. In 2005, 82% of all CHD

Electrophysiology Section, Division of Cardiovascular Medicine, Hospital of the University of Pennsylvania, 3400 Spruce Street, 9 Founders, Philadelphia, PA 19104, USA
* Corresponding author. Electrophysiology Section, Division of Cardiovascular Medicine, 3400 Spruce Street, 9 Founders Pavilion, Philadelphia, PA 19104.
E-mail address: andrew.epstein@uphs.upenn.edu

Clin Geriatr Med 28 (2012) 679–691
http://dx.doi.org/10.1016/j.cger.2012.08.001
0749-0690/12/$ – see front matter Published by Elsevier Inc.

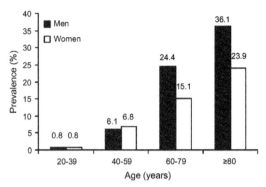

Fig. 1. Coronary heart disease in various age groups by sex. (*From* Writing Group Members, Lloyd-Jones D, Adams RJ, et al. Heart disease and stroke statistics—2010 update: a report from the American Heart Association. Circulation 2010;121(7):e46–215; with permission.)

deaths occurred in people aged 65 years and older.[2] The overall lifetime risk of developing CHD in a 70-year-old man is 34.9% and in a woman, 24.2%.[8] The predominant substrate for sudden cardiac arrest (SCA) is CHD.[9] Myocardial infarction (MI) rates increase as the population ages as well. Comparing people aged 35 to 44 years with those aged 65 to 74 years, men have an increased rate of MI from 1.0 to 10 per 1000 person-years and women from less than 0.1 to 5.4 per 1000 person-years.[10] Heart failure (HF) also increases with age. Nearly 2 decades ago, the Framingham Heart Study found an increasing prevalence of HF with increasing age in both men and women.[11] By 2009, the prevalence of HF was 8 per 1000 for men and women aged 50 to 59 years, increasing to 66 per 1000 for men and 79 per 1000 for women aged 80 to 89 years, and 80% of patients hospitalized for HF were elderly.[12] In patients with HF, death results from both progressive pump failure and SCA.[13,14] Given increasing rates of CHD, MI, SCA, and HF in the elderly, more ventricular arrhythmias will be observed, and management will almost certainly include both device implantation and catheter ablation.

DEVICE THERAPY

In accordance with American College of Cardiology/American Heart Association/Heart Rhythm Society guidelines, an implantable cardioverter-defibrillator (ICD) is recommended for patients who have survived an episode of SCA or who have symptomatic ventricular tachycardia (VT) (secondary prevention).[15] Because of the risk of SCD, ICDs are also recommended for patients with reduced left ventricular function attributable to either ischemic or nonischemic causes (primary prevention). For patients with ischemic cardiomyopathy (CM), the MI must have occurred at least 40 days before implantation, and if revascularization was done (either percutaneously or surgically), the waiting period is 3 months. For patients with ischemic CM, the left ventricular ejection fraction (LVEF) must be 35% or less when the New York Heart Association (NYHA) heart-failure class is II or III, and 30% or less when the NYHA heart-failure class is I (Class I guideline indications).[15] For patients with nonischemic CM, a LVEF of 35% or less, and NYHA heart failure class II or III, ICD implantation is a Class I recommendation. When the NYHA heart failure class is I, the recommendation is Class IIb.[15] Some of the major trials discussed in this review are summarized in **Table 1**.

Table 1
Major trials of device therapy

Trial, Year	N	Study Population	No. of Older Patients (% and Definition)
MADIT-II,[34] 2002	1232	Prior MI, LVEF ≤30%	436 (35%, ≥70 y)
DEFINITE,[35] 2004	458	NICM, PVCs or NSVT; LVEF <36%	157 (34%, ≥65 y)
DINAMIT,[36] 2004	674	6–40 d post MI, LVEF ≤35%, impaired HRV	399 (59%, ≥60 y)
COMPANION,[44] 2004	1520	Ischemic or NICM, NYHA III or IV, LVEF ≤35%, QRS duration ≥120 ms	853 (56%, ≥65 y)
CARE-HF,[45] 2005	813	NYHA III or IV, LVEF ≤35%, LVEDD ≥30 mm, QRS duration ≥120 ms	277 (34%, >70 y)
SCD-HeFT,[37] 2005	2521	Ischemic or NICM, LVEF ≤35% NYHA II or III	578 (23%, ≥65 y)
IRIS,[38] 2009	898	MI within 5–31 d, and either heart rate ≥90 beats/min and LVEF ≤40% or NSVT ≥150 beats/min	418 (47%, ≥65 y)
MADIT-CRT,[43] 2011	1820	Ischemic or NICM, LVEF ≤30%, QRS duration ≥130 ms, and NYHA I or II	331 (18%, ≥75 y)

Abbreviations: CARE-HF, Cardiac Resynchronization Heart Failure Study; COMPANION, Comparison of Medical Therapy, Pacing, and Defibrillation in Heart Failure Trial; DEFINITE, Defibrillators in Non-Ischemic Cardiomyopathy Treatment Evaluation; DINAMIT, Defibrillator in Acute Myocardial Infarction Trial; HRV, heart-rate variability; IRIS, Immediate Risk Stratification Improves Survival; LVEDD, left ventricular end-diastolic dimension; LVEF, left ventricular ejection fraction; MADIT-CRT, Multicenter Automatic Defibrillator Implantation—Cardiac Resynchronization Therapy Trial; MADIT-II, Multicenter Automatic Defibrillator Implantation Trial II; MI, myocardial infarction; NICM, nonischemic cardiomyopathy; NSVT, nonsustained ventricular tachycardia; NYHA, New York Heart Association functional class; PVCs, premature ventricular contractions; SCD-HeFT, Sudden Cardiac Death in Heart Failure Trial.

It is important to recognize that patients in clinical trials may not be the same as patients in the community. For example, the mean age of patients in HF trials conducted between 1988 and 1995 was 61 years, but the average age of patients with HF in the community is 77 years.[16] Given likely differences in comorbidities, anticipated benefits with respect to competing mortalities and complications must be considered. Such differences dilute the benefit of device therapy afforded to younger patients.

Using the Amiodarone Trial Meta-Analysis (ATMA), investigators sought to determine the effect of age on the mode of death.[17] ATMA showed that as patients (N = 6252) age, the rates of both SCA and noncardiac death increase. Furthermore, the rate of noncardiac death increased faster than the rate of SCA. For patients aged 80 years or older, only 26% of deaths were classified as SCA. The overall proportion of patients who had SCA versus noncardiac death was 41%; however, the proportion was 51% for patients younger than 50 years.

Examining the PREMIER Prospective Comparative Database (N = 26,887), investigators found that in patients who received an ICD, 17.5% (n = 4694) were aged 80 years or older, and of those 21.1% (n = 992) were 85 years or older.[18] Significant predictors of device-implantation complications were female sex, black race/ethnicity, high comorbidity score, and use of intravenous inotropic therapy. Predictors of in-hospital mortality were age 80 years or older, other comorbidities, and use of inotropes. There was increased usage of cardiac resynchronization therapy with pacing (CRT-P) among the elderly, with 21.1% receiving CRT-P if older than 85 years compared with 5.1% for those aged 19 to 79 years and 12.7% for those aged 80 to 85 years. There was likely a selection bias in choosing CRT-P for the age group older than 85 years; whether this was driven by patient and physician discussion or by physician biases is unknown. The comorbidity score for patients aged 80 years and older was slightly lower than that for the younger patients, and fewer were receiving inotropic drugs. Older patients were also less likely to have another cardiac procedure during the same hospital visit, likely indicating some selection bias. Despite these differences, older patients still had higher in-hospital mortality than those who were younger. A substudy of MADIT-II showed that although patients aged 75 years and older had a proportional reduction in mortality compared with those who were younger, the older patient group did have an increased 1-year mortality rate.[19] This large registry showed that elderly patients, despite having lower comorbidities, had higher in-patient mortality in comparison with younger patients.

Another study examined periprocedural complication rates using the National Cardiovascular Data Registry (NCDR) for ICDs.[20] This study is one the largest real-world registries. Patients receiving ICDs for primary prevention (N = 150,624) were examined, with the primary end point being any adverse event or in-hospital mortality. Those aged 65 years or older (61%, n = 91,863) had higher rates of diabetes, HF, atrial fibrillation, renal disease, and CHD. Patients who were 70 years or older comprised 46.6% (n = 47,378) of the study group. Despite adjusting for clinical conditions, multivariate analysis found that elderly patients had small but real increases in rates of complications when stratified by age: 75 to 79 years (relative risk [RR] 1.14, 95% confidence interval [CI] 1.03–1.25), 80 to 84 years (RR 1.22, 95% CI 1.10–1.36), and 85 years and older (RR 1.15, 95% CI 1.01–1.32) compared with patients younger than 65 years. Comorbid conditions were also found to increase the risk of complications with renal failure, type of device (cardiac resynchronization with defibrillation [CRT-D] device vs single-chamber ICD, dual-chamber vs single-chamber ICD), female sex, being admitted for a reason other than device implantation, and implantation by a nonelectrophysiologist. Even for patients older than 80 years, complication rates were less than 5%. This study examined the more modern era of device implantation from January 2006 to December 2008. Other studies have shown that complication rates in older patients are higher, ranging from 10% to 40%.[21–25] However, these studies used older data. When devices are implanted by electrophysiologists and more experienced physicians, complication rates are reduced.[26] Again these data are subject to referral bias, as elderly patients may not be referred or be declined ICD implantation given their age. A smaller study examined older patients (N = 199) who underwent ICD implantation and divided them into 3 groups: age 70 to 74 years (n = 88), 75 to 79 years (n = 67), and 80 years and older (n = 44).[27] The oldest patients did not show increased perioperative complications.

The Advancements in ICD Therapy (ACT) Registry included 4566 patients who underwent first ICD or CRT-D implantation.[28] Patients aged 70 years and older comprised 41.0% of the population. Of note, despite the indication for implantation being primary prevention in 75% of the cases, only 25% of the population received single-chamber devices, the type of device used predominantly in the primary prevention trials. It is also noteworthy that only 78% of elderly patients who received CRT-D devices and for whom the QRS duration and NYHA functional class data were available met accepted implantation criteria. There were no differences in terms of age for risk of sudden cardiac death; however, older patients had an increased odds ratio of noncardiac death compared with younger patients. Follow-up was conducted at 6-month intervals, with 75% of patients having 24-month follow-up.

A meta-analysis examining secondary prevention trials among the elderly found that patients aged 75 years and older did not benefit from ICD implantation in terms of reducing all-cause and arrhythmic death.[29] This study compared ICD with amiodarone therapy for secondary prevention and included the Antiarrhythmics Versus Implantable Defibrillators (AVID) study,[30] the Cardiac Arrest Study—Hamburg (CASH),[31] and the Canadian Implantable Defibrillator Study (CIDS).[32] There were only 252 patients who were 75 years or older in the combined analysis, with a total of 1866 limiting the conclusions that can be drawn. Compared with younger patients, those aged 75 years or older were more likely to die from both arrhythmic causes (6.73% per year vs 3.84%, $P = .03$) and nonarrhythmic causes (13.46% vs 5.47%, $P = .001$). In younger patients there was a reduction in all-cause mortality (hazard ratio [HR] 0.69, 95% CI 0.56–0.85, $P<.0001$) and arrhythmic death (HR 0.44, 95% CI 0.32–0.62, $P<.0001$), but this benefit was not seen in older patients (HR 1.06, 95% CI 0.69–1.64, $P = .79$; and HR 0.90, 95% CI 0.42–1.95, $P = .79$). A clear benefit of ICD implantation in improving survival in elderly patients for secondary prevention has not been demonstrated.

For primary prevention, a single-center study examined ICD implantation in patients aged 80 years and older.[33] It included 84 patients, and all survived the first year. Of note, 9.4% of patients had periprocedural complications, lead dislodgments and hematomas. Two patients had inappropriate therapy and did not die. The predicted 5-year survival rate was 60%, with the only variable found to predict survival being the type of device implanted, ICD versus CRT-D. Patients with CRT-D devices lived longer, likely as a result of either hidden confounders or the benefit of resynchronization therapy. Appropriate device therapy and survival of these patients was also high, with 87% survival. Overall, appropriate device therapy did not correlate with improved survival.

A large meta-analysis of primary prevention trials (Multicenter Automatic Defibrillator Implantation Trial II [MADIT-II],[34] Defibrillators in Non-Ischemic Cardiomyopathy Treatment Evaluation [DEFINITE],[35] Defibrillator in Acute Myocardial Infarction Trial [DINAMIT],[36] Sudden Cardiac Death in Heart Failure Trial [SCD-HeFT],[37] and Immediate Risk Stratification Improves Survival [IRIS][38]) evaluated the benefit of ICD implantation in elderly patients.[39] In DEFINITE, SCD-HeFT, and IRIS patients were considered "elderly" if they were aged 65 years or older, and in MADIT-II and DINAMIT if they were aged 60 years or more. Because DINAMIT and IRIS enrolled patients early after MI, these studies were analyzed separately because these patients are not currently considered for device therapy as a result of the trials themselves. In the older patient group, ICDs did not reduce mortality (HR 0.81, 95% CI 0.62–1.05, $P = .11$). Conversely, ICDs did reduce mortality in the younger group (HR 0.65, CI 0.50–0.83, $P<.001$). Inclusion of DINAMIT and IRIS did not change these results. Moreover, there was no change in the analysis results when comparing ischemic and nonischemic cardiomyopathies.

Another meta-analysis examined all randomized controlled trials for primary prevention for patients greater than or equal to 65 years old and 75 years old.[40] The 5 trials included in the analysis were MADIT-I,[41] the Multicenter Unsustained Tachycardia Trial (MUSTT),[42] MADIT-II,[34] DEFINITE,[35] and SCD-HeFT (**Fig. 2**).[37] In both groups, there was benefit of ICD implantation compared with the younger groups. The inclusion of differing trials confounds comparison of this meta-analysis with the study of Santangeli and colleagues.[39] The addition of MADIT-I and MUSTT may have resulted in the positive result of this meta-analysis. Of note, despite contacting the principal investigators of MADIT-I, Santangeli and colleagues were unable to obtain additional data regarding that trial. MUSTT was not included in their analysis, as they did not believe it was specifically designed to test ICD therapy against placebo.

The benefit afforded to elderly patients by cardiac resynchronization therapy (CRT) was examined using data from the MADIT-CRT study.[43] Patients were divided into

Study name	Statistics for each study					Hazard ratio and 95% CI
	Hazard ratio	Lower limit	Upper limit	Z-Value	P-Value	
MADIT-I (1996)	0.460	0.259	0.817	-2.650	0.008	
MUSTT (1999)	0.450	0.321	0.631	-4.621	0.000	
MADIT-II (2002)	0.690	0.511	0.932	-2.421	0.015	
DEFINITE (2004)	0.650	0.399	1.058	-1.733	0.083	
SCD-HeFT (2005)	0.770	0.636	0.932	-2.680	0.007	
	0.618	0.491	0.777	-4.106	0.000	

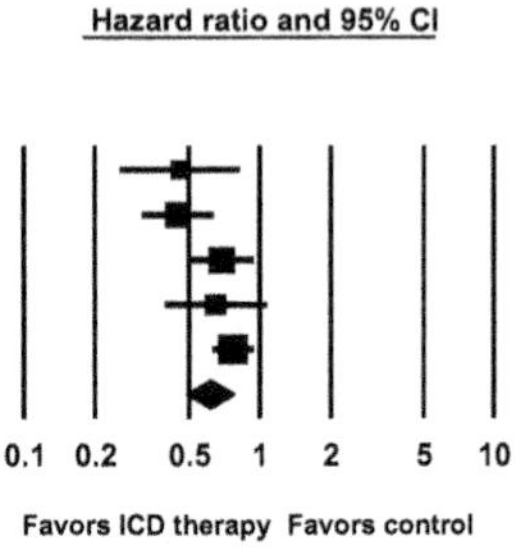

0.1　0.2　0.5　1　2　5　10

Favors ICD therapy　Favors control

Fig. 2. Hazard ratios for all-cause mortality in patients aged 65 years and older. (*From* Kong MH, Al-Khatib SM, Sanders GD, et al. Use of implantable cardioverter-defibrillators for primary prevention in older patients: a systematic literature review and meta-analysis. Cardiol J 2011;18(5):503–14; with permission. [Corrected figure courtesy of the authors.])

3 categories: younger than 60 years (n = 548), 60 to 74 years (n = 941), and 75 years and older (n = 331). Ischemic heart disease, hypertension, diabetes mellitus, history of atrial fibrillation, and impaired renal function were more prevalent in older patients. Younger patients had larger ventricles, were more likely to smoke, and were more likely to be prescribed β-blockers, angiotensin-converting enzyme inhibitors, and aldosterone antagonists. Elderly patients did not experience more complications. The benefit of CRT was of the same magnitude in the most elderly group (HR 0.57, CI 0.37–0.87, P = .010) and in the 60- to 74-year group (HR 0.55, CI 0.41–0.72, P<.001). Of interest, the youngest group (HR 0.80, CI 0.52–1.23, P = .310) did not derive the same degree of benefit. The Comparison of Medical Therapy, Pacing, and Defibrillation in Heart Failure (COMPANION) Trial[44] and the Cardiac Resynchronization-Heart Failure (CARE-HF) Study[45] examined patients aged 65 years and older and 66.4 years and older, respectively, and also showed a benefit compared with younger patients. Subgroup analyses of these trials with even older patients have not yet been published.[43] Because of the smaller sample size, analysis of those older than 80 years was not undertaken in this study.

Further analysis in older patients was undertaken, comparing patients 80 years and older who received an ICD for primary prevention (n = 99) with patients who did not receive a device but were also 80 years and older with similarly low LVEF (n = 53).[46] Comorbidities were also ranked according the Charlson Comorbidity Index (CCI), which assigns numerical values depending on the severity of the medical condition. After using a multivariate Cox model, the only significant predictors of mortality were glomerular filtration rate (GFR) and age. Implantation of an ICD did not reduce the risk of mortality in this study, nor did a higher CCI predict mortality. The only predictors of mortality were age and GFR. Another examination of patients aged 80 years and older that attempted to determine predictors of mortality in patients receiving ICDs[47] was a 2-center study with 225 patients. Multivariate analysis showed that patients with an LVEF of 20% or less and lack of β-blocker at the time of discharge had increased mortality. Renal function was not an independent predictor of mortality. There were no significant factors found that predicted time to first appropriate ICD therapy (shock or antitachycardia pacing). The proportion of patients who received appropriate therapy was 24.4%.

A study examining biases in physician attitudes to ICD implantation in the elderly (hypothetical scenarios including patients aged 50–80 years), sex, or race was conducted.[48] Four clinical scenarios with varying ICD indications (guideline Class I, Class IIa, and Class III, and Class I in a noncompliant patient) were presented and age, sex, and race were randomly varied. Responses from 1210 physicians were obtained, which did not show any biases in terms of sex and race. When the clinical scenario used an 80-year-old patient, physicians were less likely to recommend an ICD in comparison with scenarios using 50-year-old patients.

Table 2 summarizes the articles discussed in this section, and their conclusions.

CATHETER ABLATION

Catheter ablation of VT is an important option for patients with medically refractory arrhythmias.[49] Large trials akin to those related to ICD implantation are not available for catheter ablation of VT in elderly patients. One of the largest series examining catheter ablation of VT in older patients with ischemic cardiomyopathy included 285 patients followed over 9 years.[50] The patients were divided into 2 groups, 74 years and younger and 75 years and older. The younger group included 213 patients while the older group had 72 patients. There were proportionally more women in the older group; however, other clinical characteristics such as LVEF and number of VTs induced were the same. Outcomes, including complications, were the same in both groups. As in all retrospective studies, there is always the potential for referral bias. No study is available regarding patients with nonischemic cardiomyopathy. The investigators comment that ventricular function was similar between both groups but that there was a trend toward slower and more hemodynamically tolerated VT in the older patient group, and suggest that this was potentially due to referral bias.

An older study examined patients presenting for ablations of various types, including atrioventricular (AV) node and supraventricular tachycardia (SVT) as well as VT.[51] Here 695 patients were grouped into age younger than 60 years (n = 383), 60 to 79 years (n = 275) and 80 years and older (n = 37). Although the small number of those aged 80 years and older somewhat limits interpretation, procedural success was comparable in all groups, and there were remarkably no complications in the oldest age group. In terms of ablation safety, another study examined patients aged 75 years and older (n = 42) and those younger (n = 234) who presented for AV nodal reentry tachycardia ablation.[52] Another study examining SVT ablation in patients included 454 patients, of whom 67 patients 70 years or older did not have increased complications; however the cases were mostly right-sided procedures.[53] A larger study compared left-sided accessory pathway ablations in patients aged 65 years and older with those done in younger patients.[54] It also examined AV nodal reentrant tachycardia ablation along with other accessory-pathway ablations; however, there was no significant difference between the groups. Four out of 29 patients had serious complications in the elderly patient group undergoing left-sided accessory pathway ablation including tamponade, aortic dissection, acute aortic valve regurgitation- and stroke, in comparison with no complications in the younger group. However, the population with ischemic cardiomyopathy undergoing VT ablation is usually older. A large multicenter trial that examined 231 patients with a median age of 68 years found that in multivariate analysis there was no association between age and procedural success.[55] On the other hand, when complications occur, it is reasonable to postulate that changes in arterial and cardiac chamber stiffness and atherosclerotic changes likely contribute to increased risk.[56–58]

The guidelines state that VT ablation should be considered in patients with sustained monomorphic VT that recurs despite an antiarrhythmic drug or when the drug is not tolerated, for control of VT that is not due to a reversible cause, for VT or PVCs that are presumed to cause ventricular dysfunction, and for ventricular fibrillation or polymorphic VT that is caused by a trigger that is not controllable with

Table 2
Studies and outcomes discussed in this review

Study, Year	N	Description	Analysis
ATMA,[17] 2004	6252	Database examination of age on mode of death	Older patients (age ≥80) had increased rates of SCA and noncardiac death but noncardiac death increased faster than SCA
PREMIER Prospective Comparative Database,[18] 2010	26887	Database examination of device implantation	Older patients (age 80–85 and >85) had higher complications than younger patients despite having fewer comorbidities
MADIT-II Substudy,[19] 2007	1232	Substudy examining older patients from MADIT-II	Older patients (age ≥75) had higher inpatient mortality but did have proportional reduction in mortality compared with younger patients
NCDR analysis,[20] 2011	150624	Primary prevention of ICD complications	Older patients (ages ≥85, 80–84, 75–79) had increased complications compared with younger patients even when controlling for comorbid conditions
Daniels et al,[27] 2010	199	Retrospective review of older patients undergoing implant	Oldest age group (ages ≥80, 75–79, 70–74) did not show increased complications
ACT Registry,[28] 2009	4566	Database of device implants with 2-y follow-up	Oldest age group (≥70) had no increased risk of SCA but had increased risk of noncardiac comorbidity
Healey et al,[29] 2007 meta-analysis	1866	AVID, CASH, CIDS included (secondary prevention trials)	No benefit for older patients (age ≥75) in reduction of mortality

Strimel et al,[33] 2011	84	Single-center chart review of >80 patients undergoing implantation	Noted CRT improved survival over predicted survival
Santangeli et al,[39] 2010 meta-analysis	5783	MADIT-II, DEFINITE, DINAMIT, SCD-HeFT, IRIS included	Variable definition of elderly (age ≥60 for MADIT-II and DINAMIT; ≥65 DEFINITE, SCD-HeFT, IRIS) but no mortality benefit
Kong et al,[40] 2011 meta-analysis	3562	MADIT-I, MADIT-II, MUSTT, DEFINITE, SCD-HeFT	Two different definitions of elderly used for analysis (ages ≥65 and ≥75) but both groups had mortality benefit
MADIT-CRT,[43] 2011	1820	MADIT-CRT subgroup analysis	Ages <60, 60–74, and ≥75 with benefit of CRT to all groups with elderly not experiencing more complications from implantation
Mezu et al,[46] 2011	152	Single-center case control, patients undergoing primary prevention	Age ≥80 who had ICDs matched with others who did not, ICD implantation did not have a mortality benefit
Ertel et al,[47] 2010	225	Two-center study examining predictors of mortality	Age ≥80 with ICD implantation, LVEF <20% biggest predictor of mortality
Al-Khatib et al,[48] 2011 survey	1210	Survey examining physician attitudes to ICD implantation (age, race, sex)	Physicians less likely to implant 80-y-old patients vs 50-y-old patients despite the same scenario

Abbreviations: ACT Registry, Advancements in ICD Therapy; ATMA, Amiodarone Trial Meta-Analysis; AVID, Antiarrhythmics Versus Implantable Defibrillators; CASH, Cardiac Arrest Study—Hamburg; CIDS, Canadian Implantable Defibrillator Study; CRT, cardiac resynchronization therapy; DEFINITE, Defibrillators in Non-Ischemic Cardiomyopathy Treatment Evaluation; DINAMIT, Defibrillator in Acute Myocardial Infarction Trial; ICD, implantable cardioverter-defibrillator; IRIS, Immediate Risk Stratification Improves Survival; LVEF, left ventricular ejection fraction; MADIT-CRT, Multicenter Automatic Defibrillator Implantation Trial with Cardiac Resynchronization Therapy; MADIT-I, Multicenter Automatic Defibrillator Implantation Trial I; MADIT-II, Multicenter Automatic Defibrillator Implantation Trial II; MUSTT, Multicenter Unsustained Tachycardia Trial; NCDR, National Cardiac Data Registry; SCA, sudden cardiac arrest; SCD-HeFT, Sudden Cardiac Death in Heart Failure Trial.

medication.[49] However, risks and benefits of this procedure must be considered on an individual basis.

SUMMARY

Despite a growing elderly patient population there are few randomized, well-controlled studies to guide decision making with respect to the treatment of ventricular arrhythmias with either device implantation or catheter ablation. Using registries, subgroup analyses of existing trials and retrospective data may be misleading because of the lack of randomization, referral and inclusion bias, inhomogeneity, and small numbers. Although some data may be conflicting, there appears to be some degree of risk in treating the elderly; however, increased risk for these patients is in part a consequence of age itself and comorbid conditions. In terms of benefit, although the data may be mixed, there are ample data to suggest that age should not contraindicate seemingly aggressive treatment when accepted indications for intervention exist.

REFERENCES

1. Bureau USC. U.S. population projections: 2010 to 2050. Available from: http://www.census.gov/population/www/projections/summarytables.html. Accessed February 26, 2012.
2. Lloyd-Jones D, Adams RJ, Brown TM, et al. Heart disease and stroke statistics—2010 update: a report from the American Heart Association. Circulation 2010; 121(7):e46–215.
3. Alexander KP, Newby LK, Armstrong PW, et al. Acute coronary care in the elderly, part II: ST-segment-elevation myocardial infarction: a scientific statement for healthcare professionals from the American Heart Association Council on Clinical Cardiology: in collaboration with the Society of Geriatric Cardiology. Circulation 2007;115(19):2570–89.
4. Jugdutt BI. Aging and remodeling during healing of the wounded heart: current therapies and novel drug targets. Curr Drug Targets 2008;9(4):325–44.
5. Jugdutt BI. Heart failure in the elderly: advances and challenges. Expert Rev Cardiovasc Ther 2010;8(5):695–715.
6. Jugdutt BI. Aging and heart failure: changing demographics and implications for therapy in the elderly. Heart Fail Rev 2010;15(5):401–5.
7. U.S. Census Bureau. The older population: 2010. 2011 [cited February 26th, 2012]. Available at: http://www.census.gov/prod/cen2010/briefs/c2010br-09.pdf.
8. Lloyd-Jones DM, Larson MG, Beiser A, et al. Lifetime risk of developing coronary heart disease. Lancet 1999;353(9147):89–92.
9. Centers for Disease Control and Prevention (CDC). State-specific mortality from sudden cardiac death—United States, 1999. MMWR Morb Mortal Wkly Rep 2002;51(6):123–6.
10. Lerner DJ, Kannel WB. Patterns of coronary heart disease morbidity and mortality in the sexes: a 26-year follow-up of the Framingham population. Am Heart J 1986; 111(2):383–90.
11. Ho KK, Pinsky JL, Kannel WB, et al. The epidemiology of heart failure: the Framingham Study. J Am Coll Cardiol 1993;22(4 Suppl A):6A–13A.
12. Hunt SA, Abraham WT, Chin MH, et al. 2009 focused update incorporated into the ACC/AHA 2005 Guidelines for the Diagnosis and Management of Heart Failure in Adults: a report of the American College of Cardiology Foundation/American Heart Association Task Force on Practice Guidelines: developed in collaboration

with the International Society for Heart and Lung Transplantation. Circulation 2009;119(14):e391–479.

13. The CONSENSUS Trial Study Group. Effects of enalapril on mortality in severe congestive heart failure. Results of the Cooperative North Scandinavian Enalapril Survival Study (CONSENSUS). N Engl J Med 1987;316(23):1429–35.

14. The SOLVD Investigators. Effect of enalapril on survival in patients with reduced left ventricular ejection fractions and congestive heart failure. N Engl J Med 1991; 325(5):293–302.

15. Epstein AE, DiMarco JP, Ellenbogen KA, et al. ACC/AHA/HRS 2008 Guidelines for Device-Based Therapy of Cardiac Rhythm Abnormalities: a report of the American College of Cardiology/American Heart Association Task Force on Practice Guidelines (Writing Committee to Revise the ACC/AHA/NASPE 2002 Guideline Update for Implantation of Cardiac Pacemakers and Antiarrhythmia Devices): developed in collaboration with the American Association for Thoracic Surgery and Society of Thoracic Surgeons. Circulation 2008;117(21):e350–408.

16. Heiat A, Gross CP, Krumholz HM, et al. Representation of the elderly, women, and minorities in heart failure clinical trials. Arch Intern Med 2002;162(15):1682–8.

17. Krahn AD, Connolly SJ, Roberts RS, et al. Diminishing proportional risk of sudden death with advancing age: implications for prevention of sudden death. Am Heart J 2004;147(5):837–40.

18. Swindle JP, Rich MW, McCann P, et al. Implantable cardiac device procedures in older patients: use and in-hospital outcomes. Arch Intern Med 2010;170(7):631–7.

19. Huang DT, Sesselberg HW, McNitt S, et al. Improved survival associated with prophylactic implantable defibrillators in elderly patients with prior myocardial infarction and depressed ventricular function: a MADIT-II substudy. J Cardiovasc Electrophysiol 2007;18(8):833–8.

20. Tsai V, Goldstein MK, Hsia HH, et al. Influence of age on perioperative complications among patients undergoing implantable cardioverter-defibrillators for primary prevention in the United States. Circ Cardiovasc Qual Outcomes 2011; 4(5):549–56.

21. Reynolds MR, Cohen DJ, Kugelmass AD, et al. The frequency and incremental cost of major complications among Medicare beneficiaries receiving implantable cardioverter-defibrillators. J Am Coll Cardiol 2006;47(12):2493–7.

22. Groeneveld PW, Farmer SA, Suh JJ, et al. Outcomes and costs of implantable cardioverter-defibrillators for primary prevention of sudden cardiac death among the elderly. Heart Rhythm 2008;5(5):646–53.

23. Grimm W, Stula A, Sharkova J, et al. Outcomes of elderly recipients of implantable cardioverter defibrillators. Pacing Clin Electrophysiol 2007;30(Suppl 1):S134–8.

24. Duray G, Richter S, Manegold J, et al. Efficacy and safety of ICD therapy in a population of elderly patients treated with optimal background medication. J Interv Card Electrophysiol 2005;14(3):169–73.

25. Noseworthy PA, Lashevsky I, Dorian P, et al. Feasibility of implantable cardioverter defibrillator use in elderly patients: a case series of octogenarians. Pacing Clin Electrophysiol 2004;27(3):373–8.

26. Al-Khatib SM, Greiner MA, Peterson ED, et al. Patient and implanting physician factors associated with mortality and complications after implantable cardioverter-defibrillator implantation, 2002-2005. Circ Arrhythm Electrophysiol 2008;1(4):240–9.

27. Daniels JD, Saunders J, Parvathaneni S, et al. Electrocardiographic findings, device therapies, and comorbidities in octogenarian implantable defibrillator recipients. J Cardiovasc Electrophysiol 2010;21(3):236–41.

28. Epstein AE, Kay GN, Plumb VJ, et al. Implantable cardioverter-defibrillator prescription in the elderly. Heart Rhythm 2009;6(8):1136–43.

29. Healey JS, Hallstrom AP, Kuck KH, et al. Role of the implantable defibrillator among elderly patients with a history of life-threatening ventricular arrhythmias. Eur Heart J 2007;28(14):1746–9.

30. The Antiarrhythmics versus Implantable Defibrillators (AVID) Investigators. A comparison of antiarrhythmic-drug therapy with implantable defibrillators in patients resuscitated from near-fatal ventricular arrhythmias. N Engl J Med 1997;337(22):1576–84.

31. Kuck KH, Cappato R, Siebels J, et al. Randomized comparison of antiarrhythmic drug therapy with implantable defibrillators in patients resuscitated from cardiac arrest: the Cardiac Arrest Study Hamburg (CASH). Circulation 2000;102(7): 748–54.

32. Connolly SJ, Gent M, Roberts RS, et al. Canadian implantable defibrillator study (CIDS): a randomized trial of the implantable cardioverter defibrillator against amiodarone. Circulation 2000;101(11):1297–302.

33. Strimel W, Koplik S, Chen HR, et al. Safety and effectiveness of primary prevention cardioverter defibrillators in octogenarians. Pacing Clin Electrophysiol 2011;34(7): 900–6.

34. Moss AJ, Zareba W, Hall WJ, et al. Prophylactic implantation of a defibrillator in patients with myocardial infarction and reduced ejection fraction. N Engl J Med 2002;346(12):877–83.

35. Kadish A, Dyer A, Daubert JP, et al. Prophylactic defibrillator implantation in patients with nonischemic dilated cardiomyopathy. N Engl J Med 2004;350(21): 2151–8.

36. Hohnloser SH, Kuck KH, Dorian P, et al. Prophylactic use of an implantable cardioverter-defibrillator after acute myocardial infarction. N Engl J Med 2004; 351(24):2481–8.

37. Bardy GH, Lee KL, Mark DB, et al. Amiodarone or an implantable cardioverter-defibrillator for congestive heart failure. N Engl J Med 2005;352(3):225–37.

38. Steinbeck G, Andresen D, Seidl K, et al. Defibrillator implantation early after myocardial infarction. N Engl J Med 2009;361(15):1427–36.

39. Santangeli P, Di Biase L, Dello Russo A, et al. Meta-analysis: age and effectiveness of prophylactic implantable cardioverter-defibrillators. Ann Intern Med 2010;153(9):592–9.

40. Kong MH, Al-Khatib SM, Sanders GD, et al. Use of implantable cardioverter-defibrillators for primary prevention in older patients: a systematic literature review and meta-analysis. Cardiol J 2011;18(5):503–14.

41. Moss AJ, Hall WJ, Cannom DS, et al. Improved survival with an implanted defibrillator in patients with coronary disease at high risk for ventricular arrhythmia. Multicenter Automatic Defibrillator Implantation Trial Investigators. N Engl J Med 1996; 335(26):1933–40.

42. Buxton AE, Lee KL, Fisher JD, et al. A randomized study of the prevention of sudden death in patients with coronary artery disease. Multicenter Unsustained Tachycardia Trial Investigators. N Engl J Med 1999;341(25):1882–90.

43. Penn J, Goldenberg I, Moss AJ, et al. Improved outcome with preventive cardiac resynchronization therapy in the elderly: a MADIT-CRT substudy. J Cardiovasc Electrophysiol 2011;22(8):892–7.

44. Bristow MR, Saxon LA, Boehmer J, et al. Cardiac-resynchronization therapy with or without an implantable defibrillator in advanced chronic heart failure. N Engl J Med 2004;350(21):2140–50.

45. Cleland JG, Daubert JC, Erdmann E, et al. The effect of cardiac resynchronization on morbidity and mortality in heart failure. N Engl J Med 2005;352(15): 1539–49.
46. Mezu U, Adelstein E, Jain S, et al. Effectiveness of implantable defibrillators in octogenarians and nonagenarians for primary prevention of sudden cardiac death. Am J Cardiol 2011;108(5):718–22.
47. Ertel D, Phatak K, Makati K, et al. Predictors of early mortality in patients age 80 and older receiving implantable defibrillators. Pacing Clin Electrophysiol 2010; 33(8):981–7.
48. Al-Khatib SM, Sanders GD, O'Brien SM, et al. Do physicians' attitudes toward implantable cardioverter defibrillator therapy vary by patient age, gender, or race? Ann Noninvasive Electrocardiol 2011;16(1):77–84.
49. Aliot EM, Stevenson WG, Almendral-Garrote JM, et al. EHRA/HRS Expert Consensus on Catheter Ablation of Ventricular Arrhythmias: developed in a partnership with the European Heart Rhythm Association (EHRA), a Registered Branch of the European Society of Cardiology (ESC), and the Heart Rhythm Society (HRS); in collaboration with the American College of Cardiology (ACC) and the American Heart Association (AHA). Heart Rhythm 2009;6(6):886–933.
50. Inada K, Roberts-Thomson KC, Seiler J, et al. Mortality and safety of catheter ablation for antiarrhythmic drug-refractory ventricular tachycardia in elderly patients with coronary artery disease. Heart Rhythm 2010;7(6):740–4.
51. Zado ES, Callans DJ, Gottlieb CD, et al. Efficacy and safety of catheter ablation in octogenarians. J Am Coll Cardiol 2000;35(2):458–62.
52. Kihel J, Da Costa A, Kihel A, et al. Long-term efficacy and safety of radiofrequency ablation in elderly patients with atrioventricular nodal re-entrant tachycardia. Europace 2006;8(6):416–20.
53. Epstein LM, Chiesa N, Wong MN, et al. Radiofrequency catheter ablation in the treatment of supraventricular tachycardia in the elderly. J Am Coll Cardiol 1994;23(6):1356–62.
54. Chen SA, Chiang CE, Yang CJ, et al. Accessory pathway and atrioventricular node reentrant tachycardia in elderly patients: clinical features, electrophysiologic characteristics and results of radiofrequency ablation. J Am Coll Cardiol 1994;23(3):702–8.
55. Stevenson WG, Wilber DJ, Natale A, et al. Irrigated radiofrequency catheter ablation guided by electroanatomic mapping for recurrent ventricular tachycardia after myocardial infarction: the multicenter Thermocool Ventricular Tachycardia Ablation Trial. Circulation 2008;118(25):2773–82.
56. Kitzman DW, Scholz DG, Hagen PT, et al. Age-related changes in normal human hearts during the first 10 decades of life. Part II (Maturity): a quantitative anatomic study of 765 specimens from subjects 20 to 99 years old. Mayo Clin Proc 1988; 63(2):137–46.
57. Lakatta EG, Levy D. Arterial and cardiac aging: major shareholders in cardiovascular disease enterprises: part I: aging arteries: a "set up" for vascular disease. Circulation 2003;107(1):139–46.
58. Lakatta EG, Levy D. Arterial and cardiac aging: major shareholders in cardiovascular disease enterprises: part II: the aging heart in health: links to heart disease. Circulation 2003;107(2):346–54.

Quality of Life and End-Of-Life Issues for Older Patients with Implanted Cardiac Rhythm Devices

Rachel Lampert, MD

KEYWORDS

- Quality of life • End of life • Implantable cardioverter-defibrillator • Pacemaker

KEY POINTS

- Patients with implantable cardioverter-defibrillators (ICDs) demonstrate similar quality of life (QOL) to patients with other major cardiac conditions, and elderly patients may actually adjust better than younger ICD recipients.
- Pacemakers and cardiac resynchronization therapy can improve QOL for appropriately selected older patients with symptomatic bradyarrhythmias or heart failure, respectively.
- Shocks at the end of life, however, can have a significant negative impact on QOL for patients and families. Deactivation of the shock function of the ICD is legal and ethical, and can improve QOL at the end of life.
- Proactive communication between health care providers and patients and families is critical to maximizing QOL and minimizing distress as patients approach the end of their lives.

QUALITY OF LIFE

In general, patients with ICDs enjoy QOL similar to individuals with other cardiac diseases. In one early study,[1] the Medical Outcomes Study 36-Item Short Form Health Survey (SF-36) was used to compare 24 patients with ICDs with 73 patients with other cardiac diseases. There were no significant differences in mental health, emotional limitations, social functioning, vitality, health perception, pain, physical limitations, or physical function. As described by Schron and colleagues,[2] in the Antiarrhythmics Versus Implanted Defibrillators (AVID) trial of ICDs versus antiarrhythmic drugs for patients suffering life-threatening ventricular arrhythmias (secondary prevention), baseline QOL measured by SF-36 in ICD patients was similar to that of elderly patients with recent myocardial infarction or severe heart failure (HF), but less than for ambulatory patients

Department of Internal Medicine, Section of Cardiology, Yale University School of Medicine, 789 Howard Avenue, Dana 319, New Haven, CT 06510, USA
E-mail address: rachel.lampert@yale.edu

Clin Geriatr Med 28 (2012) 693–702
http://dx.doi.org/10.1016/j.cger.2012.07.005   geriatric.theclinics.com
0749-0690/12/$ – see front matter © 2012 Elsevier Inc. All rights reserved.

with HF, implying a moderately severe impairment in QOL. In this study, the physical component score improved significantly over the year following implant, although the mental component score did not. In both of the aforementioned studies, patients treated with antiarrhythmic drugs showed poorer QOL than those receiving ICDs.

In a more recent study from Iceland comparing pacemaker patients and ICD patients,[3] there were no differences between pacemaker and ICD recipients on a large number of psychometric measures, including depression and anxiety. In this study, using the Icelandic QOL questionnaire, not only did ICD patients not differ from pacemaker patients, they also did not differ in most measures from previously reported scores for the general population. The better QOL seen in this study compared with earlier studies may be due to the inclusion of less sick patients receiving an ICD for primary prevention.

Factors that affect QOL for ICD patients are the subject of ongoing investigation. Most studies suggest that receipt of frequent shocks affects QOL negatively. In the Canadian Implantable Defibrillator (CIDs) trial, also a secondary prevention study, Irvine and colleagues[4] reported a significant difference in QOL among ICD patients depending on the number of shocks received. Shocks have been described by patients as "a blow to the body, a punch in the chest, being hit by a truck, kicked by a mule, or putting a finger in a light socket."[5] In CIDs, whereas those patients who received either no shocks or 1 to 4 shocks had significant improvement in QOL over time, those with 5 or more shocks did not improve. Similarly, in the AVID trial,[2] the occurrence of even 1 shock was associated with reduction in mental well-being and physical function, even after controlling for multiple clinical factors such as HF, index arrhythmia, and ejection fraction. Furthermore, there was greater reduction in QOL as the number of shocks increased.

Other factors, such as preexisting personality types and coping styles, also affect QOL after ICD. For example, type D or "distressed personality," that is, individuals with a combination of negative affect and social inhibition, have more difficulties,[6] as do individuals prone to somatization.[7] Not surprisingly, individuals who start with high expectations and with optimism have better QOL.[8] Low social support is also a predictor of poor QOL for patients with ICDs,[9,10] in particular the absence of a spouse. In studies that evaluated the effects of both shocks and psychosocial factors, many found that psychosocial factors, such as underlying personality traits, play a larger role than shocks in determining QOL for ICD patients.[11] Thus, it is likely that shocks interact with psychosocial factors such as personality traits and social support in influencing QOL for patients with ICDs.

Several studies have evaluated specifically how age affects psychosocial adjustment and QOL after ICD implant. Sears and colleagues[12] found that psychosocial variables including depression, anxiety, optimism, and social support all affect QOL after ICD implant. Furthermore, these variables explained more of the variance in outcomes for mental and general QOL than did age and ejection fraction together, suggesting that it is not age but psychological make-up that determines a patient's QOL after ICD. Indeed, older patients may do better than younger patients after ICD placement. Younger adults may have more difficulty adjusting to the ICD,[13] including more anxiety, depression, and sleep disturbances, with overall worse QOL than older patients.[14] Hamilton and Carroll[15] compared younger ICD recipients, age 18 to 62 with a mean age of 51 years, with older recipients, 63 to 84 with a mean age of 75 years. Although physical QOL was better in the younger patients, mental QOL did not differ between older and younger recipients of ICDs. Anxiety was initially higher in the younger patients but the difference resolved over time, and other mood states showed no differences between age groups.

Whereas the impact of ICDs on QOL is modest, especially in the absence of shocks, patients undergoing cardiac resynchronization therapy (CRT) often experience reduced symptom burden and improved QOL. Overall, the CRT randomized trials showed significant improvements in QOL as measured by the Minnesota Living with HF Questionnaire, which quantifies the patient's symptoms and cardiac disability. Patients enrolled in these trials had baseline scores consistent with moderate to severely impaired QOL. Patients randomized to CRT in the 3 major trials of this modality—Miracle, Miracle ICD, and Companion—showed improvements in QOL, with reductions in impairment-related scores by about a third.[16–18] This finding is in stark contrast to those in trials of medications. Despite documented improvements in mortality, morbidity, and indices of left ventricular remodeling, valsartan, metoprolol, and carvedilol have not been associated with improved Minnesota Living with HF scores. Although few patients in the randomized trials of CRT were elderly, observational studies have demonstrated similar improvements in clinical parameters and QOL in CRT recipients older than 70 to 75 years in comparison with younger patients.[19,20]

CRT delivered in a pacing-only device without defibrillation capacity (CRT-P) has also been shown to improve clinical outcomes in some studies,[21] and may be appropriate in older patients who desire symptom relief without the possibility of defibrillator shocks. CRT-P has been used in up to one-fifth of those older than 80 years receiving an ICD or CRT device.[22]

Although there are few data on ICDs and CRT in the very elderly (>80–90 years), conventional pacemakers often improve QOL in both the elderly[23] and very elderly.[24] Shen and colleagues[24] compared outcomes in 157 octogenarians and nonagenarians receiving pacemakers to age- and sex-matched controls from the general population. While underlying heart disease and other comorbidities were strong predictors of functional status, after controlling for these factors there were no differences in functional outcomes between those with and without pacemakers.

END-OF-LIFE ISSUES
Case 1

An interview with a family member of a recently deceased ICD patient:

His defibrillator kept going off...It went off 12 times in one night...He went in and they looked at it...they said they adjusted it and they sent him back home. The next day we had to take him back because it was happening again. It kept going off and going off and it wouldn't stop going off.[25]

Case 2

A 65-year-old man received an ICD 10 years ago following an arrest. Ejection fraction was 30%. He had shock-treated ventricular tachycardia at 250 bpm 4 times in the last 10 years. He was last seen 8 months ago, and followed transtelephonically in the meantime. His wife called his electrophysiologist: F.G. was currently on the oncology floor, having been diagnosed 4 months ago with metastatic cancer. Despite multiple rounds of chemotherapy, he had continued lesions in brain and bone. He was to be discharged to hospice the following day on a morphine drip. The patient and family requested that ICD therapies be turned off. The EP team deactivated therapies, and F.G. died in hospice two days later, 'peacefully' according to his wife.[26]

These contrasting cases illustrate the potential impact of ICD shocks on QOL in patients at the end of their lives. Despite the life-saving properties of an ICD, all patients will ultimately reach the end of their lives, whether because of their under-lying heart condition or other comorbidities. As one study reported, 20% of ICD patients receive shocks in the last weeks of their lives, as illustrated by case 1.[25] Although device deactivation can facilitate a more peaceful death, as illustrated by case 2, few patients or families discuss the option with their physicians, even among patients with "do not resuscitate" orders.[25] Likewise, few clinicians initiate discus-sions with patients or family members regarding device deactivations, even during terminal situations. To address the uncertainties surrounding device deactivation and provide direction for clinicians in these difficult circumstances, the Heart Rhythm Society published recommendations regarding deactivation, with input from electro-physiologists, patients, and representatives from the fields of geriatrics, palliative care, psychiatry, nursing, law, ethics, and divinity, as well as industry and patient groups.[27]

The ethical and legal bases for deactivation of ICDs are clear cut. Informed consent, the most important legal doctrine in the clinician-patient relationship and the principle that underlies device deactivation, derives from the ethical principle of respect for persons: autonomy is maximized when patients understand the nature of their diag-noses and treatment options, and participate in decisions about their care.[28] Clini-cians are ethically and legally obligated to ensure that patients are informed about their diagnoses and treatment options.[29,30]

United States courts have ruled that the right to make decisions about medical treatments is both a common-law (derived from court decisions) right based on bodily integrity and self-determination and a constitutional right based on privacy and liberty.[31] A corollary to informed consent is informed refusal. A patient has the right to refuse any treatment, even if the treatment prolongs life or if death would follow treatment refusal. A patient also has the right to refuse a previously consented treat-ment if the treatment no longer meets the patient's health care goals because either those goals have changed (eg, from prolonging life to minimizing discomforts), or the perceived burdens of the patient's illness (eg, QOL) and ongoing treatment outweigh the perceived benefits of ongoing therapy. United States courts have consistently upheld the right of a patient to withdraw life-sustaining therapies.[31–34] In none of these cases did the courts distinguish between types of life-sustaining treat-ments. The law applies to the person, and informed consent is a right of the patient: it is not specific to any one medical intervention.[31,35–37] Thus, even though the Supreme Court has not specifically commented on the question of pacemaker or ICD deactiva-tion, because devices deliver life-sustaining therapies, discontinuation of these thera-pies is clearly addressed by Supreme Court precedents upholding the right to discontinue life-sustaining treatment.

Although the impact of ICD shocks on dying patients is well described, and the ethical and legal bases for deactivation are well established, few patients with ICDs discuss device deactivation with their clinicians or know that device deactivation is an available option.[25,38–40] Advanced care planning conversations improve outcomes for both patients and their families,[41] as patients with ICDs who engage in advance care planning are less likely to experience shocks while dying because ICD deactiva-tion has occurred.[42] Studies show that patients and families desire conversations about end-of-life care in general.[43–45] Some patient surveys have suggested that patients with ICDs would not consider deactivation even in the setting of hypothetical states such as terminal cancer,[46] constant dyspnea,[47] or receipt of frequent shocks.[47,48] However, a more recent study,[49] which incorporated an informational description of the potential benefits and burdens of the shock function of ICDs, found that more than 70% of ICD patients would want ICD deactivation in at least one of several hypothetical scenarios that are common in patients approaching the end of life, such as memory loss or advanced incurable illness.

This study highlights the importance of proactive, informative communication between physicians and ICD patients regarding the option of device deactivation. These goal-directed conversations should include a discussion of QOL, functional status, perceptions of dignity, and both current and potential future symptoms, as each of these elements can influence how patients set goals for their health care. These conversations should follow the model of "shared decision making," in which clinicians work together with patients and families to ensure that patients understand the benefits and burdens of a particular treatment and the potential outcomes that may occur as a result of its continued use or discontinuation.[50]

An important role for the clinician is to provide factual and understandable information concerning the beneficial and negative effects of continuing device therapy. The patient can then assess how the benefits and burdens of continued therapy fit with his or her ongoing health care goals. Data show that some patients with ICDs do not understand the role that the device plays in their health, particularly in terms of care at the end of life.[51] It is also vital for both the health care provider and the patient to have an accurate understanding of the expected consequences of device deactivation. While there are some cases, such as patients who are pacemaker dependent, whereby this may be relatively straightforward, in many situations it will be difficult to predict a patient's clinical course after deactivation. The timing and lethality of tachyarrhythmias is unpredictable, and bradyarrhythmias may manifest with syncope, HF, angina, fatigue, or sudden death. Consultation with a clinical electrophysiologist may help clarify the clinical picture, although in many cases significant uncertainty will remain.

Consultations with other members of the patient's multidisciplinary care team can also be helpful. Psychiatric consultation is not required, but can be helpful if care providers or families have concerns that a particular psychiatric disorder such as major depression or paranoid delusions may be interfering with the patient's ability to make informed decisions. Because changing settings or deactivating a device can result in gradual worsening of chronic symptoms or onset of new symptoms, it may be helpful to obtain palliative care consultation before devices settings are altered. Nurses, social workers, and clergy often play a key role in helping patients understand the device in terms of the overall context of their health and in helping them better comprehend aspects of their care related to device management.

Many elderly patients spend the last weeks or even years of their lives in facilities such as nursing homes or hospices. Surprisingly, a recent survey of hospices revealed that only 10% had an item regarding the presence of an implanted device on the intake form.[52] Facility intake forms should include history of ICD or pacemaker implant, as well as inspection for the presence of a generator in the right or left infraclavicular region on the physical examination.[53] The presence of an ICD should initiate prompt discussion regarding the patient's wishes for ICD activation or deactivation in the context of goals of care and resuscitation status.

Once the decision to deactivate a patient's ICD is made, the Heart Rhythm Society recommends a series of procedures that should be consistently applied,[27] although the logistical aspects of achieving deactivation will vary depending on the patient's location, whether in a hospital, facility, or at home. First, the patient's decision-making capacity should be confirmed, and the legal surrogate identified if decision-making capacity is lacking. The courts have determined that the right to refuse treatment extends to those without capacity, through a legal surrogate.[34,35,54] Next, the attending physician should contact the physician responsible for following the patient's device for consultation as to which therapies should be deactivated. Most patients will wish to have the shock function deactivated, but deactivation of pacing or CRT is also possible. A written order should be placed in the medical record, and documentation should confirm: (1) that the patient (or legal surrogate) has requested device deactivation; (2) the capacity of the patient to make the decision, or identification of the appropriate surrogate; (3) that alternative therapies have been discussed if relevant; (4) that consequences of deactivation have been discussed; (5) the specific device therapies to be deactivated; and (6) notification of family if consistent with the patient's wishes.[27]

For patients in long-term care facilities without on-site electrophysiological expertise and who are unable to travel, deactivation should be performed by medical personnel (such as a physician or nurse) with guidance from industry-employed allied professionals.[55] Although the institution of policies designed to improve proactive communication will reduce unwanted shocks in a dying patient, emergent situations may still occur. All ICDs can be deactivated by placing a doughnut magnet directly over the device. As devices differ in response when the magnet is removed, the magnet should be left in place until appropriate device function is confirmed and/or a programmer is available. All facilities should have doughnut magnets on site and readily available.

DEACTIVATION OF PACEMAKERS

Although pacemakers do not actively impair QOL or prolong the dying process, patients may determine that the benefits of the device no longer outweigh its burdens, and may request deactivation of a pacemaker or the bradycardia-pacing functions of an ICD. Although some have debated whether there are moral or philosophic distinctions between pacemaker and ICD deactivation,[56–58] particularly in a pacemaker-dependent patient, legally patients have the same right to deactivate a pacemaker as any other life-sustaining therapy.[27] Appropriate communication regarding the benefits and burdens of continuing versus discontinuing pacing therapy is imperative, as is confirming understanding of the consequences of deactivation. For those choosing pacemaker deactivation, palliative interventions should be in place.

As described in the American Medical Association Code of Medical Ethics, physicians (or other medical personnel) should not be compelled to perform device deactivations if they view the procedure as inconsistent with their personal values. However, the clinician should not impose his or her values on or abandon the patient. Instead, the clinician and patient should work to achieve a mutually agreed-upon care plan. If such a plan cannot be achieved, the primary clinician should involve a second clinician who is willing to comanage the patient and provide legally permissible care and procedures including device deactivation.[59]

SUMMARY

Patients with ICDs demonstrate similar QOL to patients with other major cardiac conditions, and elderly patients may actually adjust better than younger ICD recipients. Pacemakers and CRT can improve QOL for appropriately selected older patients with symptomatic bradyarrhythmias or HF, respectively. Shocks at the end of life, however, can have a significant negative impact on QOL for patients and families. Deactivation of the shock function of the ICD is legal and ethical, and can improve QOL at the end of life. Proactive communication between health care providers and patients and families is critical to maximizing QOL and minimizing distress as patients approach the end of their lives.

REFERENCES

1. Herbst JH, Goodman M, Feldstein S, et al. Health-related quality-of-life assessment of patients with life-threatening ventricular arrhythmias. Pacing Clin Electrophysiol 1999;22:915–26.
2. Schron E, Exner D, Yao Q, et al. Quality of life in the antiarrhythmics versus implantable defibrillators. Circulation 2002;105:589–94.
3. Leosdottir M, Sigurdsson E, Reimarsdottir G, et al. Health-related quality of life of patients with implantable cardioverter defibrillators compared with that of pacemaker recipients. Europace 2006;8:168–74.
4. Irvine J, Dorian P, Baker B, et al. Quality of life in the Canadian implantable defibrillator study (CIDS). Am Heart J 2002;144:282–9.
5. Ahmad M, Bloomstein L, Roelke M. Patients' attitudes toward implanted defibrillator shocks. PACE 2000;23:934–8.
6. Pedersen SS, van Domburg RT, Theuns DA, et al. Type D personality is associated with increased anxiety and depressive symptoms in patients with an implantable cardioverter defibrillator and their partners. Psychosom Med 2004; 66:714–9.
7. Godemann F, Butter C, Lampe F, et al. Determinants of the quality of life (QoL) in patients with an implantable cardioverter/defibrillator (ICD). Qual Life Res 2004; 13:411–6.
8. Sears SF, Serber ER, Lewis TS, et al. Do positive health expectations and optimism relate to quality-of-life outcomes for the patient with an implantable cardioverter defibrillator? J Cardiopulm Rehabil 2004;24:324–31.
9. Wallace RL, Sears SF Jr, Lewis TS, et al. Predictors of quality of life in long-term recipients of implantable cardioverter defibrillators. J Cardiopulm Rehabil 2002; 22:278–81.
10. Luyster FS, Hughes JW, Waechter D, et al. Resource loss predicts depression and anxiety among patients treated with an implantable cardioverter defibrillator. Psychosom Med 2006;68:794–800.
11. Pedersen SS, Van Den Broek KC, Van Den Berg M, et al. Shock as a determinant of poor patient-centered outcomes in implantable cardioverter defibrillator patients: is there more to it than meets the eye? Pacing Clin Electrophysiol 2010;33:1430–6.
12. Sears SF, Lewis TS, Kuhl EA, et al. Predictors of quality of life in patients with implantable cardioverter defibrillators. Psychosomatics 2005;46:451–7.
13. Sears SF Jr, Burns JL, Handberg E, et al. Young at heart: understanding the unique psychosocial adjustment of young implantable cardioverter defibrillator recipients. Pacing Clin Electrophysiol 2001;24:1113–7.
14. Friedmann E, Thomas SA, Inguito P, et al. Quality of life and psychological status of patients with implantable cardioverter defibrillators. J Interv Card Electrophysiol 2006;17:65–72.
15. Hamilton GA, Carroll DL. The effects of age on quality of life in implantable cardioverter defibrillator recipients. J Clin Nurs 2004;13:194–200.
16. Abraham WT, Fisher WG, Smith AL, et al. Cardiac resynchronization in chronic heart failure. N Engl J Med 2002;346:1845–53.
17. Young JB, Abraham WT, Smith AL, et al. Combined cardiac resynchronization and implantable cardioversion defibrillation in advanced chronic heart failure: the MIRACLE ICD Trial. JAMA 2003;289:2685–94.
18. Bristow MR, Saxon LA, Boehmer J, et al. Cardiac-resynchronization therapy with or without an implantable defibrillator in advanced chronic heart failure. N Engl J Med 2004;350:2140–50.

19. Bleeker GB, Schalij MJ, Molhoek SG, et al. Comparison of effectiveness of cardiac resynchronization therapy in patients <70 versus > or = 70 years of age. Am J Cardiol 2005;96:420–2.

20. Delnoy PP, Ottervanger JP, Luttikhuis HO, et al. Clinical response of cardiac resynchronization therapy in the elderly. Am Heart J 2008;155:746–51.

21. Cleland JG, Daubert JC, Erdmann E, et al. The effect of cardiac resynchronization on morbidity and mortality in heart failure. N Engl J Med 2005;352:1539–49.

22. Swindle JP, Rich MW, McCann P, et al. Implantable cardiac device procedures in older patients: use and in-hospital outcomes. Arch Intern Med 2010;170:631–7.

23. Lamas GA, Orav EJ, Stambler BS, et al. Quality of life and clinical outcomes in elderly patients treated with ventricular pacing as compared with dual-chamber pacing. Pacemaker Selection in the Elderly Investigators. N Engl J Med 1998; 338:1097–104.

24. Shen WK, Hayes DL, Hammill SC, et al. Survival and functional independence after implantation of a permanent pacemaker in octogenarians and nonagenarians. A population-based study. Ann Intern Med 1996;125:476–80.

25. Goldstein NE, Lampert R, Bradley E, et al. Management of implantable cardioverter defibrillators in end-of-life care. Ann Intern Med 2004;141:835–8.

26. Lampert R, Hayes DL. Ethical issues. In: Ellenbogen KA, Kay GN, Lau CP, et al, editors. Clinical cardiac pacing, defibrillation, and resynchronization therapy. Philadelphia: Elsevier; 2011. p. 1040–9.

27. Lampert R, Hayes DL, Annas GJ, et al. HRS expert consensus statement on the management of Cardiovascular Implantable Electronic Devices (CIEDs) in patients nearing end of life or requesting withdrawal of therapy. Heart Rhythm 2010;7:1008–26.

28. Beauchamp TL. Principles of biomedical ethics. 6th edition. New York: Oxford University Press; 2009.

29. Snyder L, Leffler C. Ethics manual: fifth edition. Ann Intern Med 2005;142:560–82.

30. AMA Council on Ethical and Judicial Affairs. AMA 2008–2009. Code of medical ethics: current opinions and annotations. 2008-2009 edition. Chicago: AMA Press; 2010.

31. Annas GJ. The rights of patients: the authoritative ACLU guide to the rights of patients. 3rd edition. New York: New York University Press; 2004.

32. Pellegrino ED. Decisions to withdraw life-sustaining treatment: a moral algorithm. JAMA 2000;283:1065–7.

33. Rhymes JA, McCullough LB, Luchi RJ, et al. Withdrawing very low-burden interventions in chronically ill patients. JAMA 2000;283:1061–3.

34. Quill TE, Barold SS, Sussman BL. Discontinuing an implantable cardioverter defibrillator as a life-sustaining treatment. Am J Cardiol 1994;74:205–7.

35. Annas GJ. "Culture of life" politics at the bedside—the case of Terri Schiavo. N Engl J Med 2005;352:1710–5.

36. Burt RA. Death is that man taking names. Berkeley (CA): University of California Press; 2002.

37. Schneider C. The practice of autonomy: patients, doctors, and medical decisions. New York: Oxford University Press; 1998.

38. Strachan PH, Carroll SL, de Laat S, et al. Patients' perspectives on end-of-life issues and implantable cardioverter defibrillators. J Palliat Care 2011;27:6–11.

39. Goldstein N, Bradley E, Zeidman J, et al. Barriers to conversations about deactivation of implantable defibrillators in seriously ill patients: results of a nationwide survey comparing cardiology specialists to primary care physicians. J Am Coll Cardiol 2009;54:371–3.

40. Goldstein NE, Mehta D, Teitelbaum E, et al. "It's like crossing a bridge" complexities preventing physicians from discussing deactivation of implantable defibrillators at the end of life. J Gen Intern Med 2008;1:2–6.
41. Wright AA, Zhang B, Ray A, et al. Associations between end-of-life discussions, patient mental health, medical care near death, and caregiver bereavement adjustment. JAMA 2008;300:1665–73.
42. Lewis WR, Luebke DL, Johnson NJ, et al. Withdrawing implantable defibrillator shock therapy in terminally ill patients. Am J Med 2006;119:892–6.
43. Singer PA, Martin DK, Kelner M. Quality end-of-life care: patients' perspectives. JAMA 1999;281:163–8.
44. Nicolasora N, Pannala R, Mountantonakis S, et al. If asked, hospitalized patients will choose whether to receive life-sustaining therapies. J Hosp Med 2006;1: 161–7.
45. Fried TR, O'Leary JR. Using the experiences of bereaved caregivers to inform patient- and caregiver-centered advance care planning. J Gen Intern Med 2008;23:1602–7.
46. Kobza R, Erne P. End of life decisions in patients with malignant tumors. PACE 2007;30:845–9.
47. Stewart GC, Weintraub JR, Pratibhu PP, et al. Patient expectations from implantable defibrillators to prevent death in heart failure. J Card Fail 2010;16:106–13.
48. Raphael CE, Koa-Wing M, Stain N, et al. Implantable cardioverter-defibrillator recipient attitudes towards device deactivation: how much do patients want to know? Pacing Clin Electrophysiol 2011;34:1628–33.
49. Dodson JA, Fried TR, Van Ness PH, et al. Patient preferences for deactivation of implantable cardioverter defibrillators. Archives of Internal Medicine, in press.
50. Goldstein NE, Back AL, Morrison RS. Titrating guidance: a model to guide physicians in assisting patients and family members who are facing complex decisions. Arch Intern Med 2008;168:1733–9.
51. Goldstein NE, Mehta D, Siddiqui S, et al. "That's like an act of suicide" patients' attitudes toward deactivation of implantable defibrillators. J Gen Intern Med 2008; 1:7–12.
52. Goldstein N, Carlson M, Livote E, et al. Brief communication: management of implantable cardioverter-defibrillators in hospice: a nationwide survey. Ann Intern Med 2010;152:296–9.
53. Goldstein N, Carlson M, Livote E, et al. 2010. Online appendix: sample ICD deactivation policy. Available at: http://www.ncbi.nlm.nih.gov/pmc/articles/PMC2832227/?tool=pubmed#SM. Accessed March 12, 2011.
54. Wiegand DL, Kalowes PG. Withdrawal of cardiac medications and devices. AACN Advanced Critical Care 2007;18:415–25.
55. Lindsay BD, Estes NA 3rd, Maloney JD, et al, Heart Rhythm Society. Heart Rhythm Society Policy Statement Update: recommendations on the Role of Industry Employed Allied Professionals (IEAPs). Heart Rhythm 2008;5:e8–10 [Epub 2008 Sep 24].
56. Kay GN, Bittner GT. Should implantable cardioverter-defibrillators and permanent pacemakers in patients with terminal illness be deactivated? Deactivating implantable cardioverter-defibrillators and permanent pacemakers in patients with terminal illness. An ethical distinction. Circ Arrhythm Electrophysiol 2009;2: 336–9.
57. Zellner RA, Aulisio MP, Lewis WR. Deactivating permanent pacemakers in patients with terminal illness; patient autonomy is paramount. Circ Arrhythm Electrophysiol 2009;2:340–4.

58. Mueller PS, Jenkins SM, Bramstedt KA, et al. Deactivating implanted cardiac devices in terminally ill patients: practices and attitudes. Pacing Clin Electrophysiol 2008;31:560–8.
59. AMA Council on Ethical and Judicial Affairs. Physician objection to treatment and individual patient discrimination: CEJA report 6-A-07. AMA council on ethical and judicial affairs. Chicago: AMA Press; 2007.

Bradyarrhythmias in the Elderly

Preetham Kumar, MD[a], Fred M. Kusumoto, MD[a],*,
Nora Goldschlager, MD[b,c]

KEYWORDS

- Bradyarrhythmias • Elderly • Sinus node dysfunction • Management

KEY POINTS

- With the dramatic increase in the number of elderly people in the United States and in most parts of the world, including China, India, and Europe, there will be an accompanying increase in patients with sinus node dysfunction (SND) and atrioventricular (AV) block; therefore, it will be essential for health care personnel to have a basic knowledge of bradyarrhythmias and the special considerations required for managing these rhythms in elderly patients.
- Comprehensive assessment before decisions on medical and device-based management is critical and must take into account social issues and the presence of comorbid conditions that are so commonly observed in this patient group.
- When management decisions are considered, life expectancy, social support, physical and cognitive capacity to follow basic maintenance strategies and follow-up options need to be assessed and individualized. Consideration must also be given to psychological health and wellbeing, along with clear education and clarification of expectations regarding the potential benefits and adverse effects associated with the available treatment options.
- In patients with SND, maintaining AV synchrony reduces the likelihood of developing atrial fibrillation, particularly in those patients without a history of this arrhythmia; reduces the incidence of pacemaker syndrome; and may reduce the likelihood of heart failure hospitalizations. Thus, dual-chamber pacing may be preferred over single-chamber atrial pacing as the initial pacing strategy.

In the most recent US census performed in 2010, 12.7% of the population was older than 65 years, and it is projected that this demographic group will increase to almost 20% of the population by 2030.[1] Moreover, it has been predicted that most developed countries will also experience increases in their elderly population similar to the United States.[2] For example, a separate analysis from the United Nations has estimated that by 2050 people older than 60 years would account for more than 30% of people living in the United States and in Europe and reach 40% in Italy and Japan.[2] Because bradyarrhythmias are the most common arrhythmias identified in older patients, a significant increase in the prevalence of bradyarrhythmias is likely.

[a] Electrophysiology and Pacing Service, Division of Cardiovascular disease, Department of Medicine, Mayo Clinic, 4500 San Pablo Avenue, Jacksonville, FL 32224, USA; [b] Cardiology Division, Department of Medicine, San Francisco General Hospital, San Francisco, CA 94110, USA; [c] Department of Medicine, University of California, 505 Parnassus, San Francisco, CA 94143, USA
* Corresponding author.
E-mail address: Kusumoto.fred@mayo.edu

Clin Geriatr Med 28 (2012) 703–715
http://dx.doi.org/10.1016/j.cger.2012.08.004
0749-0690/12/$ – see front matter © 2012 Elsevier Inc. All rights reserved.

PREVALENCE AND PATHOPHYSIOLOGY OF BRADYARRHYTHMIAS IN THE ELDERLY

Bradyarrhythmias are a group of rhythm disorders that can be generally divided into abnormalities of impulse generation or impulse conduction (**Fig. 1**). Abnormalities of impulse generation and conduction can be caused by decreased automaticity of the sinus node and/or delayed or blocked impulse conduction within the sinoatrial node; in either case, abnormal rates of atrial muscle depolarization (P waves) are observed on the electrocardiogram (ECG). The ECG manifestations of sinus node dysfunction (SND) are diverse and include sinus bradycardia; ectopic atrial and junctional rhythms (which are often escape rhythms); sinus pauses; and, if the bradycardia-tachycardia syndrome is present, periods of rapid heart rhythms, such as atrial fibrillation and atrial tachycardia interspersed with the slower rhythms (**Fig. 2**).

Sinus rhythm

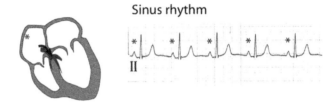

Sinus node dysfunction with junctional escape rhythm

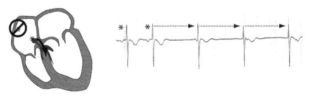

AV block with junctional escape rhythm

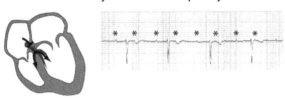

Fig. 1. Types of bradyarrhythmias. Top: In normal sinus rhythm, the sinus node generates an impulse at a normal physiologic rate that is conducted to the ventricles via the AV node–His-Purkinje system. Middle: In sinus node dysfunction (SND), the sinus node either does not generate an impulse or the impulse is generated but does not exit the sinus node to depolarize the atria, and a subsidiary pacemaker originating in the AV node region depolarizes the ventricles (junctional rhythm). Bottom: In AV block, the sinus node functions normally but AV conduction is blocked. In this example a junctional focus below the site of AV block depolarizes the ventricles (junctional rhythm). Notice that in both SND and AV block, junctional rhythm is present; but in SND, there are not enough P waves, whereas in AV block there are enough P waves. AV, atrioventricular. (*Adapted from* Kusumoto FM, ECG interpretation: from pathophysiology to clinical application. New York: Springer; 2009; with permission.)

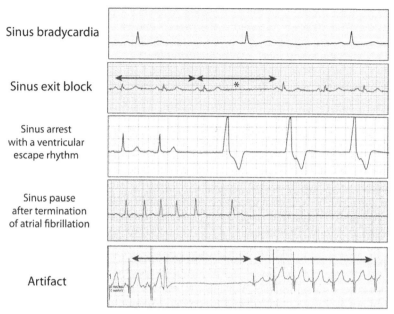

Fig. 2. ECG manifestations of SND. All rhythm strips display lead II from the ECG. In sinus node exit block the interval between the P waves is relatively constant (*double-headed arrows*) and absence of a P wave (*asterisk*) is caused by block of the sinus impulse from the sinus node to atrial tissue. An example of artifact caused by a loose lead electrode causing an apparent sinus pause is also shown (*bottom*). In this case, the PP intervals remain constant but several P waves are not observed along with loss of QRST complex amplitude and integrity. In this case, changes in the QRS- and T-wave morphology caused by poor electrical integrity help the clinician distinguish artifact from a true sinus pause.

A delay or block in conduction can occur at any part of the sinoatrial and atrioventricular (AV) nodes and His-Purkinje system. However, because the AV node and the His bundle form a single conduction axis between the atria and the ventricles, blocked conduction at either of these critical anatomic locations may lead to slow ventricular rates; regardless of the specific site of block, this condition defines AV block. A delay or block in impulse conduction can also occur in the left or right bundle branches or in the left anterior or posterior fascicles. In bundle branch or fascicular block, if the ventricles can be depolarized by one of the remaining bundle branches or fascicles, slow ventricular rates will not be observed, although the QRS complexes may be wider than normal because of abnormal intraventricular conduction.

The resting heart rate does not change dramatically with normal aging, although after autonomic blockade with beta blockers and atropine the intrinsic heart rate is decreased, suggesting that changes in autonomic balance may be important for maintaining a relatively constant heart rate.[3,4] However, starting in early adulthood the maximal heart rate achieved with exercise decreases by approximately 0.7 beats per minute every year.[5] This normal decrease in maximal achieved heart rate is not appreciably changed with exercise training and is the single most important reason for the decrease in exercise capacity associated with the normal aging process. In addition to the decrease in maximal achieved heart rate, the response of the sinus node to other forms of stress also seems to diminish with age. In particular, there may be delayed recovery of the sinus node following a period of supraventricular tachycardia. This delayed recovery is the reason that sinus pauses, which may be quite prolonged, are frequently observed on termination of atrial tachyarrhythmias in the elderly with the brady-tachy syndrome (see **Fig. 2**).

Anatomic studies have demonstrated increases in fibrous and fatty tissue in the AV node and His bundle with aging.[6,7] In one pathology series of hearts from 150 adults of different ages, almost all patients had the development of fibrofatty tissue and about 50% displayed calcification in this region.[7] In 7 hearts, calcium deposition was so extensive that it impinged on a portion of the AV conduction system.[7] The impact of these pathoanatomic changes on AV node function is uncertain; in fact, one small clinical study found that refractory periods of the AV node prolonged only slightly once adulthood was reached.[8] However, as discussed later, large population studies have consistently demonstrated progressive delay in AV conduction with age. It may be that aging has different effects on refractoriness and conduction velocity properties of the AV conduction system. Finally, an anatomic study has described a decrease in autonomic innervation of the AV conduction system with aging, thereby potentially reducing the usual and expected effects of autonomic input to the heart.[9]

The severity of AV block is generally classified electrocardiographically as 1° AV block, 2° AV block, or advanced or 3° AV block (**Fig. 3**). In 1° AV block, every P wave leads to a QRS complex but the PR interval is prolonged. In 2° AV block, some but not all P waves lead to a QRS complex. Second-degree AV block is further

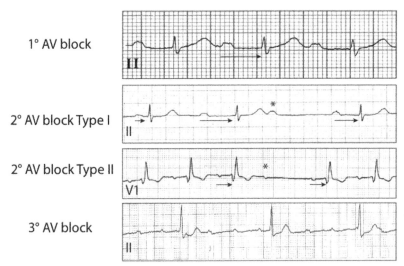

Fig. 3. Different forms of AV block. In 1° AV block (*top strip*), the PR interval is prolonged (*arrow*) but the 1:1 relationship between P waves and QRS complexes is maintained. In 2° AV block, some but not all of the P waves are conducted to the ventricles. For this reason, in most cases of 2° AV block, the QRS complexes will be regularly irregular. The only exception is 2° AV block with 2:1 conduction in which every other P wave leads to a QRS complex. A 2° AV block is further classified as Mobitz type I if the PR interval (*arrows, second strip*) lengthens before the dropped QRS complex (*asterisk*) or Mobitz type II if the PR interval (*arrows, third strip*) is constant before and after the P wave associated with the dropped QRS (*asterisk*). In 3° AV block (*bottom strip*), there is dissociation between the P waves and the QRS complexes; note that the P waves and QRS complexes are regular but the PR interval is highly variable.

subdivided into Mobitz type I (also often called Wenckebach block) if the PR interval gradually prolongs before the QRS complex is dropped (P wave without a QRS complex) and Mobitz type II if the PR interval remains constant before and after the dropped QRS complex. This distinction is important because Mobitz type I 2° AV block is generally caused by a block within the AV node, whereas Mobitz type II 2° AV block is in the His bundle region or His-Purkinje system. Mobitz type II 2° AV block and advanced or complete AV block in which no P waves are conducted to the ventricles are associated with a worse prognosis, in part because patients can develop severe symptoms of cerebral hypoperfusion because of the unreliability and slow rates of subsidiary pacemakers that originate in ventricular tissue. Importantly, the degree of AV block may change, which is a feature that may be related to changes in autonomic tone or the effects of medications.

Clinical studies have reported a gradual increase in the prevalence of SND and AV block with age, identified by ECG monitoring in both symptomatic patients and large population cohorts. In one study of 167 patients with unexplained syncope who underwent prolonged monitoring with an implantable loop recorder, 106 patients had recurrent syncope. Significant bradycardia was the most commonly recorded abnormal rhythm, occurring in 33% of cases, whereas tachycardia accounted for only 9% of the cases.[10] The Cardiovascular Health Study was a large population-based study of 5201 adults older than 65 years from 4 different regions in the United States.[11] A randomly selected subset of 1372 patients underwent 24-hour ambulatory electrocardiography as part of their initial evaluation. In this group of patients, evidence for SND (defined as sinus pause >3 seconds or heart rate <40 beats per minute) was observed in 1.8% of women and 5% of men. Evidence for significant AV block (2° type II or complete AV block) was less common: 0.4% in women and 1.1% in men. The prevalence of significant bradycardia seemed to be affected not only by age but also by gender, with almost 10% of men older than 80 years having documented bradycardia compared with 2% of women in the same age group. The likelihood of developing significant AV block seems to progress further with advanced aging. In a study comparing 32 Japanese centenarians with a control group of older Japanese men and women with an average age of 75 years, although sinus rates were similar, first- or second-degree AV block was observed in 25% of the centenarians compared with 7% of the elderly controls.[12] In another study that compared AV conduction characteristics between a group of young adults (average age of 30 years) and a group of healthy older adults (average age of 79 years), atrial pacing at a fixed rate of 120 beats per minute led to a longer PR interval in the older patients (PR interval 0.18 seconds) compared with younger patients (PR interval 0.15 seconds), and this difference was still present after complete autonomic blockade, providing evidence that changes in AV conduction properties are probably caused by structural changes rather than to changes in autonomic tone.[13]

The incidence and prevalence of bundle branch block (BBB) increases with age. In a cohort study of 855 men initially evaluated at 50 years of age and subsequently followed for 30 years, the prevalence of BBB increased from 1% to 17%.[14] Right bundle branch block (RBBB) was more commonly observed than left bundle branch block (LBBB) at both 50 years of age (RBBB 0.8% vs LBBB 0.4%) and 80 years of age (RBBB 11.3% vs LBBB 5.7%). These observations have been confirmed in other large cohorts. In a group of 110 000 patients screened by the Irish Heart Foundation, isolated RBBB was observed more frequently than isolated LBBB (0.18% vs 0.1%, respectively) with an increase with age from 0.4% in the cohort 45 to 54 years of age to 1.3% in the patients older than 64 years.[15] Finally, gender differences were noted in the Framingham Heart Study in which complete LBBB or RBBB was observed in 11% of men but only 5% of women older than 60 years.[16]

CAUSE

The pathophysiology of bradyarrhythmias is complex and diverse. SND can be primarily caused by intrinsic cardiac conditions or systemic conditions or illnesses. Idiopathic degeneration of the sinus node caused by aging is probably the most common cause of SND. Myocardial ischemia, infiltrative diseases, infectious diseases, trauma, collagen vascular diseases, myotonic muscular dystrophy, and familial diseases are known to be associated with SND. Genetic studies of families with SND have generally described mutations that affect sodium (Na^+) channel function, although families with mutations in potassium (K^+) channels and ankyrin-B (a protein important for cellular architecture) have also been reported. Similarly, although progressive fibrosis and fatty infiltration can be observed in the septum at the region of the AV node and His bundle in almost all patients beginning in their forties, this process can be accelerated by comorbid conditions, such as diabetes, hypertension, or coronary artery disease.

For both SND and AV block, potentially reversible and iatrogenic causes, such as electrolyte imbalance, hypothermia, hypothyroidism, or the use of certain pharmacologic agents, must be considered in determining the cause. The elderly are particularly susceptible to side effects from drugs for several reasons. First, the elderly are more likely to be receiving calcium channel blockers, beta-blockers, and antiarrhythmic medications for coexisting cardiovascular conditions, especially hypertension, heart failure, and atrial fibrillation. With the increasing prevalence of dementia in the elderly, there has been an increase in the use of medications to manage the dementia that have cholinergic properties that can affect both sinus nodal and AV nodal function. In a population-based cohort study, patients with dementia receiving cholinesterase inhibitors were more likely to be hospitalized for syncope (hazard ratio 1.76) or symptomatic bradycardia (hazard ratio 1.69) and to undergo pacemaker implantation (hazard ratio 1.49).[17] Polypharmacy is also much more likely to be present in the elderly because of the presence of multiple chronic problems, thereby increasing the risk of untoward drug interactions. Second, aging is often associated with complex and unpredictable changes in medication pharmacokinetics and pharmacodynamics. Elderly patients have reduced first-pass metabolism, which can increase the bioavailability of some drugs, such as propranolol. With aging there is a reduction in muscle mass and, hence, decreased water content in the body; hydrophilic (water soluble) medications, such as digoxin, may thereby reach higher serum concentrations even when given at lower doses. Worsening renal function observed in some elderly patients compounds the problem of higher-than-desired serum concentrations, leading to adverse or toxic effects at standard doses. Third, different medications within the same class may have different effects in elderly populations. In the Cardiac Insufficiency Bisoprolol Study in the Elderly, 883 patients with an average age of 73 years and heart failure were randomized to bisoprolol or carvedilol in an effort to evaluate tolerability.[18] Although the overall incidence of side effects was similar in both groups (24%–25%), bisoprolol was associated with a greater reduction in heart rate and more dose-limiting bradycardia (bisoprolol 16% vs carvedilol 11%), whereas carvedilol was associated with more pulmonary adverse events, such as bronchospasm or development of shortness of breath (bisoprolol 4% vs carvedilol 10%). Finally, even though bradycardias are often related to medications, the association may not be causal. In a natural history study of 169 patients with AV block, 92 (54%) were taking rate-slowing medications; although AV block resolved in 35% of the group when the drug was discontinued, AV block often recurred. On final analysis, rate-slowing medication was causal for the observed AV block in only 14 out of 92 patients (15%).

CLINICAL MANIFESTATIONS, DIAGNOSIS, AND INITIAL EVALUATION

The clinical manifestations of bradyarrhythmia can range from an asymptomatic state to symptoms of skipped heart beat, sensation of pauses in cardiac rhythm, fatigue, light-headedness, dizziness, syncope, and even death. Diminished perfusion to the brain and the inability to meet oxygen demands at rest or during activity may lead to symptoms of presyncope or frank syncope or, commonly, exercise intolerance (chronotropic incompetence). In elderly patients, loss of AV synchrony caused by AV block with AV dissociation can cause elevated left atrial and pulmonary venous pressures with the consequent development of pulmonary congestive symptoms, such as exertional dyspnea.[19] Cerebral hypoperfusion as a cause of symptoms may go unrecognized or be misinterpreted by patients, making it challenging to correlate symptoms with bradyarrhythmias.[20] Importantly, bradyarrhythmias are often transient, so that correlation of symptoms with a specific rhythm disorder may be particularly difficult.

The presence and significance of AV block may also be difficult to evaluate in elderly patients. Although the diagnosis of AV block can occasionally be easily confirmed by the presence of 2° or 3° AV block on the ECG or suspected by the presence of PR interval prolongation (especially if infra-His conduction disease manifested as BBB is present), not infrequently the diagnosis is more difficult because of the intermittent nature of higher grades of AV block. In some cases, extended ECG monitoring is required using either an external event recorder or an implantable loop recorder. Even in the presence of AV block, however, the evaluation of symptoms can be difficult. For example, because of the progression of AV block may be gradual, symptoms may be ascribed to normal aging or, in some cases, not recognized at all. Similarly, although the presence of first-degree AV block or BBB often constitutes a clue to the possibility of symptomatic intermittent high degrees of AV block, the findings could also be spurious and merely reflect normal aging.

To summarize, elderly patients present unique challenges both in the diagnosis and management of bradyarrhythmias. Elderly patients often have higher incidences of comorbidities, drug-drug interactions, and altered pharmacokinetic and pharmacodynamic profiles; they may also manifest cardiopulmonary signs and symptoms not necessarily resulting from bradycardia. When management decisions are considered, life expectancy, social support, and the physical and cognitive capacity to follow basic maintenance strategies and follow-up options need to be assessed and individualized. Consideration must also be given to psychological health and wellbeing, along with clear education and clarification of expectations regarding the potential benefits and adverse effects associated with the available treatment options.

PROGNOSIS OF BRADYARRHYTHMIAS IN THE ELDERLY

Untreated SND has been associated with significant adverse outcomes, such as syncope, tachycardia-bradycardia syndrome, and decreased ejection fraction. Age is a powerful predictor for unfavorable cardiovascular outcomes in patients with untreated SND. In a small study of 35 patients that evaluated the natural history of untreated SND, after a 17-month follow-up, 20 patients (57%) developed a major cardiovascular event defined as syncope, heart failure, or atrial fibrillation.[21] On multivariate analysis, age of more than 65 years was the most important predictor of a major cardiovascular event (hazard ratio 7.80), followed by ejection fraction less than 55% (hazard ratio 3.7), and echocardiographic left ventricular diastolic diameter more than 52 mm (hazard ratio 2.9).[21]

The natural history of AV block has been evaluated in several studies. In patients with 1° AV block, the prognosis seems to be excellent. In a 30-year longitudinal study of 176 patients with first-degree AV block, only 2 patients developed higher grades of AV block.[22] Patients with 2° AV block within the AV node also have a good prognosis if other forms of heart disease, such as ischemia or left ventricular hypertrophy, are not present. In one study of 56 patients with 2° AV block documented by electrophysiology study to be due to block within the AV node, only one of nineteen patients without associated heart disease (age range 18–83 years, 3 patients older than 60 years) required implantation of a permanent pacemaker during a 3 year follow-up period.[23] However, in the 37 patients with associated heart disease, during the same time period, pacemakers were required in 10 patients and 16 patients died, including 5 who had undergone permanent pacemaker implantation. In almost all patients with symptomatic AV block, permanent pacing is the only effective long-term therapy.

PACEMAKER THERAPY

Only one randomized trial has evaluated the use of medical therapy for SND. In the Oral Theophylline versus Permanent Pacemaker in Sick Sinus Syndrome study, 107 patients with SND and an average age of 73 years were randomized to cardiac pacing therapy, oral theophylline, or no therapy. After a mean follow-up period of 19 months, cardiac pacing was associated with a decrease in syncope and heart failure.[24] For this reason, once the clinician is certain that symptomatic SND is present, permanent cardiac pacing is the preferred treatment.

The aim of pacemaker therapy is to prevent adverse outcomes associated with bradycardia and to maximize functional outcomes, such as quality of life, exercise capacity, and sense of wellbeing. Because the primary function of permanent cardiac pacing is to provide ventricular rate support, pacing options for patients with SND include single-chamber atrial pacing and dual-chamber pacing (**Fig. 4**).

For patients with AV block, either single-chamber ventricular pacing or dual-chamber pacing provide rate support. Over the past decades, several large randomized trials have evaluated the effect of pacing mode on patient outcomes. Pacing mode will determine whether AV synchrony is maintained if atrial rhythms other than fibrillation are present, and specific programming choices are critical for optimizing hemodynamic and clinical outcomes in these patients. Although dual-chamber pacing systems provide the greatest flexibility for programming, they are more complex and are associated with higher periprocedural complication rates.[20]

Several large randomized trials have evaluated the effect of pacing mode specifically in patients with SND. In the largest of these trials, the Mode Selection Trial (MOST), 2010 patients with SND (median age of 74 years) were randomized to a dual-chamber pacing mode or a ventricular pacing–only mode (although pacing systems with both atrial and ventricular leads were implanted in all patients).[25] The primary end point of MOST was a composite of nonfatal stroke and death from any cause. After an average follow-up of almost 3 years, the primary end point was reached in 22% of patients, with no significant difference between the two pacing modes. However, dual-chamber pacing was associated with a small but significant reduction in the incidence of heart failure hospitalizations (dual chamber 10% vs single chamber 12%; $P = .021$) and a significant reduction in the development of pacemaker syndrome. This syndrome consists of a constellation of symptoms related to loss of AV synchrony, retrograde ventriculoatrial conduction in some patients, and an inability to increase pacing rate in response to increased metabolic needs. Symptoms include light-headedness, fatigue, effort intolerance, presyncope, and sometimes frank syncope. Pacemaker syndrome is essentially eliminated with appropriately programmed dual-chamber

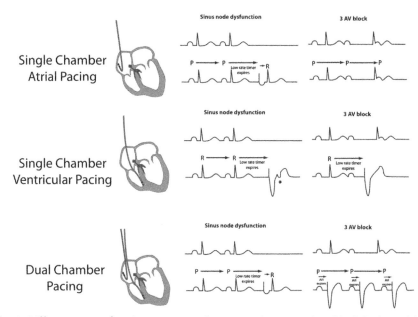

Fig. 4. Different types of pacing systems and responses in SND and AV block (3° heart block in this example). Top: In single-chamber atrial pacing, a single lead is placed in the right atrium. For patients with SND, bradycardia will be prevented as long as AV block is not present. However, in 3° AV block, ventricular rate support is not provided because there is no ventricular lead. Middle: In single-chamber ventricular pacing, a single lead is placed in the right ventricle. In SND, a ventricular stimulus is provided when the low rate timer expires, which may be associated with a retrograde P wave. In the setting of 3° AV block, ventricular pacing provides rate support but AV synchrony is not maintained. Bottom: In dual-chamber pacing, a lead is placed in the right atrium and a second lead is placed in the right ventricle. In both SND and AV block, dual-chamber pacing provides ventricular rate support and maintains AV synchrony.

pacing parameters, including the rate response feature in appropriate patients. Maintaining AV synchrony with dual-chamber pacing also seems to be important for decreasing the likelihood of developing atrial fibrillation (AF). In MOST, patients with a history of AF had a nonsignificant 14% decrease in incident AF with dual-chamber pacing. In contrast, among patients without a history of AF, dual-chamber pacing was associated with a 50% reduction in incident AF compared with single-chamber ventricular pacing.

The concurrently performed Canadian Trial of Physiologic Pacing (CTOPP) also addressed the issue of the importance of maintaining AV synchrony (with single-chamber atrial pacing or dual-chamber pacing) in patients with symptomatic bradycardia caused by SND or AV block.[26] In this study, approximately 40% of the 2500 randomized patients had SND and the remaining 60% had AV block. The CTOPP study found a marginally significant decrease in the annual risk of AF associated with pacing modes that maintained AV synchrony (AV synchrony 5.3% vs ventricular pacing 6.6%; $P = .05$).

A recently published trial provided additional information on differences in outcomes between single-chamber atrial pacing and dual-chamber pacing in SND. In the Danish Multicenter Randomized Trial on Single Atrial Pacing versus Dual Chamber Pacing in Sick Sinus Syndrome, 1415 patients with SND and an average age of 73 years were randomized to single-chamber atrial pacing (AAIR) or dual-chamber pacing (DDDR).[27] After a mean follow-up of 5.4 years, death (27%–29%) and development of AF (23%–28%) was observed at similar rates in both groups. Patients in the single-chamber atrial pacing group were almost twice as likely to require reoperation as the dual-chamber pacing group (AAIR 22.1% vs DDDR 11.9%; $P<.0001$) because of the development of AV block.

In summary, data from the randomized trials are reasonably consistent. In patients with SND, maintaining AV synchrony reduces the likelihood of developing AF, particularly in those patients without a history of this arrhythmia; reduces the incidence of pacemaker syndrome; and may reduce the likelihood of heart failure hospitalizations. Thus, dual-chamber pacing may be preferred over single-chamber atrial pacing as the initial pacing strategy.

There are less data on the effects of pacing mode in patients with AV block. Because the primary function of permanent pacemakers is to provide ventricular rate support, single-chamber ventricular pacing and dual-chamber pacing are the only two viable options in this condition. In the United Kingdom Pacing and Cardiovascular Events (UKPace) trial, almost 2000 patients older than 70 years with high-grade (2° or 3°) AV block were randomized to single-chamber ventricular pacing or dual-chamber pacing.[28] The mean age of the study group was almost 80 years, and 60% of patients were judged to have persistent AV block and 40% intermittent bradycardia. After a median follow-up of 4.6 years, mortality was similar in both groups (ventricular pacing 7.2% vs dual-chamber pacing 7.4%). There was no difference in rates of AF, stroke, or heart failure between the two groups. UKPace was a well-designed trial but has been criticized because of possible selection bias because only 50% of eligible patients were randomized and because of the relatively high percentage of ventricular pacing in the dual-chamber pacing group (99%) compared with the single-chamber ventricular pacing group (94%).[29] This last point is particularly important because several lines of evidence have demonstrated the detrimental effects of right ventricular (particularly apical) pacing. For example, in a secondary analysis of the MOST study, increased right ventricular pacing was associated with an increased likelihood of heart failure hospitalization regardless of pacing mode; cumulative ventricular pacing greater than 40% was associated with a 2.5- to 3.0-fold increase in heart failure hospitalization in both the dual-chamber and single-chamber pacing groups.[30]

Similarly, in the Dual Chamber and VVI Implantable Defibrillator Trial, 506 patients with an ejection fraction less than 0.40 were randomized to backup single-chamber ventricular pacing (VVI, programmed rate of 40 beats per minute [ie, essentially no pacing]) or rate-responsive dual-chamber pacing (DDDR) programmed to a rate of 70 beats per minute.[31] At 1 year, dual-chamber pacing was associated with a 50% increase in heart failure hospitalizations (DDDR 23% vs VVI 13%). The mechanism for increased heart failure is thought to be the functional LBBB and resultant cardiac dyssynchrony associated with single-site right ventricular pacing. Newly designed algorithms have been developed by all manufacturers to minimize ventricular pacing in patients with SND or AV block. In general, maintaining AV synchrony with dual-chamber pacing systems is preferable in most patients with AV block; however, the results of the UKPace trial do suggest that single-chamber ventricular pacing may be a reasonable option in older patients, particularly if they have only intermittent episodes of AV block.

PACEMAKER THERAPY IN THE ELDERLY: COMPLICATIONS AND PROGRAMMING CONSIDERATIONS

Link and colleagues[32] analyzed the complication rate of dual-chamber permanent pacing in the Pacemaker Selection in the Elderly study, one of the early trials that evaluated the effects of pacing mode in patients older than 60 years who had SND. The most common periprocedural complication was lead dislodgement, which was seen in 2.2% of patients. Pneumothorax occurred in 2.0%, cardiac perforation in 1.0%, and subclavian vein thrombosis in 0.5%; the total periprocedural complication rate was 6.2%, a value similar to historical rates.[32] However, there was a trend toward a higher risk of pneumothorax in patients older than 75 years, in women, and in patients with low body weight. Complications after the periprocedural period did not seem to be dependent on age. For example, the incidence of infection at the pocket site or pacemaker lead was 0.25% in both younger and older patients. Similar results were reported in a recently published meta-analysis of 4814 patients from the randomized trials on pacing therapy.[33] Early complications were more common in patients older than 75 years (5.1%) when compared with those younger than 75 years (3.4%), a difference that was mainly caused by an increased incidence of pneumothorax and a higher likelihood of lead dislodgement. After an average follow-up of 5 years, the risk of lead fracture was lower in older patients (≥75 years 2.7% vs <75 years 3.6%). Generally, the risks of pacemaker implantation are similar in younger and older patients, but pneumothorax and lead dislodgement are somewhat more common in older patients.

Once implanted, pacemaker programming should aim for appropriate rate support but minimize the amount of right ventricular pacing with its resulting functional LBBB. Because pacing from the right ventricle, especially the apex, is inferior to intrinsic ventricular depolarization, special pacing algorithms or increasing the programmed AV delay may be helpful for facilitating ventricular depolarization via the native His-Purkinje system. In addition to appropriate programming, changes in the patient's medication regimen may be required for optimum management. For example, worsening renal function in patients receiving digoxin could lead to an increase in the percent of ventricular pacing through production of AV block, which in turn could trigger the development of heart failure symptoms.

The pacing system should be interrogated routinely for the presence and duration of atrial arrhythmias, specifically AF, which could lead to consideration for anticoagulation therapy. In the Asymptomatic AF and Stroke Evaluation in Pacemaker Patients and the AF Reduction Atrial Pacing Trial, 2580 patients older than 65 years who had hypertension and no history of AF were followed for 2.5 years. Approximately 10% of patients had subclinical AF identified by the device, and at follow-up these patients had a 6-fold increase in the likelihood of developing symptomatic AF and a 2.5-fold increased risk of stroke or thromboembolism.[34] Although it is not clear whether treatment of subclinical AF with anticoagulants to reduce stroke is beneficial, it is important for the clinician to be aware of this risk and factor it into the decision on whether or not to initiate treatment.

Remote monitoring methods may be a particularly attractive option for pacemaker follow-up in elderly patients who are less mobile. In the Pacemaker Remote Follow-up Evaluation and Review study, 897 patients with a clinical indication for permanent pacing (33% for SND and 67% for AV block) were randomized to either a remote monitoring group (office visit at 1 year and remote interrogation every 3 months) or a control group (office visits at 6 and 12 months combined with traditional transtelephonic monitoring every 2 months).[35] Issues leading to clinical intervention, such as changing pacing parameters or medications, were identified 2 months earlier in the remote monitoring group.

SUMMARY

Over the next decade, there will be a dramatic increase in the number of elderly people in the United States and in most parts of the world, including China, India, and Europe, and people older than 80 years already represent the fastest growing subgroup in the United States. With this increase in lifespan, there will be an accompanying increase in patients with SND and AV block; therefore, it will be essential for health care personnel to have a basic knowledge of bradyarrhythmias and the special considerations required for managing these rhythms in elderly patients. In particular, comprehensive assessment before decisions on medical and device-based management is critical and must take into account social issues and the presence of comorbid conditions that are so commonly observed in this patient group.

REFERENCES

1. United States census data 2010; United States Census Bureau. Available at: www.census.gov/2010census/. Accessed July 20, 2012.
2. United Nations, world populations prospects: the 2008 revision (medium scenario). 2009. Available at: www.un.org/esa/population/./wpp2008/wpp2008_text_tables.pdf. Accessed July 20, 2012.
3. Brubaker PH, Kitzman DW. Chronotropic incompetence: causes, consequences, and management. Circulation 2011;123(9):1010–20.
4. Ogawa T, Spina RJ, Martin WH, et al. Effects of aging, sex, and physical training on cardiovascular responses to exercise. Circulation 1992;86(2):494–503.
5. Gulati M, Shaw LJ, Thisted RA, et al. Heart rate response to exercise stress testing in asymptomatic women: the St. James Women Take Heart Project. Circulation 2010;122:130–7.
6. Bharati S, Lev M. The pathologic changes in the conduction system beyond the age of ninety. Am Heart J 1992;124(2):486–96.
7. Song Y, Laaksonen H, Saukko P, et al. Histopathological findings of cardiac conduction system of 150 finns. Forensic Sci Int 2001;119(3):310–7.
8. Kuo CT, Wu JM, Lin KH, et al. The effects of aging on AV nodal recovery properties. Pacing Clin Electrophysiol 2001;24(2):194–8.
9. Chow LT, Chow SS, Anderson RH, et al. Autonomic innervation of the human cardiac conduction system: changes from infancy to senility–an immunohistochemical and histochemical analysis. Anat Rec 2001;264(2):169–82.
10. Assar MD, Krahn AD, Klein GJ, et al. Optimal duration of monitoring in patients with unexplained syncope. Am J Cardiol 2003;92:1231–3.
11. Manolio TA, Furberg CD, Rautaharju PM, et al. Cardiac arrhythmias on 24-hour ambulatory electrocardiography in older women and men: the Cardiovascular Health Study. J Am Coll Cardiol 1994;23:916–25.
12. Wakida Y, Okamoto Y, Iwa T, et al. Arrhythmias in centenarians. Pacing Clin Electrophysiol 1994;17(11 Pt 2):2217–21.
13. Craft N, Schwartz JB. Effects of age on intrinsic heart rate, heart rate variability, and AV conduction in healthy humans. Am J Physiol 1995;268(4 Pt 2):H1441–52.
14. Eriksson P, Hansson PO, Eriksson H, et al. Bundle-branch block in a general male population: the study of men born 1913. Circulation 1998;98:2494–500.
15. Fahy GJ, Pinski SL, Miller DP, et al. Natural history of isolated bundle branch block. Am J Cardiol 1996;77:1185–90.
16. Kreger BE, Anderson KM, Kannel WB. Prevalence of intra-ventricular block in the general population. The Framingham Study. Am Heart J 1989;117:903–10.
17. Gill SS, Anderson GM, Fischer HD, et al. Syncope and its consequences in patients with dementia receiving cholinesterase inhibitors: a population-based cohort study. Arch Intern Med 2009;169(9):867–73.

18. Dungen HD, Apostolovic S, Inkrot S, et al. Titration to target dose of bisoprolol vs. carvedilol in elderly patients with heart failure: the CIBIS-ELD Trial. Eur J Heart Fail 2011;13:670–80.

19. Goldschlager N. Conduction disorders & cardiac pacing. In: Michael Crawford, editor. Current diagnosis & treatment: cardiology. New York: McGraw Hill; 2011. p. 222–7.

20. Kusumoto FM, Goldschlager N. Cardiac pacing. N Engl J Med 1996;334(2): 89–97.

21. Menozzi C, Brignole M, Alboni P, et al. The natural course of untreated sick sinus syndrome and identification of the variables predictive of unfavorable outcome. Am J Cardiol 1998;82:1205–8.

22. Mymin D, Mathewson FA, Tate RB, et al. The natural history of primary first-degree atrioventricular heart block. N Engl J Med 1986;315:1183–7.

23. Zeltser D, Justo D, Halkin A, et al. Drug-induced atrioventricular block: prognosis after discontinuation of the culprit drug. J Am Coll Cardiol 2004;44:105–8.

24. Alboni P, Menozzi C, Brignole M, et al. Effects of permanent pacemaker and oral theophylline in sick sinus syndrome the THEOPACE study: a randomized controlled trial. Circulation 1997;96(1):260–6.

25. Lamas GA, Lee K, Sweeney M, et al. The Mode Selection Trial (MOST) in sinus node dysfunction: design, rationale, and baseline characteristics of the first 1000 patients. Am Heart J 2000;140:541–51.

26. Kerr CR, Connolly SJ, Abdollah H, et al. Canadian trial of physiological pacing: effects of physiological pacing during long-term follow-up. Circulation 2004; 109:357–62.

27. Nielsen JC, Thomsen POB, Hojberg S, et al. A comparison of single-lead atrial pacing with dual-chamber pacing in sick sinus syndrome. Eur Heart J 2011;32: 686–96.

28. Toff WD, Camm AJ, Skehan JD. Single-chamber versus dual-chamber pacing for high-grade atrioventricular block. N Engl J Med 2005;353:145–55. UKPACE.

29. Heist EK, Harthorne JW, Sinhgh JP. Pacing for AV block. N Engl J Med 2005;353: 1742–4.

30. Sweeney MO, Hellkamp AS, Ellenbogen KA, et al. Adverse effect of ventricular pacing on heart failure and atrial fibrillation among patients with normal baseline QRS duration in a clinical trial of pacemaker therapy for sinus node dysfunction. Circulation 2003;107:2932–7.

31. Wilkoff BL, Cook JR, Epstein AE, et al. Dual chamber and VVI implantable defibrillator trial inestigators. JAMA 2002;288:3115–23.

32. Link MS, Estes NA 3rd, Griffin JJ, et al. Complications of dual chamber pacemaker implantation in the elderly. Pacemaker Selection in the Elderly (PASE) investigators. J Interv Card Electrophysiol 1998;2:175–9.

33. Armaganijan LV, Toff WD, Nielsen JC, et al. Are elderly patients at increased risk of complications following pacemaker implantation? A meta-analysis of randomized trials. Pacing Clin Electrophysiol 2012;35(2):131–4.

34. Healey JS, Connolly SJ, Gold MR, et al, ASSERT Investigators. Subclinical atrial fibrillation and the risk of stroke. N Engl J Med 2012;366(2):120–9.

35. Crossley GH, Chen J, Choucair W, et al. Clinical benefits of remote versus transtelephonic monitoring of implanted pacemakers. J Am Coll Cardiol 2009;54: 2012–9.

Syncope
Evaluation and Management in the Geriatric Patient

Blair P. Grubb, MD[a],*, Beverly Karabin, RN, MSN, PhD[b]

KEYWORDS

- Syncope • Elderly • Falls • Loss of consciousness

KEY POINTS

- Syncope is a common clinical problem accounting for 3% of all emergency room visits and 1% to 6% of all hospital admissions.
- Both a sign and a symptom, syncope can be caused by a wide variety of conditions.
- Syncope in the geriatric patient can be a particularly challenging problem because of the coexistence of multiple possible causative pathologies in the same individual.

INTRODUCTION

Syncope, which is defined as the transient loss of consciousness and postural tone with spontaneous recovery, is a common clinical problem. Current estimates are that in the United States alone syncope accounts for about 3% of all emergency department visits and close to 6% of all hospital admissions.[1–4] Of these, around 80% are 65 years of age or older.[5–7] Syncope can be considered as both a sign and a symptom. Syncope can occur from a wide variety of causes ranging from benign to life-threatening. Indeed, syncope may be the sole warning of an impending episode of sudden cardiac death. However, even if the cause of syncope is benign, the consequences of the resultant fall may not be. Significant injuries sustained during a syncopal event occur in 17% to 35% of patients, and fractures of bone occur in 5% to 7% of elderly patients.[7–9] Motor vehicle accidents have occurred because of syncope in 1% to 5% of patients.[1] Syncope, which is recurrent and unpredictable, leads to levels of functional impairment akin to those observed with chronic debilitating disorders such as rheumatoid arthritis.[3] Thus, it is not surprising that syncope (particularly in the geriatric patient) often prompts such a profound sense of concern among patients, their families, and the physicians who care for them.

[a] College of Medicine and Life Sciences, The University of Toledo, 3000 Arlington Avenue, Toledo, OH 43614, USA; [b] College of Nursing, The University of Toledo, 3000 Arlington Avenue, Toledo, OH 43614, USA
* Corresponding author. Cardiology, The University of Toledo Medical Center, 3000 Arlington Avenue, Toledo, OH 43614.
E-mail address: Blair.Grubb@utoledo.edu

Clin Geriatr Med 28 (2012) 717–728
http://dx.doi.org/10.1016/j.cger.2012.07.002
0749-0690/12/$ – see front matter © 2012 Elsevier Inc. All rights reserved.

The epidemiology of syncope in the geriatric population is hard to access. In part, this is because of a general lack of availability of eye witness accounts and a considerable overlap with the diagnosis of falls.[10–15] Older patients, both with and without significant cognitive impairment, will have great difficulty recalling the events around a fall, and some cannot even remember falling.[14] In one study, the incidence of syncope in the institutionalized elderly was 6% annually with a recurrence rate of 30%.[13] The morbidity and mortality associated with syncope in geriatric patients is greater than in the general population because falls in older patients are more frequently complicated by bone fractures, subdural hematomas, and other serious injuries. A study of elderly patients with syncope secondary to carotid sinus hypersensitivity found that more than 50% had suffered a serious injury as a consequence of a syncopal event that resulted in fractures or other injuries of such magnitude that they required hospitalization.[11] It is important to remember that a single syncopal event can convert an independent functional geriatric patient into a patient that requires permanent nursing home placement at a tremendous cost to not only the patient and their families but to society as well.

Although syncope in younger patients is often caused by a single pathologic process, in older patients it is often multifactorial in origin. Geriatric patients seem especially prone to syncope as a consequence of age-related alterations in the cardiovascular system with respect to the control of the circulation, the concurrence of multiple different illnesses, and the use of numerous medications.

The complete spectrum of potential causes for syncope is quite broad and somewhat beyond the scope of this article. The interested reader is referred to additional sources.[1]

THE AUTONOMIC NERVOUS SYSTEM

Because many of nervous disorders result from a disturbance in normal autonomic function, it seems appropriate to briefly review some aspects of its structure and operation.[16–25]

The human nervous system has two basic components: (1) the central nervous system (CNS), made up of the brain and the spinal cord, and (2) the peripheral nervous system, which is composed of groups of neurons termed ganglia and of peripheral nerves that lie outside the brain and spinal cord. Although anatomically separate, the two systems are functionally interconnected. The peripheral nervous system is further divided into somatic and autonomic divisions. The somatic division is principally concerned with sensory information about the environment outside the body as well as muscle and limb position. The autonomic division, which is usually called the autonomic nervous system (ANS), is the motor system for the viscera, the smooth muscles of the body (especially those of the vasculature), and the exocrine glands. It is composed of three distinct parts: the sympathetic, the parasympathetic, and the enteric nervous system. The sympathetic nervous system helps control the reaction of the body to stress, whereas the parasympathetic system works to conserve the body's resources and to restore equilibrium to the resting state. The enteric system controls the function of the gut. The organ systems governed by the ANS are, for the most part, independent of volitional control (although they sometimes can be affected by volitional or emotional inputs) and include the cardiorespiratory organs, gastrointestinal, and genitourinary tracts. The autonomic system is vital to the maintenance of internal homeostasis and achieves this by mechanisms that regulate blood pressure, fluid and electrolyte balance, and body temperature.

Although representative of one of the defining aspects of the evolution of *Homo sapiens*, the adoption of upright posture presented a novel challenge to the blood pressure control system that developed to meet the requirements of an animal in the dorsal position. Indeed, the organ that defines our humanity, the brain, was placed in a somewhat precarious position with regards to vascular perfusion and oxygenation. It is the ANS that governs both the short-term and medium-term blood pressure responses to positional change. Normally, around 25% of the circulating blood volume is in the thorax. Immediately following the assumption of upright posture, gravity produces a downward displacement of roughly 500 cc of blood to the abdomen and lower extremities. Approximately 50% of this amount is redistributed within seconds after standing, and almost one-quarter of total blood volume may be involved in the process. The process causes a decrease in venous return to the heart and cardiac filling pressures, and stroke volume may decrease by 40%. The reference point for determination of these changes is known as the venous hydrostatic indifference point (HIP) and represents the part of the vascular system in which pressure is independent of posture. In humans, the venous HIP is around the level of the diaphragm and the arterial HIP is at the left ventricle. The venous HIP is somewhat dynamic in that it can be altered by changes in venous compliance brought on by muscular activity. Following standing, the normal patient achieves orthostatic stabilization in 1 minute or less. Note that the exact circulatory responses brought on by standing (an active process) are somewhat different from those brought on by head-up tilt (a passive process). In the moments following regaining of upright posture, a slow decline in arterial pressure and cardiac filling occurs. This causes activation of the high-pressure receptors of the carotid sinus and aortic arch, as well as the low-pressure receptors of the heart and lungs. The mechanoreceptors that are within the heart are linked by unmyelinated vagal afferents in both the atria and ventricles. These fibers have been found to cause continuous inhibitory actions on the cardiovascular areas of the medulla (the nuclei tractus solitarii). The decrease in venous return that results from upright posture produces less stretch on these receptors, then discharge rates decrease, and the change in input to the brain stem causes an increase in sympathetic outflow resulting in systematic vasoconstriction. At the same time, the decrease in arterial pressure while upright actuates the high-pressure receptor in the carotid sinus, which stimulates an increase in heart rate. These early steady-state adaptations to upright posture, therefore, result in a 10 to 15 beat per minute increase in heart rate, a diastolic pressure increase of 10 mm/Hg, and little or no change in systolic blood pressure. Once these adjustments are complete, compared with the supine state, during upright stance the thoracic blood volume is 30% less, as is the total cardiac output, and the mean heart rate is 10 to 15 beats per minute higher.

As a person continues to stand, there is activation of neurohumoral responses, the amount of which is dependent on the patient's volume status. As a rule, the lower the volume, the higher the degree of the renin-angiotensin-aldosterone system involvement. The inability of any of these processes to function adequately (or in a coordinated manner) can potentially result in a failure in the normal response to sudden shifts in posture (or their maintenance) with resultant hypotension that may be sufficiently great enough to result in cerebral hypoperfusion, hypoxia, and loss of consciousness.

AGE-RELATED CHANGES IN AUTONOMIC CONTROL

The sympathetic nervous system undergoes a series of changes as a person ages.[16–23] Plasma norepinephrine levels have been noted to increase, possibly due to an increased spillover from sympathetic nerve terminals as well as a decreased rate of clearance. There is a reduction of beta-adrenergic–mediated cardioacceleratory response to the sympathetic activation that is observed even though circulating norepinephrine levels are increased. There is also a reduction in beta-adrenergic vaso-dilatory and alpha-adrenergic vasoconstrictive responses. This may occur because of a reduced number of adrenergic receptors that occur due to downregulation in the face of high serum norepinephrine levels. This reduction in beta-adrenergic vasodilatory response may account, in part, for the increased peripheral vascular resistance observed in the elderly.

Although the mechanisms involved remain elusive, aging is also associated with a reduction in parasympathetic tone. These data come from observations of heart rate variability in older patients that demonstrate a reduced parasympathetic response to the Valsalva maneuver, respiration, and cough. Older syncope patients have been reported to demonstrate a lower degree of heart rate variability in response to deep breathing compared with matched controls.

Alterations in heart rate that occur in response to sudden changes in blood pressure are controlled by the baroreflex. The baroreflex seems to lose its sensitivity with age, as demonstrated by a reduced augmentation in heart rate, and with hypotension (perhaps related to the reduction in beta-adrenergic responsiveness). Although most older patients compensate for this with greater degree of vasoconstriction, this mechanism may be attenuated by hypovolemia or by vasodilatory drugs. Thus, older patients treated with vasodilators or diuretics may show an enhanced suscepti-bility to syncope.

The alterations in sympathetic and parasympathetic tone that occur with aging result in disturbed heart rate control. In addition, there is a reduction in the number of cardiac pacemaker cells in the sinus node associated with aging, as well as a gener-alized increase in collagenous and elastic tissue in the entire cardiac conduction system. It has been reported that by the age of 75 years there are less than 10% of the sinoatrial cells that were present during young adulthood.[19] This reduction in bar-oreflex control of heart rate makes vasoconstriction even more important in the compensatory responses to orthostatic stress. However, the elderly exhibit alterations in atrial natriuretic peptide, renin aldosterone levels that favor an increased rate of water and salt excretion by the kidneys.[20] In addition, the normal thirst-sensing mech-anisms diminish with age and favor states of relative dehydration.[1] Therefore, the elderly are particularly sensitive to the effects of low fluid intake, diuretics, and vaso-dilatory agents of all forms.

FACTORS THAT CONTRIBUTE TO SYNCOPE IN GERIATRIC PATIENTS

A particularly challenging aspect of the evaluation of syncope in the geriatric patient is that often several potential causes of syncope will be present in a single individual. In addition, the number of medications that the average geriatric patient consumes has grown steadily over the years. It is now estimated that the average person over the age of 65 routinely takes three or more prescribed medications.[1] At the same time, many older patients consume a variety of herbal supplements and over–the-counter medi-cations that can have significant effects on blood pressure and heart rhythm. Thus, it is not uncommon to encounter a patient in whom multiple conditions that could predispose to syncope are present. Indeed it is not infrequent that no one predispos-ing condition is sufficiently severe enough to cause syncope by itself but, in comb-ination with other predisposing factors, may be sufficient to produce loss of consciousness. There are several conditions that can lead to syncope—a complete account is beyond the scope of this article. Below is an outline of conditions that have particular relevance to the geriatric patient.

HYPERTENSION

It is presently thought that a minimum of 30% of people greater than 75 years of age manifest hypertension, most likely as a consequence of the age-related physiologic changes discussed earlier.[1,22,23] Recent evidence has demonstrated that systolic hypertension is a risk factor for developing both orthostatic and postprandial hypotension.[22] Ergo, the geriatric patients at highest risk for orthostatic hypotension are those who have systolic hypertension while supine. This relationship is not fully understood; however it is thought that it is related to hypertension's ability to reduce baroreflex sensitivity and increase both ventricular and vascular stiffness.[23] Hypertension is also known to shift the threshold of the cerebral autoregulatory curve toward higher levels of blood pressure. Therefore, there can be a decline in cerebral perfusion at higher blood pressures in hypertensive as compared with normotensive patients, leading to cerebral hypoxemia and loss of consciousness at what are usually considered normal blood pressures.

In some older patients, the arteries become quite thickened and calcified. As a result, compression of the brachial artery with a sphygmomanometer requires a cuff pressure greater than that present in the artery. The net effect of this is termed pseudohypertension, in which the systolic and diastolic blood pressures measured from the sphygmomanometer are higher than the directly measured intraarterial pressures.[1] Pseudohypertension should be suspected if there is severe hypertension in the absence of end-organ damage, if there is severe calcification of the brachial arteries on radiologic examination, and if antihypertensive therapy induces symptoms compatible with cerebral hypoperfusion (eg, dizziness and weakness) in the absence of an excessive reduction in blood pressure. Some studies have reported that, when one or more of these findings are present, the incidence of true pseudohypertension may be between 25% and 50%.[1] Unfortunately, the diagnosis of pseudohypertension can only be definitively confirmed by direct measurement of intraarterial pressure; however, some investigators have suggested that the Osler maneuver may sometimes suggest the diagnosis.[26] This is performed by inflating the sphygmomanometer to a level above the systolic blood pressure, which should collapse the brachial artery. In this setting, the radial artery will only be palpable because the arterial wall is markedly stiffened and thick. Unfortunately, the results of the Osler maneuver are inadequately reproducible and demonstrate significant intraobserver variability.

DISORDERS OF ORTHOSTATIC CONTROL

The psychological changes that occur with aging, combined with the effects of acute or chronic illness, poor physical tone, prolonged bed rest, dehydration, and the effects of various medications (and occasional alcohol) may combine together and result in significant hypotension sufficient to lead to loss of consciousness.

There are a variety of disturbances in the body's orthostatic control mechanisms that can lead to profound hypotension.

REFLEX SYNCOPE

The reflex syncopes are those characterized by sudden abrupt decreases in blood pressure and often in heart rate as well. These include neurocardiogenic (vasovagal), carotid sinus hypersensitive, micturition, cough, and defecation syncope.[27] There is usually a quick recovery and prolonged postictal states are rare. Each of these states is characterized by hypersensitive response to various stimuli.[28] Neurocardiogenic syncope occurs in response to prolonged orthostatic or emotional stress. This increases venous pooling enough that venous return to the right ventricle decreases and a dramatic increase in ventricular inotropy occurs. This causes activation of mechanoreceptors that would normally fire only during stretch. This sudden increase in neural traffic to the brain stem is thought to mimic the conditions normally seen with hypertension, thereby activating an apparently paradoxic decrease in sympathetic output that leads to hypotension, bradycardia, and loss of consciousness. It should be kept in mind that activation of other mechanoreceptor beds (eg, bladder, rectum, or carotid sinus) or stimuli such as profound emotion or an epileptic discharge may cause identical responses.[29] This suggests that these patients have an inherent predisposition to these stimuli. During head-up tilt table testing these patients demonstrate a sudden dramatic decrease in blood pressure that is often followed by a decrease in heart rate (occasionally producing prolonged periods of asystole). What seems to distinguish these illnesses from the other forms of autonomic insufficiency is that, between the episodes of decompensation, these individuals seem to be healthy (exhibiting few, if any, other symptoms) and have relatively normal day-to-day autonomic function in spite of their hypersensitive predisposition. This is as compared with situations in which the autonomic system seems to fail.[30]

CHRONIC DISORDERS

Chronic autonomic failure was first reported in 1925 by Bradbury and Eggleston[31] who described it as "idiopathic orthostatic hypotension" because of a presumed lack of other neurologic deficits. Since that time, however, it has been realized that these patients suffer from a chronic state of autonomic failure characterized by alterations in thermoregulatory, bowel, bladder, sexual, and sudomotor function. The American Autonomic Society has now termed this disorder pure autonomic failure (PAF).[32] Although the cause of PAF remains obscure, some researchers have suggested that a progressive degeneration of peripheral postganglionic autonomic neurons may be to blame.

A second type of autonomic failure syndrome was reported by Shy and Drager[33] in 1960. As opposed to PAF, they described a condition that was much more severe, characterized by profound orthostatic hypotension, loss of sweating, rectal and urinary incontinence, impotence, external ocular palsy, rigidity, and tremor. Distal muscle wasting and fasciculations may be seen in the disorder. The American Autonomic Society has termed this condition multiple symptom atrophy (MSA) and has subdivided it into three types.[34] The first group displays a tremor that can be remarkably similar to that seen in Parkinson disease (some investigators refer to this group as having striatonigral degeneration). The second group seems to have principally cerebellar and/or pyramidal symptoms (also known as the olivopontocerebellar degeneration group). The third type seems to be a mixture of these two. MSA may seem similar to Parkinson disease. An autopsy study performed in the United Kingdom found that between 7% and 22% of subjects thought to be suffering from Parkinson disease during life had neuropathologic evidence for MSA instead.[35] Most cases begin between ages 50 and 70 and follow a progressive down-hill course. Death usually occurs between 7 and 9 years after onset of symptoms, usually from respiratory failure.[36]

A milder form of chronic autonomic insufficiency has recently been referred to as the postural orthostatic tachycardia syndrome (POTS). The defining feature here is a marked tachycardia that occurs while the patient is upright that can reach rates above 160 beats per minute.[37] Patients with POTS often complain of lightheadedness, severe fatigue, exercise intolerance, dizziness, and near syncope. During head-up tilt table testing, patients with POTS will have a sudden increase in heart rate of more than 30 beats per minute in the first 5 minutes upright, or will achieve a rate of greater than 120 beats per minute associated with only modest reductions in blood pressure.

The most common pathophysiological mechanism that causes POTS is a failure of the peripheral vasculature to adequately vasoconstrict during orthostatic stress. A second form of POTS has been identified that seems to result from an excessive production of norepinephrine due to a genetic defect in a norepinephrine transporter protein.

SECONDARY AUTONOMIC DISORDERS

A large variety of diseases and conditions may cause disturbances in normal autonomic function. The physician should keep in mind that autonomic symptoms may be but one manifestation of a greater disorder. Conditions such as diabetes mellitus, cancer, amyloidosis, and autoimmune disorders may all affect autonomic function.[36] Nearly one-third of patients with Parkinson will develop autonomic involvement. Recent data suggest that orthostatic hypotension may accompany the development of senile dementia.[38]

CARDIOVASCULAR SYNCOPE

Between 21% and 34% of syncope in geriatric patients has a cardiovascular cause.[1,7] Of these, various cardiac arrhythmias cause 16%; brady-tachy syndrome, 3% to 6%; aortic stenosis, 4% to 5%; myocardial infarction, 2% to 6%; and heart block, 1% to 3%.[13] Pulmonary embolism is an unrecognized cause of syncope, particularly in the elderly who have undergone surgery.

EVALUATION AND MANAGEMENT

The single-most important aspect of the evaluation is the history and physical examination. Particular attention should be paid to a description of the syncopal event itself, the frequency, and the setting in which it occurs. Sometimes the elderly will have difficulty remembering the circumstances around the syncopal event. In these cases, bystander eye witness accounts are of great importance. A detailed physical examination should follow with special attention paid to the cardiovascular and neurologic systems. Blood pressure and heart rate should be obtained supine, sitting, and standing. In the authors' clinic, all geriatric syncope patients have a 12-lead ECG performed. Thereafter, further testing should proceed according to the physician's clinical suspicions. Many of the older patients the authors see undergo ECG to access cardiac function.

Arrhythmic causes of syncope have been difficult to determine because true confirmation requires some sort of ECG monitoring during a syncopal episode. However, because episodes are often unpredictable and of varying frequency, prolonged ECG monitoring may have a low diagnostic yield. Monitoring devices that require that the patient activate a recording mechanism are often difficult for many elderly patients to use. Also, many older patients will be amnestic to the event. The development of the implantable loop recorder (ILR) has greatly enhanced the ability to detect arrhythmias in a real-world setting. These small rectangular devices measure $62 \times 19 \times 8$ mm and they weigh approximately 17 g.[39] They are implanted under the skin through a small incision. The device operates by continually recording ECGs loops, replacing prior ECG recordings with new recordings. Current devices can automatically detect and record periods of tachycardia, bradycardia, or atrial fibrillation. In addition the patient can cause the device to record using a small hand activator. Episodes recorded are stored in the device for download in an office setting or transtelephonically (**Fig. 1**). Therapy based on ILR data is far more successful than treatment by conventional approaches. Although there has been some controversy on the role of permanent cardiac pacing in the prevention of reflex (vasovagal) syncope, the recent ISSUE-3 Trial demonstrated that the ILR-based placement of pacemakers in patients with asystole markedly reduced rates of recurrent syncope.[40]

Tilt table testing can be a valuable tool in accessing orthostatic causes of syncope in select patients.[41] Details regarding tilt table testing can be found elsewhere.[29]

TREATMENT

The treatments of syncope in the geriatric patient are as diverse as its causes. Cardiovascular causes are treated by modalities appropriate to the illness (ie, valve replacement in patients with aortic stenosis). These are treated in greater detail elsewhere.[35,36]

With respect to the treatment of autonomic disorders, one of the most critical points is establishing a diagnosis and then determining if the syncope is primary or secondary in nature. Educating both the patient and the family about the nature of the problem and the avoidance of situations that aggravate the condition is of critical importance.

Nonpharmacologic therapies include biofeedback, sleeping with the head of the bed elevated, and elastic support hose. Pharmacotherapy should be used carefully and cautiously and should be adapted to meet the needs of each patient. Several pharmacotherapies have been used. In classic neurocardiogenic syncope, beta-adrenergic–blocking agents have long been considered the mainstay of therapy. They supposedly work via a combination of their negative inotropic actions, which

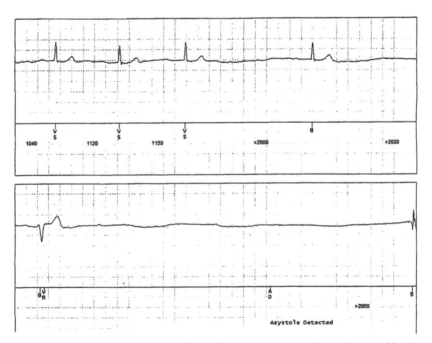

Fig. 1. An episode of asystole detected by an ILR causing syncope in an 80-year-old patient.

lessen the degree of mechanoreceptor activation, and the increase in peripheral vascular resistance, which accompanies unopposed beta-receptor blockade. Although they are of little use in younger patients, they seem effective in older patients. A useful therapy in many patients is the mineral corticoid agent fludrocortisone. The mechanism by which it raises blood pressure seems to be twofold in that it not only promotes fluid and sodium retention but it also seems to cause sensitization of peripheral vascular alpha-receptors, thus promoting a vasoconstrictive state. When using fludrocortisone, serum magnesium and potassium levels should be followed.

Because failure of the peripheral vasculature to constrict appropriately seems common to these disorders, drugs that promote vasoconstriction are frequently used. At first, drugs such as dextroamphetamine and methylphenidate were successfully used, but problems with CNS stimulation, abuse, and dependence have limited their utility.[42] An excellent alternative is the pure alpha-1–stimulating agent midodrine hydrochloride. It has little or no CNS or cardiac effects and provides significant constriction of the peripheral vasculature. Several studies have demonstrated its utility in the treatment of autonomic disorders associated with orthostatic intolerance.[43,44]

Clonidine, an alpha-2–receptor agonist that is usually used to treat hypertension can actually be used to raise blood pressure in people whose hypotension is secondary to a severe postganglionic sympathetic lesion.[45] In individuals who suffer from severe autonomic failure it is thought that the postjunctional vascular alpha-2–receptors (that are densely packed throughout the venous beds) become hypersensitive. Whereas in normal patients clonidine causes a reduction in sympathic output (and, therefore, blood pressure), patients with autonomic-failure seem to have markedly reduced sympathetic output; therefore, the peripheral effects of the drug are greater.

Many patients with autonomic failure will be anemic. A landmark report by Hoeldtke and Streeten[46] demonstrated that subcutaneous injections of erythropoietin while raising blood count will also produce dramatic increases in blood pressure. This pressure effect seems to occur independently of the red cell effect, (but does seem to increase in parallel with blood counts).[47]

A series of animal and human studies have demonstrated that neurotransmitter serotonin (5-hydroxytrypamine) plays an essential role in the central regulation of blood pressure and heart rate.[48] It has been postulated that some patients with autonomic disorders may have disturbances in central serotonin production or regulation. Supporting this concept is the observation that the serotonin reuptake inhibitors can be effective in the treatment of both neurocardiogenic syncope and orthostatic hypotension.[49]

The somatostatin analogue octreotide has proven useful in the treatment of refractory orthostatic disorders.[36] The role of permanent pacemaker therapy in the treatment of neurocardiogenic syncope has been controversial.[50] Initial open-label trials showed a benefit. However subsequent double-blind trials did not show a benefit from pacing. However, pacing in these trials was not based on ILR recordings of actual clinical events. The recently completed ISSUE-3 trial was a double-blind, prospective, randomized, placebo-controlled trail of pacemaker therapy placed in patients with ILR document asystole associated with clinical syncopal events.[40] After 2 years of follow-up, the group of patients with the pacemakers turned on had a syncope recurrence rate of 25%, while the group with pacing turned off had a recurrence rate of 57%. Thus, pacing based on ILR-guided therapy seems beneficial.

However, standard cardiac pacemakers sense only heart rate and many syncopal episodes are associated with drops in blood pressure that precede any changes in heart rate. Thus, standard pacing may not be activated until the syncopal process is well underway. Recent developments may have addressed this issue. A pacemaker has been developed that has the capability to sense blood pressure (indirectly) via changes in an electrical impedance current sent from the pacemaker lead tip to the can of the pacemaker pulse generator, a process referred to as closed-loop stimulation (CLS). Preliminary data from these separate trials suggest that CLS pacers, which can pace based on changes in blood pressure, are clearly superior to standard pacemakers in patients with neurocardiogenic syncope.[51,52] Further prospective trials will be necessary to better clarify these findings.

It should be kept in mind that, in dysautonomic disorders (as opposed to the reflex syncopes) hypotensive syncope is just one aspect of a broader constellation of symptoms relating to a generalized state of autonomic failure. The physician should, therefore, not give the patient unrealistic expectations as to what symptoms can and cannot be eliminated. Both physician and patient should remain cognizant that these disorders can be progressive in nature and that therapies may have to be altered over time.

SUMMARY

Syncope in the geriatric patient can be both dangerous for the individual affected and a diagnostic challenge to the physician. Careful attention to details of the events, a meticulous physical examination, and directed laboratory examinations can often reveal the responsible cause. Therapy can then be successfully instituted to help prevent future events.

REFERENCES

1. Lipsitz L, Grubb BP. Syncope in the elderly. In: Grubb BP, Olshansky B, editors. Syncope: mechanisms and management. Malden (MA): Blackwell-Futura; 2005. p. 301–14.
2. Calkins H, Byrne M, El-Atassi R, et al. The economic burden of unrecognized vasodepressor syncope. Am J Med 1993;95:473–9.
3. Linzer M, Pontinen M, Gold GT. Impairment of physical and psychological function in recurrent syncope. J Clin Epidemiol 1991;44:1037–43.
4. Hori S. Diagnosis of patients with syncope in emergency room. Keio J Med 1994; 43:185–91.
5. Day SC, Cook EF, Funkenstein H, et al. Evaluation and outcome of emergency room patients with transient loss of consciousness. Am J Med 1982;73:15–23.
6. Kapoor WN. Evaluation and outcome of patients with syncope. Medicine 1990; 69:16–175.
7. Kapoor WN, Karpf M, Wieand S, et al. A prospective evaluation and follow-up of patients with syncope. N Engl J Med 1983;309:197–308.
8. Eagle KA, Black HR, Cook EF, et al. Evaluation of prognostic classifications of patients with syncope. Am J Med 1985;79:455–60.
9. Kapoor WN, Karpf M, Maher Y, et al. Syncope of unknown origin: the need for cost effective approach to its diagnostic evaluation. JAMA 1982;247:2687–91.
10. Campbell AJ, Reinken J, Allan BC, et al. Falls in old age: a study of frequency and related clinical factors. Age Ageing 1981;10:264–70.
11. Nevitt MC, Cummings SR, Hudes ES. Risk factors for injurious falls: a prospective study. J Gerontol 1991;46:M164–70.
12. Savage DD, Corwin L, McGee DL, et al. Epidemiologic features of isolated syncope: the Framingham Study. Stroke 1985;16:626–8.
13. Lipsitz LA. Syncope in the elderly. Ann Intern Med 1983;99:92–104.

14. Kenny R. Syncope in the older patient. London: Chapman and Hall Medical; 1996.
15. Linares OA, Halter JB. Sympathochromaffin system activity in the elderly. J Clin Endocrinol Metab 1987;65:508–11.
16. Morrow LA, Linares OA, Hill TJ, et al. Age differences in plasma clearance mechanisms for epinephrine and norepinephrine in humans. J Clin Endocrinol Metab 1987;65:508–11.
17. Supiano MA, Linares OA, Smith MJ, et al. Age-related difference in norepinephrine kinetics: effect of posture and sodium-restricted diet. Am J Phys 1990;259: E422–31.
18. Rowe JW, Troen BR. Sympathetic nervous system and aging in man. Endocr Rev 1980;1:167–79.
19. Hogikyan RV, Supiano MA. Arterial a-adrenergic responsiveness is decreased and SNS activity is increased in older humans. Am J Phys 1994;266:E717–24.
20. Pan HYM, Blaschke TF. Decline in beta-adrenergic receptor-mediated vascular relaxation with aging in man. J Pharmacol Exp Ther 1986;239:802–7.
21. Brodde OE, Zerkowski HR, Schranz D, et al. Age-dependent changes in the beta-adrenoceptor-G-protein(s)-adenylyl cyclase system in human right atrium. J Cardiovasc Pharmacol 1995;26:20–6.
22. Shimada K, Kitazumi T, Ogura H, et al. Differences in age-independent effects on blood pressure on baroreflex sensitivity between normal and hypertensive subjects. Clin Sci 1986;70:489–94.
23. Gribbin B, Pickering TG, Sleight P, et al. Effect of age and high blood pressure on baroreflex sensitivity in man. Circ Res 1971;29:424–31.
24. Benarroch E. The central autonomic network: functional organization, dysfunction, and perspective. Mayo Clin Proc 1993;68:988–1001.
25. Weiling W, Lieshout J. Maintenance of postural normotension in humans. In: Low P, editor. Clinical autonomic disorders. Philadelphia: Little Brown Co; 1993. p. 69–73.
26. Messerli FH, Ventura HO, Amodeo C. Osler's maneuver and pseudohypertension. N Engl J Med 1985;312(24):1548–51.
27. Kosinski D, Grubb BP, Temesy-Armos P. Pathophysiological aspects of neurocardiogenic syncope. Pacing Clin Electrophysiol 1995;18:716–21.
28. Sutton R, Peterson M. The clinical spectrum of neurocardiogenic syncope. J Cardiovasc Electrophysiol 1995;6:569–76.
29. Grubb BP. Neurocardiogenic syncope. In: Grubb BP, Olshansky B, editors. Syncope: mechanisms and management. Malden (MA): Blackwell/Futura Press; 2005. p. 47–71.
30. Grubb BP. Neurocardiogenic syncope and related disorders of orthostatic intolerance. Circulation 2005;111:2997–3006.
31. Bradbury S, Eggleston C. Postural hypotension: a report of three cases. Am Heart J 1925;1:73–86.
32. Robertson D, Biaggioni I, Burnstock G, et al, editors. A primer on the autonomic nervous system. San Diego (CA): Academic Press; 2011.
33. Shy GM, Drager GA. A neurologic syndrome associated with hypotension. Arch Neurol 1960;3:511–27.
34. Mathias CJ. The classification and nomenclature of autonomic disorders: ending chaos, restoring conflict, and hopefully achieving clarity. Clin Auton Res 1995;5: 307–10.
35. Grubb BP. Dysautonomic (orthostatic) syncope. In: Grubb BP, Olshansky B, editors. Syncope: mechanisms and management. Malden (MA): Blackwell/Futura Press; 2005. p. 72–91.

36. Grubb BP, Kanjwal Y, Karabin B, et al. Orthostatic hypotension and autonomic failure: a concise guide to diagnosis and management. Clin Med Cardiol 2008; 2:279–91.

37. Grubb BP. Postural tachycardia syndrome. Circulation 2008;117:2814–7.

38. Passant V, Warkentin S, Karlson, et al. Orthostatic hypotension in organic dementia: relationship between blood pressure, cortical blood flow and symptoms. Clin Auton Res 1996;6:29–36.

39. Kanjwal K, Figueredo V, Karabin K, et al. The implantable loop recorder: current uses future directions. J Innov Cardiac Rhythm Management 2011;2:215–22.

40. Brignole M, Menozzi C, Moy A, et al. Pacemaker therapy in patients with neurally mediated syncope and documented asystole: Third International Study on Syncope of Uncertain Etiology (ISSUE-3): a randomized trial. Circulation 2012; 125:2566–71.

41. Grubb BP, Kosinski D. Tilt table testing: concepts and limitations. Pacing Clin Electrophysiol 1997;20(Pt II):781–7.

42. Grubb BP, Kosinski D, Mouhaffel A, et al. The use of methylphenidate in the treatment of refractory neurocardiogenic syncope. Pacing Clin Electrophysiol 1996; 19:836–40.

43. Low P, Gilden J, Freeman R, et al. Efficacy of midodrine vs. placebo in neurocardiogenic orthostatic hypotension. JAMA 1997;277:1046–51.

44. Sra J, Magio C, Biehl M, et al. Efficacy of midodrine hydrochloride in neurocardiogenic syncope refractory to standard therapy. J Cardiovasc Electrophysiol 1997; 8:42–6.

45. Robertson D, Dabis TL. Recent advances in the treatment of orthostatic hypotension. Neurology 1995;5:526–32.

46. Hoeldtke RD, Streeton DH. Treatment of orthostatic hypotension with erythropoietin. N Engl J Med 1993;329:611–5.

47. Kanjwal K, Bilal S, Karabin B, et al. Erythropoietin in the treatment of postural tachycardia syndrome. Am J Ther 2012;19:92–5.

48. Grubb BP, Kosinski D. Serotonin and syncope: an emerging connection? Eur J Cardiac Pacing Electrophysiol 1996;5:306–14.

49. Grubb BP, Samoil D, Kosinski D, et al. Fluoxetine hydrochloride for the treatment of severe refractory orthostatic hypotension. Pacing Clin Electrophysiol 1993;16: 801–5.

50. Benditt D, Peterson ME, Lurie KG, et al. Cardiac pacing for prevention of recurrent vasovagal syncope. Ann Intern Med 1995;122:204–9.

51. Kanjwal K, Karabin B, Kanjwal Y, et al. Preliminary observations of the use of closed-loop cardiac pacing in patients with refractory neurocardiogenic syncope. J Interv Card Electrophysiol 2010;27:69–73.

52. Palmisano P, Zaccaria M, Luzzi G, et al. Closed-loop cardiac pacing vs. conventional dual-chamber pacing with specialized sensing and pacing algorithms for syncope prevention in patients with refractory vasovagal syncope: results of a long-term follow-up. Europace 2012;14:1036–43.

Management of Arrhythmias in the Perioperative Setting

Rowlens M. Melduni, MD, MPH[a],*, Yuki Koshino, MD, PhD[a],
Win-Kuang Shen, MD[b]

KEYWORDS

- Arrhythmia • Postoperative atrial fibrillation • Surgery • Elderly

KEY POINTS

- Data from several studies suggest that the incidence of postoperative arrhythmia after cardiothoracic surgery is approximately 30% to 40%, with postoperative atrial fibrillation (AF) being most common dysrhythmia.[1–3] For noncardiothoracic procedures, the incidence ranges from 4% to 20%, depending on the type of surgery performed.[4–6]
- Bradyarrhythmias are common after cardiac surgery and occur most frequently in the early postoperative period. These arrhythmias, in part, are related to the fluctuation of vagal tone caused direct surgical injury and local edema.
- The initial management of patients with perioperative atrial arrhythmia depends on the hemodynamic effect of the arrhythmia on the patient's clinical status. The first step in managing these patients is to eliminate any potential precipitating factors.
- Multiple studies have demonstrated that beta blocker reduces the risk of AF by up to 61% compared with placebo. Therefore, routine administration of beta blocker after cardiac surgery should be the standard of care to prevent AF.[7,8]
- Sustained monomorphic or polymorphic ventricular arrhythmias are uncommon with approximately 1% to 3% of patients usually within the first week after surgery.

INTRODUCTION

Perioperative arrhythmias, which often reflect the presence of underlying cardiopulmonary disease or metabolic imbalances, are a common complication of surgery, particularly in the elderly.[9] Thousands of patients undergo major surgery each year and a major complication of these procedures is the occurrence of perioperative arrhythmia. There is a considerable body of literature regarding the subject in cardiothoracic patients, with little work in noncardiothoracic surgical patients. The immediate postoperative period after surgery is a dynamic period, with elevated levels of

[a] Division of Cardiovascular Diseases, 200 First Street SW, Rochester, MN 55905, USA; [b] Division of Cardiovascular Diseases, Mayo Clinic, 13400 E. Shea Boulevard, Scottsdale, AZ 85259, USA
* Corresponding author. Division of Cardiovascular Diseases, Mayo Clinic, 200 First Street Southwest, Rochester, MN 55905.
E-mail address: melduni.rowlens@mayo.edu

Clin Geriatr Med 28 (2012) 729–743
http://dx.doi.org/10.1016/j.cger.2012.08.006   **geriatric.theclinics.com**

circulating catecholamines, fluctuation of intravascular volume, alterations in sympathetic and parasympathetic activity, metabolic and electrolyte abnormalities, new surgical wound and cannulation sites on or near myocardial tissue, increased levels of inflammatory mediators, and the frequent presence of pericarditis, all of which have been implicated in the development of postoperative arrhythmias.[10] Data from several studies suggest that the incidence of postoperative arrhythmia after cardiothoracic surgery is approximately 30% to 40%, with postoperative atrial fibrillation (AF) being the most common dysrhythmia.[1-3] For noncardiothoracic procedures, the incidence ranges from 4% to 20%, depending on the type of surgery performed.[4-6] Among patients undergoing major vascular interventions, the reported incidence ranges from 10% to 20%.[11] The presence of postoperative AF is associated with increased morbidity, ICU stay, length of hospitalization, and hospital costs.[2] The burdens associated with perioperative arrhythmias are expected to rise in the future, given that the population undergoing cardiac surgery is getting older and sicker, thus making it imperative for clinicians managing these patients to be up-to-date on current management of these arrhythmias. In this article, we aim to accomplish the following objectives: (1) to review the prevalence, causes, and management of perioperative bradyarrhythmias, (2) to discuss the mechanisms and therapeutic options for perioperative atrial arrhythmias with a focus on AF, and (3) to review the prevalence and management of perioperative ventricular arrhythmias **Box 1**.

Bradyarrhythmias

Bradyarrhythmias are common after cardiac surgery and occur most frequently in the early postoperative period. These arrhythmias, in part, are related to the fluctuation of vagal tone caused by direct surgical injury and local edema.

The hemodynamic physiologic effects of perioperative bradyarrhythmia may be influenced by the type of arrhythmia, ventricular response, its duration, and the patient's volume status. Bradyarrhythmias, if associated with a loss of atrial synchronous contraction, can dramatically decrease cardiac output, particularly in elderly patients who often have relatively fixed stroke volumes due to underlying diastolic dysfunction. The result is hypotension, decrease coronary perfusion pressure, and myocardial ischemia. In the POISE multicenter randomized controlled trial,[12] which investigated the effects of perioperative beta-blockers in patients undergoing noncardiac surgery, significant hypotension occurred in 15% of treated patients. Preoperative left bundle branch block, concomitant left ventricular aneurysmectomy,

---

Box 1
Common risk factors for perioperative arrhythmia

Advanced age	Electrolyte abnormalities
Left atrial enlargement	Heightened adrenergic state
*Myocardial ischemia	Drug toxicity (*proarrhythmia)
Hypoxia	*Myocardial infarction
Hypovolemia	*Acute graft closure
Hemodynamic instability	*Reperfusion after cessation of bypass
Valvular heart disease	*Female sex
Hypertension	Hypoglycemia or hyperglycemia
Pulmonary disease	*Cardiomyopathy
Inflammation due to serositis	Beta-blocker withdrawal

* More specific for ventricular arrhythmias.

and age greater than 64 years are independent predictors of severe and prolonged postoperative bradyarrhythmias. The most common abnormalities are complete atrioventricular block with a narrow or wide complex escape rhythm, sinus node dysfunction, and a nodal rhythm. In patients undergoing cardiothoracic surgery, temporary epicardial atrial and ventricular pacing wires placed at the time of surgery usually facilitate temporary pacing in the early postoperative period. Postoperative bradyarrhythmias requiring permanent pacemaker implantation is more common after valve surgery (3%–9%) than after isolated coronary artery bypass grafting (0.8%).[13–16]

The need for long-term pacing may be unpredictable, although postoperative complete atrioventricular block is the most important predictor of pacemaker dependency, enabling an earlier decision on permanent pacemaker implantation (no later than postoperative days 6 and 9 for wide-complex and narrow-complex escape, respectively).[17] The need for permanent pacing in patients with transient postoperative atrioventricular block and residual bifascicular block has not been established, although patients with atrioventricular conduction that returns to normal have a favorable prognosis. The American College of Cardiology/American Heart Association/Heart Rhythm Society (ACC/AHA) *2008 Guidelines for device-based therapy of cardiac rhythm abnormalities* established that permanent pacemaker implantation is indicated for third-degree and advanced second-degree atrioventricular block at any anatomic level associated with postoperative atrioventricular block that is not expected to resolve after cardiac surgery.[18]

MECHANISM OF PERIOPERATIVE AF AND ATRIAL ARRHYTHMIAS

The pathophysiology of perioperative AF (POAF) is complex and is incompletely understood. However, POAF seem to require a trigger and an atrial substrate. During diastole, the left atrium is directly exposed to pressures in the left ventricle that can increase with abnormal relaxation and decreased compliance. Left atrial pressure increases to maintain adequate filling, and the increased atrial wall tension leads to atrial electrical and structural remodeling, including stretching, dilatation, and fibrosis of the atrial myocardium, providing a vulnerable substrate for AF. Normally, the left atrium is a highly compliant structure that maintains relatively low pressures despite mild volume shifts. Under conditions of pathophysiological stress or aging, the myocardium becomes progressively stiff and fibrotic.[19,20] This leads to abnormalities in ventricular relaxation and increased filling pressures characteristic of diastolic dysfunction.[3,21] As ventricular filling pressures increase, the left atrium becomes progressively distended and the atrial stretch distorts the electrical activity of the pulmonary veins, thus triggering POAF.[22,23] The muscular wall of the left atrium may extend up to a few centimeters around the pulmonary veins.[24] In the setting of an additional substrate in the atria, the atrial tissue in the pulmonary veins is often the initiating focus for AF[25] and has relatively short refractory periods compared with other parts of the atria.[26] When superimposed by the acute stress of surgical intervention,[27] the initial trigger, in the setting of heterogeneity of conduction and refractoriness, may facilitate the development of a substrate for reentry, favoring an environment for the perpetuation of POAF. These mechanisms are complex and involve a dynamic interplay between the triggers and substrate abnormalities. In patients undergoing major vascular surgery (eg, thoracic aortic), arrhythmias are presumed to involve disruption of the aortic fat pad, leading to reduced cardiac vagal tone, which may predispose to postoperative arrhythmias.[11] Other common factors in the perioperative period that may contribute to the development of POAF include increased sympathetic activation and outflow due to metabolic and hemodynamic perturbations such as blood loss, fluid shifts, pain, beta-blocker withdrawal, hypoglycemia or hyperglycemia and electrolyte disturbances.[28,29] Because the incidence of AF is highest 2 to 3 days after surgery, inflammatory mechanisms have also been proposed.[30] Clinical and mechanical factors associated with increased risk of AF after cardiothoracic surgery are summarized in **Fig. 1**.

MANAGEMENT OF POAF AND ATRIAL ARRHYTHMIA

The initial management of patients with perioperative atrial arrhythmia depends on the hemodynamic effect of the arrhythmia and the patient's clinical status. The first step in managing these patients is to eliminate any potential precipitating factors. Electrolyte abnormalities should be corrected. Optimization of intravascular fluid balance and correction of electrolyte abnormalities, hypoxia, and severe anemia, should be undertaken as a standard protocol in all patients. Pain control and sedation for comfort are important to reduce significant fluctuation of autonomic tone. Timely transfusion of patients with serum hemoglobin levels less than 7 g/dL may reduce perioperative cardiac morbidity (exacerbation of myocardial ischemia and heart failure).[31,32] Appropriate steps should be implemented to assess and treat any symptoms or signs of heart failure, ischemia, or infection.

The strategies for managing patients with postoperative atrial arrhythmias are generally divided into rate or rhythm control and anticoagulation. Rate control is thought to improve hemodynamic stability and ventricular filling. Rhythm control is generally used for acute management of patients who are hemodynamically compromised (ie, hypotension, angina, or HF) or significantly symptomatic from the arrhythmia itself. Control may be accomplished by electrical or pharmacologic cardioversion.

RATE CONTROL

Most postoperative arrhythmias are transient and typically short-lived. In a study of Olmsted County patients who underwent cardiac surgery at the Mayo Clinic 2000 to 2005, the incidence of POAF peaked at a median of 2 days (range, 0–28 days), which corresponded to time to peak inflammation and volume overload due to mobilization of fluid that had "third spaced" postoperatively.[30,33] POAF lasted a median of 2 days (range, 0.04–18 days).[3] In principle, rate control intervention with pharmacologic therapy should be initiated while or after optimizing the patient's general clinical status.

Beta-blockers, nondihydropyridine calcium channel blockers (diltiazem, verapamil), or digoxin are generally accepted as the mainstay of therapy for rate control (**Table 1**). Digoxin alone is not as effective as other atrioventricular nodal blocking agents are; beta-blockers are the most effective agent for controlling the ventricular response during POAF[34] and may even accelerate the conversion of postoperative supraventricular arrhythmias to sinus rhythm.[35] Elderly patients are at increased risk for digitalis toxicity related in part to decreased renal excretion. Because digoxin is predominantly excreted by the kidneys, it is common practice to decrease the initial and maintenance doses of digitalis in the elderly.[36]

Note that, although nondihydropyridine calcium channel blockers possess negative chronotropic effects to lower heart rate without significantly affecting systemic vascular resistance or arterial blood pressure, they also have negative inotropic effects and should be avoided or used cautiously in individuals with left ventricular dysfunction or signs of heart failure.[37] Moreover, nondihydropyridine calcium channel

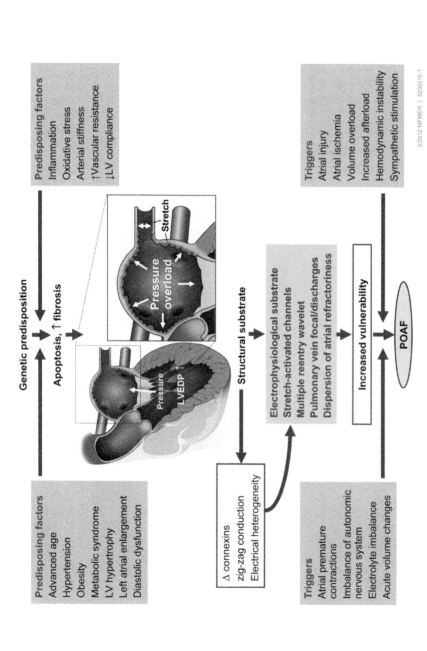

Fig. 1. Pathogenesis of perioperative AF. LV, left ventricle; LVEDP, left ventricular end-diastolic pressure; POAF, postoperative atrial fibrillation. (*Courtesy of Mayo Clinic, Rochester, MN.*)

Table 1
Intravenous and orally administered pharmacologic agents for heart rate control in patients with AF

Drug[a]	Loading Dose	Onset	Maintenance Dose	Major Side Effects
Acute Setting				
1. Heart rate control in patients without accessory pathway				
Esmolol[a,b]	0.5 mg/kg over 1 min	5 min	0.06–0.2 mg/kg/min	Hypotension, heart block, bradycardia, asthma, HF
Metoprolol[b]	2.5–5 mg IV bolus over 2 min; up to 3 doses	5 min	NA	Hypotension, heart block bradycardia, asthma, HF
Propranolol[b]	0.15 mg/kg	5 min	NA	Hypotension, heart block, bradycardia, asthma, HF
Diltiazem	0.25 mg/kg IV over 2 min	2–7 min	5–15 mg/h infusion	Hypotension, heart block, HF
Verapamil	0.075–0.15 mg/kg over 2 min	3–5 min	NA	Hypotension, heart block, HF
2. Heart rate control in patients with accessory pathway[d]				
Amiodarone[c,e]	150 mg over 10 min	Days	0.5–1.0 mg/min	Hypotension, heart block, pulmonary toxicity, warfarin interaction, sinus bradycardia; and chronically, skin discoloration, hypothyroidism, hyperthyroidism, corneal deposits, optic neuropathy
3. Heart rate control in patients with heart failure and without accessory pathway				
Digoxin	0.25 mg every 2 h, up to 1.5 mg	2 h	0.125–0.25 mg/d	Digitalis toxicity, heart block, bradycardia
Amiodarone[c]	150 mg over 10 min	Days	0.5–1.0 mg/min	See "Major side effects" of amiodarone
Nonacute Setting And Chronic Maintenance Therapy[f]				
1. Heart rate control				
Metoprolol[b]	25–100 mg bid, orally	4–6 h	25–100 mg bid, orally	Hypotension, heart block bradycardia, asthma, HF
Propranolol[b]	80–240 mg/d in divided doses, orally	60–90 min	80–240 mg/d in divided doses, orally	Hypotension, heart block, bradycardia, asthma, HF

Diltiazem	120–360 mg/d; slow release available, orally	2–4 h	120–360 mg/d; slow release available, orally	Hypotension, heart block, HF
Verapamil	120–360 mg/d; slow release available	1–2 h	120–360 mg/d; slow release available, orally	Hypotension, heart block, HF
2. Heart rate control in patients with heart failure and without accessory pathway				
Digoxin	0.5 mg/d by mouth	2 days	0.125–0.375 mg/d, orally	Digitalis toxicity, heart block, bradycardia
Amiodarone[c]	800 mg/d for 1 wk, then 600 mg/d for 1 wk, then 400 mg/d for 4–6 wk, orally	1–3 wk	200 mg/d, orally	Hypotension, heart block, pulmonary toxicity, skin discoloration, hypothyroidism, hyperthyroidism, corneal deposits, optic neuropathy, warfarin interaction, sinus bradycardia

Abbreviations: HF, heart failure; IV, intravenous; NA, not applicable.

[a] Onset is variable and some effect occurs earlier.

[b] Only representative members of the type of beta-adrenergic antagonist drugs are included. Other, similar, agents could be used for this indication in appropriate doses. Beta-blockers are grouped in an order preceding the alphabetical listing of drugs.

[c] Amiodarone can be useful to control the heart rate in patients with AF when other measures are unsuccessful or contraindicated.

[d] Conversion to sinus rhythm and catheter ablation of the accessory pathway are generally recommended; pharmacologic therapy for rate control may be appropriate in certain patients.

[e] If rhythm cannot be converted or ablated and rate control is needed, IV amiodarone is recommended.

[f] Adequacy of heart rate control should be assessed during physical activity as well as at rest.

Adapted from Fuster V, Ryden LE, Cannom DS, et al. ACC/AHA/ESC 2006 guidelines for the management of patients with atrial fibrillation: a report of the American College of Cardiology/American Heart Association Task Force on Practice Guidelines and the European Society of Cardiology Committee for Practice Guidelines (Writing Committee to Revise the 2001 Guidelines for the Management of Patients with Atrial Fibrillation). J Am Coll Cardiol 2006;48:e149.

blockers exert their electrophysiological effects by blocking the slow calcium channel, slowing propagating action potentials, and prolonging the antegrade and retrograde refractory periods of the atrioventricular node in a dose-dependent fashion.[38] This results in a negative chronotropic effect, or a lowering of heart rate, but increases the potential for heart block.[39] There are no established guidelines for what constitutes a target heart rate in patients with perioperative arrhythmias. The target heart rate is usually guided by patient's comfort and hemodynamic parameters such as blood pressure, cardiac, and renal outputs. In stable patients with POAF, heart rates of 70 to 100 beats per minute are generally considered acceptable.

RHYTHM CONTROL

Current guidelines recommend restoration of sinus rhythm (preferably via electrical cardioversion) for acute management of patients with hemodynamic compromise or who are symptomatic from sustained AF.[40] Electrical cardioversion should be attempted in any patient with life-threatening hemodynamic instability, regardless of the duration of the arrhythmia. Generally, cardioversion should be attempted in patients whose AF persists more than 24 but less than 48 hours, so that anticoagulation therapy can be avoided.

In selected circumstances when it is desirable to avoid anesthesia, pharmacologic cardioversion is preferred. Pharmacologic cardioversion is most often used for AF of short duration in symptomatic patients without structural heart disease. The efficacy of antiarrhythmic drugs for reversion of POAF is similar to that in AF not related to surgery.[7,8,41,42] There are several classes of agents that are effective for pharmacologic cardioversion (**Table 2**). Class IC agents (flecainide and propafenone) are sodium channel blockers. They may be used for early cardioversion in patients with minimal or no structural heart disease. Class IC drugs are contraindicated in patients with coronary artery disease or heart failure. The success rate of cardioversion after one initial oral loading dose of flecainide (300 mg) or propafenone (600 mg) is approximately 70% to 80%. Ibutilide and amiodarone are Class III agents that inhibit potassium channels. Both drugs can be administered intravenously. Ibutilide is effective in cardioversion of recent-onset AF and atrial flutter with a success rate in the 70% range. It is contraindicated in patient with left ventricular systolic dysfunction, prolonged QT interval, or hypokalemia due to risk of torsades de pointes ventricular tachycardia. Amiodarone has an added advantage of slowing the ventricular rate during AF due to its atrioventricular-nodal blocking effects mediated through beta-receptor and calcium channel antagonism.

For patients who have failed electrical cardioversion, an option is to pretreat them with a class IC (flecainide or propafenone) or class III antiarrhythmic (eg, ibutilide, dofetilide, or amiodarone) agent before repeating the procedure, thereby enhancing cardioversion success rates.[43] Ibutilide, in particular, has been shown to facilitate successful cardioversion in patients for whom direct-current cardioversion has failed.[44] In a study of 100 patients with AF for 117 ± 201 days who were randomly assigned to undergo transthoracic cardioversion with or without pretreatment ibutilide (1 mg intravenous), conversion to sinus rhythm occurred in all 50 out of 50 (100%) patients who received ibutilide compared with 36 out of 50 (72%) of those who did not receive ibutilide (P<.001). In all 14 patients in whom transthoracic cardioversion alone failed, sinus rhythm was restored when cardioversion was attempted again after pretreatment with ibutilide. Sustained polymorphic ventricular tachycardia occurred in 2 out of 64 (3%) of patients who received ibutilide, both of whom had an ejection fraction of less than or equal to 20%.

Table 2
Recommended doses of drugs (listed alphabetically) proven effective for pharmacologic cardioversion of AF

Drug	Route of Administration	Dosage[a]	Potential Adverse Effects
Amiodarone	Oral	Inpatient: 1.2–1.8/d in divided dose until 10 g total, then 200–400 mg/d single dose Outpatient 600–800 mg/d divided dose until 10 g total, then 200–400 mg/d maintenance	Hypotension, bradycardia, QT prolongation, torsade de pointes (rare), GI upset, constipation, phlebitis (IV use)
	Intravenous (IV)/oral	5–7 mg/kg over 30–60 min, then 1.2–1.8 g/d continuous IV or in divided oral doses until 10 g total, then 200–400 mg/d maintenance	
Dofetilide	Oral	Creatinine clearance (mL/min): Greater than 60: 500 mcg bid 40–60: 250 mcg bid 20–40: 125 mcg bid Less than 20: contraindicated	QT prolongation, torsade de pointes; adjust dose for renal function, body size, age
Flecainide	Oral	200–300 mg[b]	Hypotension, rapidly conducting atrial flutter
	Intravenous	1.5–3.0 m/kg over 10–20 min	
Ibutilide	Intravenous	1 mg over 10 min; repeat 1 mg if necessary	QT prolongation, torsade de pointes
Propafenone	Oral	450–600 mg	Hypotension, rapidly conducting atrial flutter
	Intravenous	1.5–2.0 mg/kg over 10–20 min	

Abbreviations: GI, gastrointestinal; IV, intravenous.
  [a] Dosages given in the table may differ from those recommended by the manufacturers.
  [b] Insufficient data are available on which to base specific recommendations for the use of one loading regimen over another for patients with ischemic heart disease or impaired left ventricular function; these drugs should be used cautiously or not at all in such patients.
  Adapted from Fuster V, Ryden LE, Cannom DS, et al. ACC/AHA/ESC guidelines for the management of patients with atrial fibrillation. J Am Coll Cardiol 2006;48:e149.

PRIMARY AF PREVENTION

Of the many different strategies studied, beta-blockers have the most evidence to support their use for the prevention of POAF.[45,46] Multiple studies have demonstrated that beta-blockers reduce the risk of AF by up to 61% compared with placebo. Therefore, routine administration of a beta-blocker after cardiac surgery should be the standard of care to prevent AF.[45,46]

The ACC/AHA guidelines[47] recommend preoperative or early postoperative beta blocker therapy for patients undergoing cardiac surgery. The European Association for Cardio-Thoracic Surgery guidelines[48] recommends beta blockers as first choice for the prevention of POAF in all patients undergoing cardiac surgery.

Sotalol is a beta-blocker with class III antiarrhythmic properties. A meta-analysis of four trials comparing sotalol with beta blocker against postoperative AF revealed that sotalol has a statistically significant advantage over conventional beta blockers, and the number needed to treat with sotalol over beta blockers was 10.[49] In several randomized controlled trials, amiodarone was effective in reducing the incidence of AF after cardiac surgery.[46,50–53] Oral amiodarone at a dose of 600 mg daily for

7 days before surgery, then 200 mg daily until hospital discharge is the only oral regimen of amiodarone AF prophylaxis that has been shown to significantly reduce the incidence of POAF and the duration and cost of hospitalization.[51] Intravenous amiodarone, administered immediately after surgery, also reduces the incidence of POAF without significant adverse effects.[54]

Multiple studies of magnesium for prevention of AF have been published. A meta-analysis showed that magnesium may be an effective prophylactic agent for prevention of POAF. However, in a randomized trial, the addition of magnesium to postoperative beta blocker therapy did not reduce the incidence of AF.[55] Although hypomagnesemia is a risk factor for AF and magnesium may be a useful therapy, its role in preventing POAF is more controversial.

ANTICOAGULATION

Anticoagulation for AF in the postoperative setting has not been studied in large clinical trials. Although standard guidelines for nonsurgical patients should be followed, there are a few points to consider. Patients with AF for more than 48 hours are at risk of thromboembolism, particularly older patients with diabetes, hypertension, rheumatic mitral valve disease, prior thromboembolism, or heart failure. In a study of 4507 adult patients who underwent cardiac surgical procedures requiring cardiopulmonary bypass, POAF was associated with an increased incidence of postoperative stroke (3.3% vs 1.4% without AF; $P<.0005$).[56] Other studies have suggested that factors other than the arrhythmia are responsible for these cerebrovascular events.[57,58] Thus, the role of anticoagulation in the early postoperative period is undefined. Extrapolating from the guidelines for managing anticoagulation in AF that is not related to surgery, antithrombotic therapy to prevent thromboembolism is recommended for all patients with AF lasting greater than or equal to 48 hours, if bleeding risks are acceptable.[40] In most cases, anticoagulation is not warranted in the perioperative setting because AF episodes are usually transient and not recurrent. In addition, the risks of bleeding with anticoagulation in the first 1 to 2 days following major surgery may be prohibitive, particularly for neurosurgical patients.

VENTRICULAR ARRHYTHMIAS

Sustained monomorphic or polymorphic ventricular arrhythmias are uncommon, occurring in approximately 1% to 3% of patients within the first week after surgery.[59,60]

Multiple studies have shown that risk for ventricular arrhythmias among hospitalized patients is strikingly greater in women than in men, by approximately twofold.[61,62] Hypokalemia is a well-established predisposing risk factor for ventricular arrhythmias,[63,64] as is hypomagnesemia.[65,66] Bradycardia is an additional important risk factor for ventricular arrhythmias when other predisposing factors are present.[67] Simple sinus bradycardia, complete atrioventricular block, or any rhythm in which there are sudden long R-R cycles may lead to arrhythmogenic early afterdepolarizations.[68,69] Premature beats may foster the development of ventricular tachycardia.

Prevention of hypokalemia reduces the risk of ventricular arrhythmias. Standard practice after cardiac surgery is to maintain serum potassium at the upper half of the normal range (4.0–5.0 mmol/L).[48] In general, management of ventricular arrhythmia is based on the clinical significance. Isolated premature ventricular contractions during the perioperative period are usually benign in the absence of significant structural or ischemic heart disease. Patients with underlying heart disease and preexisting frequent premature ventricular contractions have increased risk of perioperative cardiac complications.[70] Ventricular arrhythmias are frequently associated with myocardial ischemia or congestive heart failure. Nonsustained ventricular tachycardia often occurs in patients after CABG and is thought to be reperfusion-induced. It is usually benign, although some patients may be at increased risk for future life-threatening arrhythmias.[71–74]

Asymptomatic and hemodynamically stable nonsustained ventricular tachycardia does not require treatment in the acute setting.[75,76] However, unstable ventricular tachycardia with hemodynamic compromise is an indication for direct current cardioversion. For hemodynamically stable patients with sustained ventricular tachycardia who are thought to be at risk of impending hemodynamic collapse, pharmacologic therapy with intravenous amiodarone or lidocaine can be considered as reasonable first options. Procainamide can be considered as an alternative, but its use is limited by hypotension and the potential for negative inotropic effects.

SUMMARY

Perioperative arrhythmias are a common complication of surgery, with incidence ranging from 4% to 20% for noncardiothoracic procedures, depending on the type of surgery performed. The immediate postoperative period is a dynamic time and is associated with many conditions conducive to the development of postoperative arrhythmias. The presence of postoperative atrial fibrillation is associated with increased morbidity, ICU stay, length of hospitalization, and hospital costs. The associated burdens are expected to rise in the future, given that the population undergoing cardiac surgery is getting older and sicker. Thousands of patients undergo major surgery each year and a major complication of these procedures is the occurrence of perioperative arrhythmia. It is imperative for clinicians to be up-to-date on current management of these arrhythmias.

REFERENCES

1. Almassi GH, Schowalter T, Nicolosi AC, et al. Atrial fibrillation after cardiac surgery: a major morbid event? Ann Surg 1997;226(4):501–11 [discussion: 511–03].
2. Aranki SF, Shaw DP, Adams DH, et al. Predictors of atrial fibrillation after coronary artery surgery. Current trends and impact on hospital resources. Circulation 1996;94(3):390–7.
3. Melduni RM, Suri RM, Seward JB, et al. Diastolic dysfunction in patients undergoing cardiac surgery: a pathophysiological mechanism underlying the initiation of new-onset post-operative atrial fibrillation. J Am Coll Cardiol 2011;58(9):953–61.
4. Brathwaite D, Weissman C. The new onset of atrial arrhythmias following major noncardiothoracic surgery is associated with increased mortality. Chest 1998;114(2):462–8.
5. Walsh SR, Oates JE, Anderson JA, et al. Postoperative arrhythmias in colorectal surgical patients: incidence and clinical correlates. Colorectal Dis 2006;8(3):212–6.
6. Christians KK, Wu B, Quebbeman EJ, et al. Postoperative atrial fibrillation in noncardiothoracic surgical patients. Am J Surg 2001;182(6):713–5.
7. Di Biasi P, Scrofani R, Paje A, et al. Intravenous amiodarone vs propafenone for atrial fibrillation and flutter after cardiac operation. Eur J Cardiothorac Surg 1995;9(10):587–91.

8. Yilmaz AT, Demirkilic U, Arslan M, et al. Long-term prevention of atrial fibrillation after coronary artery bypass surgery: comparison of quinidine, verapamil, and amiodarone in maintaining sinus rhythm. J Card Surg 1996;11(1):61–4.

9. Goldman L, Caldera DL, Nussbaum SR, et al. Multifactorial index of cardiac risk in noncardiac surgical procedures. N Engl J Med 1977;297(16):845–50.

10. Rho RW. The management of atrial fibrillation after cardiac surgery. Heart 2009; 95(5):422–9.

11. Valentine RJ, Rosen SF, Cigarroa JE, et al. The clinical course of new-onset atrial fibrillation after elective aortic operations. J Am Coll Surg 2001;193(5):499–504.

12. Group PS, Devereaux PJ, Yang H, et al. Effects of extended-release metoprolol succinate in patients undergoing non-cardiac surgery (POISE trial): a randomised controlled trial. Lancet 2008;371(9627):1839–47.

13. Emlein G, Huang SK, Pires LA, et al. Prolonged bradyarrhythmias after isolated coronary artery bypass graft surgery. Am Heart J 1993;126(5):1084–90.

14. Limongelli G, Ducceschi V, D'Andrea A, et al. Risk factors for pacemaker implantation following aortic valve replacement: a single centre experience. Heart 2003; 89(8):901–4.

15. Gordon RS, Ivanov J, Cohen G, et al. Permanent cardiac pacing after a cardiac operation: predicting the use of permanent pacemakers. Ann Thorac Surg 1998; 66(5):1698–704.

16. Dawkins S, Hobson AR, Kalra PR, et al. Permanent pacemaker implantation after isolated aortic valve replacement: incidence, indications, and predictors. Ann Thorac Surg 2008;85(1):108–12.

17. Glikson M, Dearani JA, Hyberger LK, et al. Indications, effectiveness, and long-term dependency in permanent pacing after cardiac surgery. Am J Cardiol 1997; 80(10):1309–13.

18. Epstein AE, DiMarco JP, Ellenbogen KA, et al. ACC/AHA/HRS 2008 guidelines for device-based therapy of cardiac rhythm abnormalities: a report of the American College of Cardiology/American Heart Association Task Force on Practice Guidelines (Writing Committee to Revise the ACC/AHA/NASPE 2002 guideline update for implantation of cardiac pacemakers and antiarrhythmia devices) developed in collaboration with the American Association for Thoracic Surgery and Society of Thoracic Surgeons. J Am Coll Cardiol 2008;51(21):e1–62.

19. Boldt A, Wetzel U, Lauschke J, et al. Fibrosis in left atrial tissue of patients with atrial fibrillation with and without underlying mitral valve disease. Heart 2004; 90(4):400–5.

20. Khan A, Moe GW, Nili N, et al. The cardiac atria are chambers of active remodeling and dynamic collagen turnover during evolving heart failure. J Am Coll Cardiol 2004;43(1):68–76.

21. Lam CS, Roger VL, Rodeheffer RJ, et al. Cardiac structure and ventricular-vascular function in persons with heart failure and preserved ejection fraction from Olmsted County, Minnesota. Circulation 2007;115(15):1982–90.

22. Chang SL, Chen YC, Chen YJ, et al. Mechanoelectrical feedback regulates the arrhythmogenic activity of pulmonary veins. Heart 2007;93(1):82–8.

23. Kalifa J, Jalife J, Zaitsev AV, et al. Intra-atrial pressure increases rate and organization of waves emanating from the superior pulmonary veins during atrial fibrillation. Circulation 2003;108(6):668–71.

24. Nathan H, Eliakim M. The junction between the left atrium and the pulmonary veins. An anatomic study of human hearts. Circulation 1966;34(3):412–22.

25. Chen SA, Hsieh MH, Tai CT, et al. Initiation of atrial fibrillation by ectopic beats originating from the pulmonary veins: electrophysiological characteristics,

pharmacological responses, and effects of radiofrequency ablation. Circulation 1999;100(18):1879–86.

26. Jais P, Hocini M, Macle L, et al. Distinctive electrophysiological properties of pulmonary veins in patients with atrial fibrillation. Circulation 2002;106(19): 2479–85.

27. Jais P, Peng JT, Shah DC, et al. Left ventricular diastolic dysfunction in patients with so-called lone atrial fibrillation. J Cardiovasc Electrophysiol 2000;11(6): 623–5.

28. Kalus JS, Caron MF, White CM, et al. Impact of fluid balance on incidence of atrial fibrillation after cardiothoracic surgery. Am J Cardiol 2004;94(11):1423–5.

29. Tselentakis EV, Woodford E, Chandy J, et al. Inflammation effects on the electrical properties of atrial tissue and inducibility of postoperative atrial fibrillation. J Surg Res 2006;135(1):68–75.

30. Bruins P, te Velthuis H, Yazdanbakhsh AP, et al. Activation of the complement system during and after cardiopulmonary bypass surgery: postsurgery activation involves C-reactive protein and is associated with postoperative arrhythmia. Circulation 1997;96(10):3542–8.

31. Nelson AH, Fleisher LA, Rosenbaum SH. Relationship between postoperative anemia and cardiac morbidity in high-risk vascular patients in the intensive care unit. Crit Care Med 1993;21(6):860–6.

32. Ferraris VA, Ferraris SP, Saha SP, et al. Perioperative blood transfusion and blood conservation in cardiac surgery: the society of thoracic surgeons and the society of cardiovascular anesthesiologists clinical practice guideline. Ann Thorac Surg 2007;83(Suppl 5):S27–86.

33. Ruan Q, Rao L, Middleton KJ, et al. Assessment of left ventricular diastolic function by early diastolic mitral annulus peak acceleration rate: experimental studies and clinical application. J Appl Physiol 2006;100(2):679–84.

34. Farshi R, Kistner D, Sarma JS, et al. Ventricular rate control in chronic atrial fibrillation during daily activity and programmed exercise: a crossover open-label study of five drug regimens. J Am Coll Cardiol 1999;33(2):304–10.

35. Balser JR, Martinez EA, Winters BD, et al. Beta-adrenergic blockade accelerates conversion of postoperative supraventricular tachyarrhythmias. Anesthesiology 1998;89(5):1052–9.

36. Ewy GA, Kapadia GG, Yao L, et al. Digoxin metabolism in the elderly. Circulation 1969;39(4):449–53.

37. The effect of diltiazem on mortality and reinfarction after myocardial infarction. The Multicenter Diltiazem Postinfarction Trial Research Group. N Engl J Med 1988;319(7):385–92.

38. Cranefield PF, Aronson RS, Wit AL. Effect of verapamil on the noraml action potential and on a calcium-dependent slow response of canine cardiac Purkinje fibers. Circ Res 1974;34(2):204–13.

39. Singh BN, Hecht HS, Nademanee K, et al. Electrophysiologic and hemodynamic effects of slow-channel blocking drugs. Prog Cardiovasc Dis 1982; 25(2):103–32.

40. European Heart Rhythm Association, Heart Rhythm Society, Fuster V, Rydén LE, Cannom DS, et al. ACC/AHA/ESC 2006 guidelines for the management of patients with atrial fibrillation–executive summary: a report of the American College of Cardiology/American Heart Association Task Force on Practice Guidelines and the European Society of Cardiology Committee for Practice Guidelines (Writing Committee to Revise the 2001 Guidelines for the Management of Patients With Atrial Fibrillation). J Am Coll Cardiol 2006;48(4):854–906.

41. McAlister HF, Luke RA, Whitlock RM, et al. Intravenous amiodarone bolus versus oral quinidine for atrial flutter and fibrillation after cardiac operations. J Thorac Cardiovasc Surg 1990;99(5):911–8.

42. Hjelms E. Procainamide conversion of acute atrial fibrillation after open-heart surgery compared with digoxin treatment. Scand J Thorac Cardiovasc Surg 1992;26(3):193–6.

43. Maisel WH, Rawn JD, Stevenson WG. Atrial fibrillation after cardiac surgery. Ann Intern Med 2001;135(12):1061–73.

44. Oral H, Souza JJ, Michaud GF, et al. Facilitating transthoracic cardioversion of atrial fibrillation with ibutilide pretreatment. N Engl J Med 1999;340(24):1849–54.

45. Connolly SJ, Cybulsky I, Lamy A, et al. Double-blind, placebo-controlled, randomized trial of prophylactic metoprolol for reduction of hospital length of stay after heart surgery: the beta-Blocker Length Of Stay (BLOS) study. Am Heart J 2003;145(2):226–32.

46. Crystal E, Connolly SJ, Sleik K, et al. Interventions on prevention of postoperative atrial fibrillation in patients undergoing heart surgery: a meta-analysis. Circulation 2002;106:75–80.

47. Eagle KA, Guyton RA, Davidoff R, et al. ACC/AHA 2004 guideline update for coronary artery bypass graft surgery: a report of the American College of Cardiology/American Heart Association Task Force on Practice Guidelines (Committee to Update the 1999 Guidelines for Coronary Artery Bypass Graft Surgery). Circulation 2004;110(14):e340–437.

48. Dunning J, Treasure T, Versteegh M, et al. Guidelines on the prevention and management of de novo atrial fibrillation after cardiac and thoracic surgery. Eur J Cardiothorac Surg 2006;30(6):852–72.

49. Shiga T, Wajima Z, Inoue T, et al. Magnesium prophylaxis for arrhythmias after cardiac surgery: a meta-analysis of randomized controlled trials. Am J Med 2004;117(5):325–33.

50. Dunning J, Botha P, Amanullah M. Prophylactic amiodarone effectively prevents post-operative atrial fibrillation. Interact Cardiovasc Thorac Surg 2004;3(3):510–5.

51. Daoud EG, Strickberger SA, Man KC, et al. Preoperative amiodarone as prophylaxis against atrial fibrillation after heart surgery. N Engl J Med 1997;337(25):1785–91.

52. Giri S, White CM, Dunn AB, et al. Oral amiodarone for prevention of atrial fibrillation after open heart surgery, the Atrial Fibrillation Suppression Trial (AFIST): a randomised placebo-controlled trial. Lancet 2001;357(9259):830–6.

53. Kerstein J, Soodan A, Qamar M, et al. Giving IV and oral amiodarone perioperatively for the prevention of postoperative atrial fibrillation in patients undergoing coronary artery bypass surgery: the GAP study. Chest 2004;126(3):716–24.

54. Guarnieri T, Nolan S, Gottlieb SO, et al. Intravenous amiodarone for the prevention of atrial fibrillation after open heart surgery: the Amiodarone Reduction in Coronary Heart (ARCH) trial. J Am Coll Cardiol 1999;34(2):343–7.

55. Cook RC, Humphries KH, Gin K, et al. Prophylactic intravenous magnesium sulphate in addition to oral {beta}-blockade does not prevent atrial arrhythmias after coronary artery or valvular heart surgery: a randomized, controlled trial. Circulation 2009;120(Suppl 11):S163–9.

56. Creswell LL, Schuessler RB, Rosenbloom M, et al. Hazards of postoperative atrial arrhythmias. Ann Thorac Surg 1993;56(3):539–49.

57. Hogue CW Jr, Murphy SF, Schechtman KB, et al. Risk factors for early or delayed stroke after cardiac surgery. Circulation 1999;100(6):642–7.

58. Kollar A, Lick SD, Vasquez KN, et al. Relationship of atrial fibrillation and stroke after coronary artery bypass graft surgery: when is anticoagulation indicated? Ann Thorac Surg 2006;82(2):515–23.

59. Azar RR, Berns E, Seecharran B, et al. De novo monomorphic and polymorphic ventricular tachycardia following coronary artery bypass grafting. Am J Cardiol 1997;80(1):76–8.

60. Steinberg JS, Gaur A, Sciacca R, et al. New-onset sustained ventricular tachycardia after cardiac surgery. Circulation 1999;99(7):903–8.

61. Drici MD, Clement N. Is gender a risk factor for adverse drug reactions? The example of drug-induced long QT syndrome. Drug Saf 2001;24(8):575–85.

62. Pedersen HS, Elming H, Seibaek M, et al. Risk factors and predictors of Torsade de pointes ventricular tachycardia in patients with left ventricular systolic dysfunction receiving Dofetilide. Am J Cardiol 2007;100(5):876–80.

63. Choy AM, Lang CC, Chomsky DM, et al. Normalization of acquired QT prolongation in humans by intravenous potassium. Circulation 1997;96(7):2149–54.

64. Pinto YM, van Gelder IC, Heeringa M, et al. QT lengthening and life-threatening arrhythmias associated with fexofenadine. Lancet 1999;353(9157):980.

65. Roden DM. Early after-depolarizations and torsade de pointes: implications for the control of cardiac arrhythmias by prolonging repolarization. Eur Heart J 1993;14(Suppl H):56–61.

66. Roden DM, Iansmith DH. Effects of low potassium or magnesium concentrations on isolated cardiac tissue. Am J Med 1987;82(3A):18–23.

67. Diaz-Castro O, Puchol A, Almendral J, et al. Predictors of in-hospital ventricular fibrillation or torsades de pointes in patients with acute symptomatic bradycardia. J Electrocardiol 2004;37(1):55–60.

68. Roden DM. Drug-induced prolongation of the QT interval. N Engl J Med 2004; 350(10):1013–22.

69. Drew BJ, Ackerman MJ, Funk M, et al. Prevention of torsade de pointes in hospital settings: a scientific statement from the American Heart Association and the American College of Cardiology Foundation. Circulation 2010;121(8): 1047–60.

70. Goldman L. Cardiac risks and complications of noncardiac surgery. Ann Intern Med 1983;98(4):504–13.

71. Pires LA, Wagshal AB, Lancey R, et al. Arrhythmias and conduction disturbances after coronary artery bypass graft surgery: epidemiology, management, and prognosis. Am Heart J 1995;129(4):799–808.

72. Pinto RP, Romerill DB, Nasser WK, et al. Prognosis of patients with frequent premature ventricular complexes and nonsustained ventricular tachycardia after coronary artery bypass graft surgery. Clin Cardiol 1996;19(4):321–4.

73. Wu ZK, Iivainen T, Pehkonen E, et al. Ischemic preconditioning suppresses ventricular tachyarrhythmias after myocardial revascularization. Circulation 2002;106(24):3091–6.

74. Kron IL, DiMarco JP, Harman PK, et al. Unanticipated postoperative ventricular tachyarrhythmias. Ann Thorac Surg 1984;38(4):317–22.

75. Fisher FD, Tyroler HA. Relationship between ventricular premature contractions on routine electrocardiography and subsequent sudden death from coronary heart disease. Circulation 1973;47(4):712–9.

76. Chung MK. Cardiac surgery: postoperative arrhythmias. Crit Care Med 2000; 28(Suppl 10):N136–44.

Index

Note: Page numbers of article titles are in **boldface** type.

A

Clin Geriatr Med 28 (2012) 745–749
http://dx.doi.org/10.1016/S0749-0690(12)00102-4
0749-0690/12/$ – see front matter © 2012 Elsevier Inc. All rights reserved.

geriatric.theclinics.com

United States Postal Service

Statement of Ownership, Management, and Circulation
(All Periodicals Publications Except Requester Publications)

1. Publication Title	2. Publication Number									3. Filing Date
Clinics in Geriatric Medicine	0	0	0	-	7	0	4			9/14/12

4. Issue Frequency	5. Number of Issues Published Annually	6. Annual Subscription Price
Feb, May, Aug, Nov	4	$257.00

7. Complete Mailing Address of Known Office of Publication (Not printer) (Street, city, county, state, and ZIP+4®)

Elsevier Inc.
360 Park Avenue South
New York, NY 10010-1710

Contact Person
Stephen R. Bushing
Telephone (Include area code)
215-239-3688

8. Complete Mailing Address of Headquarters or General Business Office of Publisher (Not printer)

Elsevier Inc., 360 Park Avenue South, New York, NY 10010-1710

9. Full Names and Complete Mailing Addresses of Publisher, Editor, and Managing Editor (Do not leave blank)

Publisher (Name and complete mailing address)

Kim Murphy, Elsevier, Inc., 1600 John F. Kennedy Blvd. Suite 1800, Philadelphia, PA 19103-2899

Editor (Name and complete mailing address)

Yonah Korngold, Elsevier, Inc., 1600 John F. Kennedy Blvd. Suite 1800, Philadelphia, PA 19103-2899

Managing Editor (Name and complete mailing address)

Barbara Cohen - Kligerman, Elsevier, Inc., 1600 John F. Kennedy Blvd. Suite 1800, Philadelphia, PA 19103-2899

10. Owner (Do not leave blank. If the publication is owned by a corporation, give the name and address of the corporation immediately followed by the names and addresses of all stockholders owning or holding 1 percent or more of the total amount of stock. If not owned by a corporation, give the names and addresses of the individual owners. If owned by a partnership or other unincorporated firm, give its name and address as well as those of each individual owner. If the publication is published by a nonprofit organization, give its name and address.)

Full Name	Complete Mailing Address
Wholly owned subsidiary of	1600 John F. Kennedy Blvd., Ste. 1800
Reed/Elsevier, US holdings	Philadelphia, PA 19103-2899

11. Known Bondholders, Mortgagees, and Other Security Holders Owning or Holding 1 Percent or More of Total Amount of Bonds, Mortgages, or Other Securities. If none, check box ☐ None

Full Name	Complete Mailing Address
N/A	

12. Tax Status (For completion by nonprofit organizations authorized to mail at nonprofit rates) (Check one)
The purpose, function, and nonprofit status of this organization and the exempt status for federal income tax purposes:
☐ Has Not Changed During Preceding 12 Months
☐ Has Changed During Preceding 12 Months (Publisher must submit explanation of change with this statement)

PS Form 3526, September 2007 (Page 1 of 3 (Instructions Page 3)) PSN 7530-01-000-9931 PRIVACY NOTICE: See our Privacy policy in www.usps.com

---

13. Publication Title			14. Issue Date for Circulation Data Below
Clinics in Geriatric Medicine			August 2012

15. Extent and Nature of Circulation			Average No. Copies Each Issue During Preceding 12 Months	No. Copies of Single Issue Published Nearest to Filing Date
a. Total Number of Copies (Net press run)			711	508
b. Paid Circulation (By Mail and Outside the Mail)	(1)	Mailed Outside-County Paid Subscriptions Stated on PS Form 3541. (Include paid distribution above nominal rate, advertiser's proof copies, and exchange copies)	341	308
	(2)	Mailed In-County Paid Subscriptions Stated on PS Form 3541 (Include paid distribution above nominal rate, advertiser's proof copies, and exchange copies)		
	(3)	Paid Distribution Outside the Mails Including Sales Through Dealers and Carriers, Street Vendors, Counter Sales, and Other Paid Distribution Outside USPS®	132	137
	(4)	Paid Distribution by Other Classes Mailed Through the USPS (e.g. First-Class Mail®)		
c. Total Paid Distribution (Sum of 15b (1), (2), (3), and (4))		▶	473	445
d. Free or Nominal Rate Distribution (By Mail and Outside the Mail)	(1)	Free or Nominal Rate Outside-County Copies Included on PS Form 3541	59	62
	(2)	Free or Nominal Rate In-County Copies Included on PS Form 3541		
	(3)	Free or Nominal Rate Copies Mailed at Other Classes Through the USPS (e.g. First-Class Mail)		
	(4)	Free or Nominal Rate Distribution Outside the Mail (Carriers or other means)		
e. Total Free or Nominal Rate Distribution (Sum of 15d (1), (2), (3) and (4))		▶	59	62
f. Total Distribution (Sum of 15c and 15e)		▶	532	507
g. Copies not Distributed (See instructions to publishers #4 (page #3))			179	1
h. Total (Sum of 15f and g)		▶	711	508
i. Percent Paid (15c divided by 15f times 100)			88.91%	87.77%

16. Publication of Statement of Ownership

If the publication is a general publication, publication of this statement is required. Will be printed
in the **November 2012** issue of this publication.

☐ Publication not required

17. Signature and Title of Editor, Publisher, Business Manager, or Owner		Date
Stephen R. Bushing Stephen R. Bushing - Inventory Distribution Coordinator		September 14, 2012

I certify that all information furnished on this form is true and complete. I understand that anyone who furnishes false or misleading information on this form or who omits material or information requested on the form may be subject to criminal sanctions (including fines and imprisonment) and/or civil sanctions (including civil penalties).

PS Form 3526, September 2007 (Page 2 of 3)